D0491652

Guide to Symptoms

Abdominal pain. Check for appendicitis; constipation; anxiety; diarrhoea (Chapter 13).

Blisters, on palms of hands and soles of feet. Check for hand, foot, and mouth disease (Chapter 14).

Blisters on skin. Check for chickenpox (Chapter 14).

Coughing, croaking. Check for croup (Chapter 14).

Coughing, gasping. Check for whooping cough (Chapter 14).

Coughing, wheezy. Check for asthma (Chapter 15).

Dislike of bright light. Check for meningitis (Chapter 14).

Ear, yellow discharge. Check for ear infection; burst eardrum; glue ear (Chapter 13).

Earache. Check for ear infection (Chapter 13).

Fever. Check for infectious diseases (Chapter 14).

Headache. Check for fever; cold or flu symptoms; dehydration; eye strain; meningitis (Chapters 13 and 14).

Itching skin. Check for eczema, allergic reaction (Chapter 15); chickenpox (Chapter 14).

Mouth, spots or blisters inside. Check for measles; hand, foot, and mouth disease (Chapter 14).

Neck or jaw, lump in. Check for swollen glands; mumps (Chapter 14).

Listlessness. Check for meningitis (Chapter 14).

Yellow skin (in newborn baby). Check for jaundice (Chapter 8).

Rash. See the colour insert. Check for food allergy; eczema (Chapter 15); heat rash; milia (in babies) (Chapter 8); measles; roseola; German measles; scarlet fever; slapped cheek disease (Chapter 14).

Runny nose. Check for infectious disease (Chapter 14); allergy (Chapter 15).

Skin, patches of red, rough, itchy. Check for eczema (Chapter 15).

Swollen glands. Check for infectious diseases (Chapter 14).

Throat, sore. Check for tonsillitis (Chapter 14).

Vomiting. Check for gastroenteritis (Chapter 13).

Children's Health For Dummies®

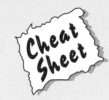

Cheat Sheet

Typical Infant Check-up Schedule

Check-up	With whom	What they look at
Weekly until 6 weeks	Health visitor	Weight, length, head circumference
6–8 weeks	GP and health visitor	Feeding and sleeping habits, vision and hearing
Every 2–4 weeks until 7–8 months	Health clinic	Weight, length, head circumference
7–8 months	Health visitor and GP	Development, hearing, physical examination

Basic Equipment for Your First Aid Cabinet

Make sure you have basic medical equipment handy in your home – but always out of reach from the children. Stock up on:

- Sticking plasters
- Bandages, gauze, and tape
- Antibacterial cleansing wipes
- Sling (or scarf for a home-made sling)
- Thermometer
- Tweezers, scissors, and safety pins
- Infant paracetamol

Turn to Chapter 19 for first aid basics.

Copyright © 2006 John Wiley & Sons, Ltd.
All rights reserved.

Item 2735-5.

For more information about John Wiley & Sons, call (+44) 1243 779777.

Wiley, the Wiley Publishing logo, For Dummies, the Dummies Man logo, the For Dummies Bestselling Book Series logo and all related trade dress are trademarks or registered trademarks of John Wiley & Sons, Inc., and/or its affiliates. All other trademarks are property of their respective owners.

For Dummies: Bestselling Book Series for Beginners

Children's Health

FOR

DUMMIES®

by Katy Holland and Dr Sarah Jarvis, GP

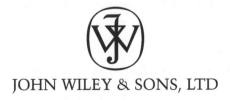

JOHN WILEY & SONS, LTD

GREENWICH LIBRARIES

3 8028 01768114 6

Children's Health For Dummies®

Published by
John Wiley & Sons, Ltd
The Atrium
Southern Gate
Chichester
West Sussex
PO19 8SQ
England

E-mail (for orders and customer service enquires): cs-books@wiley.co.uk

Visit our Home Page on www.wileyeurope.com

Copyright © 2006 by John Wiley & Sons, Ltd, Chichester, West Sussex, England.

Published by John Wiley & Sons, Ltd, Chichester, West Sussex.

All Rights Reserved. No part of this publication may be reproduced, stored in a retrieval system or transmitted in any form or by any means, electronic, mechanical, photocopying, recording, scanning or otherwise, except under the terms of the Copyright, Designs and Patents Act 1988 or under the terms of a licence issued by the Copyright Licensing Agency Ltd, 90 Tottenham Court Road, London, W1T 4LP, UK, without the permission in writing of the Publisher. Requests to the Publisher for permission should be addressed to the Legal Department, Wiley Publishing, Inc, 10475 Crosspoint Blvd, Indianapolis, Indiana 46256, United States, 317-572-3447, fax 317-572-4355, or online at www.wiley.com/go/permissions.

Trademarks: Wiley, the Wiley Publishing logo, For Dummies, the Dummies Man logo, A Reference for the Rest of Us!, The Dummies Way, Dummies Daily, The Fun and Easy Way, Dummies.com and related trade dress are trademarks or registered trademarks of John Wiley & Sons, Inc and/or its affiliates, in the United States and other countries, and may not be used without written permission. All other trademarks are the property of their respective owners. John Wiley & Sons, Ltd, is not associated with any product or vendor mentioned in this book.

LIMIT OF LIABILITY/DISCLAIMER OF WARRANTY: THE CONTENTS OF THIS WORK ARE INTENDED TO FURTHER GENERAL SCIENTIFIC RESEARCH, UNDERSTANDING, AND DISCUSSION ONLY AND ARE NOT INTENDED AND SHOULD NOT BE RELIED UPON AS RECOMMENDING OR PROMOTING A SPECIFIC METHOD, DIAGNOSIS, OR TREATMENT BY PHYSICIANS FOR ANY PARTICULAR PATIENT. THE PUBLISHER AND THE AUTHOR MAKE NO REPRESENTATIONS OR WARRANTIES WITH RESPECT TO THE ACCURACY OR COMPLETENESS OF THE CONTENTS OF THIS WORK AND SPECIFICALLY DISCLAIM ALL WARRANTIES, INCLUDING WITHOUT LIMITATION ANY IMPLIED WARRANTIES OF FITNESS FOR A PARTICULAR PURPOSE. IN VIEW OF ONGOING RESEARCH, EQUIPMENT MODIFICATIONS, CHANGES IN GOVERNMENTAL REGULATIONS, AND THE CONSTANT FLOW OF INFORMATION RELATING TO THE USE OF MEDICINES, EQUIPMENT, AND DEVICES, THE READER IS URGED TO REVIEW AND EVALUATE THE INFORMATION PROVIDED IN THE PACKAGE INSERT OR INSTRUCTIONS FOR EACH MEDICINE, EQUIPMENT, OR DEVICE FOR, AMONG OTHER THINGS, ANY CHANGES IN THE INSTRUCTIONS OR INDICATION OF USAGE AND FOR ADDED WARNINGS AND PRECAUTIONS. READERS SHOULD CONSULT WITH A SPECIALIST WHERE APPROPRIATE. THE FACT THAT AN ORGANISATION OR WEB SITE IS REFERRED TO IN THIS WORK AS A CITATION AND/OR A POTENTIAL SOURCE OF FURTHER INFORMATION DOES NOT MEAN THAT THE AUTHOR OR THE PUBLISHER ENDORSES THE INFORMATION THE ORGANISATION OR WEB SITE MAY PROVIDE OR RECOMMENDATIONS IT MAY MAKE. FURTHER, READERS SHOULD BE AWARE THAT INTERNET WEB SITES LISTED IN THIS WORK MAY HAVE CHANGED OR DISAPPEARED BETWEEN WHEN THIS WORK WAS WRITTEN AND WHEN IT IS READ. NO WARRANTY MAY BE CREATED OR EXTENDED BY ANY PROMOTIONAL STATEMENTS FOR THIS WORK. NEITHER THE PUBLISHER NOR THE AUTHOR SHALL BE LIABLE FOR ANY DAMAGES ARISING HEREFROM.

Wiley also publishes its books in a variety of electronic formats. Some content that appears in print may not be available in electronic books.

British Library Cataloguing in Publication Data: A catalogue record for this book is available from the British Library.

ISBN-13: 978-0-470-02735-6

ISBN-10: 0-470-02735-5

Printed and bound in Great Britain by Bell and Bain Ltd, Glasgow.

10 9 8 7 6 5 4 3 2 1

WILEY

About the Authors

Katy Holland lives in London with her two sons. She is Deputy Editor of *Mother & Baby* magazine, and also writes a weekly column for the *Independent on Sunday* about travelling with children.

Katy has written three books on childcare – *Your Baby from Birth to Six Months*, *Sleep*, and *Baby and Child Safety*.

Before taking up her current position on *Mother & Baby*, she was the magazine's Health Editor for two years.

Dr Sarah Jarvis is a GP and GP trainer in inner city London. She is a Fellow of, and the Women's Health spokesperson for, the Royal College of General Practitioners (RCGP). She is also a medical writer and broadcaster, and appears regularly on Radio Five Live and GMTV, as well as being the Radio 2 doctor and the regular medical advisor for ITN lunchtime news. She writes regularly for a variety of magazines, including *Good Housekeeping*, *Women's Health*, *Pregnancy*, and *Baby and You*. Her great passion (as far as work is concerned) is patient education, and she has written over 500 patient information leaflets, as well as three previous books, *A Younger Woman's Diagnose-It-Yourself Guide to Health*, *Diabetes For Dummies*, and *Pregnancy For Dummies*. Her other great passion is her family, and she loves spending time with her husband, Simon, their two children, Seth and Matilda, and their dog, Dascha.

L B OF GREENWICH LIBRARIES	Mo
017681146	
Bertrams	05.11.06
613.0432	£14.99
FAMILY MATTERS	

Dedication

To Patrick and Stanley, my fantastic boys.

–Katy

To my wonderful children, Seth and Matilda, who have taught me that the theory is all very well, but that what you really learn from is practical experience.

–Sarah

Authors' Acknowledgements

From Katy: A very special thank you to David Griffiths, for putting up with me and keeping me going. Thanks also to Rachael Chilvers and Alison Yates, who have been so amazingly supportive in the face of such adversity! Their patience, kindness, and words of encouragement have been very much appreciated. Big thanks and love also go to Abina Manning, Linda Stanfield, Nicole Rees, Tony Holland, Lesley-ann Vernon, and Alan Milford.

Publisher's Acknowledgements

We're proud of this book; please send us your comments through our Dummies online registration form located at www.dummies.com/register/.

Some of the people who helped bring this book to market include the following:

Acquisitions, Editorial, and Media Development

Project Editor: Rachael Chilvers

Development Editor: Tracy Barr

Content Editor: Steve Edwards

Commissioning Editor: Alison Yates

Executive Editor: Jason Dunne

Executive Project Editor: Martin Tribe

Copy Editor: Colette Holden

Proofreader: Anne O'Rorke

Special Help: Nicci Talbot, Jennifer Bingham

Cover Photo: © Dimitri Vervitz/Getty Images

Colour Insert Photos: 1, 4, 5, 6, 8, 9, 11: Dr P. Marazzi / Science Photo Library; 2: Chris Priest / Science Photo Library; 3: Arthur Glauberman / Science Photo Library; 7: Lowell Georgia / Science Photo Library; 10: Science Photo Library; 12: Dr H. C. Robinson / Science Photo Library

Cartoons: Ed McLachlan

Composition

Project Coordinator: Jennifer Theriot

Layout and Graphics: Carl Byers, Andrea Dahl, Denny Hager, Joyce Haughey, Stephanie Jumper, Barry Offringa, Heather Ryan, Alicia South

Proofreaders: Brian H. Walls

Indexer: Techbooks

Publishing and Editorial for Consumer Dummies

Diane Graves Steele, Vice President and Publisher, Consumer Dummies

Joyce Pepple, Acquisitions Director, Consumer Dummies

Kristin A. Cocks, Product Development Director, Consumer Dummies

Michael Spring, Vice President and Publisher, Travel

Brice Gosnell, Associate Publisher, Travel

Kelly Regan, Editorial Director, Travel

Publishing for Technology Dummies

Andy Cummings, Vice President and Publisher, Dummies Technology/General User

Composition Services

Gerry Fahey, Vice President of Production Services

Debbie Stailey, Director of Composition Services

Contents at a Glance

Table of Contents

Introduction

*B*eing a parent is fantastic – but that doesn't mean to say it's easy. Caring for your little bundle of joy and making sure he or she is healthy and safe at all times is a full time job – without the holidays – and the only way you can discover how to do this is through experience. We (Katy and Sarah) have done our fair share of mopping fevered brows, dashing to A&E at all hours, and giving lots of cuddles and kissing better. Although we can't promise to stop the panic completely, we hope this book goes a long way towards answering some of those thousands of questions and concerns that every single parent has about their child.

About This Book

We want you to think of this book as an experienced friend with a sense of humour, who cuts through the reams of mythology out there about children's health and gives you the best ways to keep your children healthy.

We want this book to entertain you as well as inform you, so we hope you enjoy the lighter tone and personal experiences throughout the book. We don't assume you know about the best ways to look after your baby; we simply assume you want the very best for him or her.

Conventions Used in This Book

To help you navigate through this book, we set up a few conventions:

- *Italics* are used for emphasis and to highlight new words, or define terms.
- **Boldfaced** text indicates the key concept in a list, or the action part of a numbered list.
- Monofont is used for Web and e-mail addresses.

We use the female pronoun 'she' in odd-numbered chapters and the male 'he' in even-numbered chapters, just to be fair to both genders! We also use metric weights and measurements, with the imperial equivalent in brackets for good measure.

How This Book Is Organised

The great thing about *For Dummies* books is that you don't have to read them all the way through. You can simply turn to the bit you're interested in and start at any point within a chapter, within a section, or even just go directly to a paragraph that interests you.

The book has six parts, with each broken into chapters. The Table of Contents and the Index help you pinpoint information within the outline explained in the next sections.

Part 1: Children's Health: The Basics

This part is an overview of your child's health and development. We include information about the health professionals you'll encounter, and the services available to your child. Head to this part if you want to find out more about vaccinations and your child's immune system.

Part II: The First Year of Life

Looking after your baby can sometimes be daunting. This part guides you through the first year of life, covering feeding and weaning your baby, and dealing with common newborn concerns from jaundice to squints.

Part III: Raising Healthy Children

You can never protect your child from every bug doing the rounds, but you can ensure optimum health by making sure your little sweeties eat well, get loads of time to run around and play, and get a good night's sleep. This part has lots of tips on tearing little eyes away from the TV and getting out and about.

Part IV: Symptoms, Illnesses, and Treatments

This part focuses on how to spot what's wrong with your child, whether it's earache, an upset tummy, or a nasty rash. We also cover emotional and behavioural health and development here.

Part V: Playing Doctors and Nurses: Looking After a Sick Child

All parents end up caring for a poorly little bundle of germs at some point – you're not alone. This part explains how to ease the burden, both for your child and yourself.

Part VI: The Part of Tens

Here you'll find a set of mini chapters about keeping your child healthy on holiday, and how to ensure your home, car, and garden are safe and child-proof. This part also lists ten tried and tested Web sites on children's health that we hope you find useful.

Icons Used in This Book

Every *For Dummies* book has a selection of icons to help you quickly and easily identify information that may be of particular interest to you, or high-light important points you shouldn't miss. Here's an explanation of each icon:

This icon alerts to you to when an illness or emergency needs medical attention.

As a parent, you can get the heebie-jeebies when your precious darling gets the sniffles, or grazes a knee. This icon acts as a soothing balm for you, as we let you know the stuff that you really don't need to worry about.

This icon draws your attention to an important point to bear in mind.

This guy is highlighting techy information that increases your knowledge about a particular topic (how a certain drug works, perhaps), but you can skip these non-essential paragraphs if you like.

When you see this icon we're trying to emphasise a bit of information that may be particularly helpful or time-saving to you.

 This icon is saying 'watch out!' When it comes to the health of your children, you need to do your best to protect them from the dangers next to this icon.

Where to Go from Here

Each chapter of this book can be approached individually, depending on your interest. Have a look at the Table of Contents and jump right into any chapter that is relevant to you and use the Index to look up particular illnesses or treatments.

If, for example, your baby is having trouble sleeping for any length of time, you could start by going straight to Chapter 11. If you want an overview of first aid so you can help your child in an emergency, then Chapter 19 is an excellent starting place.

Of course, we'd be delighted if you take the traditional route and read this book from cover to cover!

We hope you enjoy reading this book, and that it helps you to keep your children healthy and happy.

Part I
Children's Health: The Basics

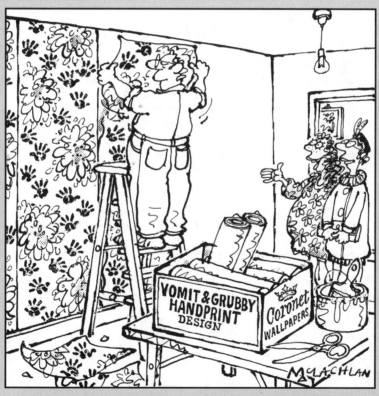

"We're just decorating the baby's bedroom for when he or she arrives"

In this part . . .

You've been through the rigours of pregnancy and labour and now you can relax with your beautiful bundle of joy, right? We sincerely hope so. But you're probably bursting with questions about what happens now concerning check-ups about your baby's development; the immunisation your child needs against all those nasty diseases; and who you can call in the middle of the night when your precious darling is feeling under the weather.

Rest assured, this part answers all these questions – and more – about the basics of your child's health.

Chapter 1

Your Child's Health in a Nutshell

*B*eing a parent is a tremendous life-changing experience: The moment your little bundle of joy arrives, you suddenly morph into a provider, a full-time caregiver, and a nurse all in one go – quite scary, to put it mildly. Along with the dirty nappies and the sleepless nights, you have fevered brows to mop and big questions to answer. Should you call an ambulance or send your child back to bed with a kiss and a little infant paracetamol? How can you make sure that she's getting the right nutrients she needs to grow big and strong, and disease-free? What can you do to reduce the risk of accidents or illness? If your child becomes sick, who should you go to and how do you navigate the healthcare system? The list of questions is endless, but the chapter ahead narrows it down to the big three, outlining the general strategies you can use to keep your child healthy, spot the signs of illness, and care for a child who's under the weather.

Keeping Your Child Healthy

Illness is one of the things we fear most for our children. It's impossible – and unnecessary – to shield your child from every bug out there, but you can help to boost her health and vitality, making her stronger and better able to fight off illnesses efficiently.

Eat, drink, and be healthy

If you want your child to eat healthily, you need to serve her a wide variety of nutritious foods for energy, growth, and development. This means giving processed and junk foods a wide berth – but it doesn't mean not being flexible. Food isn't worth arguing over, and if your child insists on eating curly cheesy crisps, that's fine – as long as they don't form her staple diet. If most of the food your child eats is nutritious, you'll be keeping her in tip-top condition. Try doing the following to make sure that she eats well:

✔ **Give your child at least five helpings of fruit and vegetables a day – fresh, frozen, canned, dried, or juiced.** You're probably already aware of this important point, but there's no harm in stressing it again. Fruit and veg contain the crucial nutrients needed to maintain a healthy digestive system, create new body tissue, fight infections, and a lot more. Try to offer your child at least one orange and one green fruit or vegetable every day, as they are known to be particularly beneficial and may help to prevent cancer and other serious diseases.

Fruit or vegetable juice only makes up one of her daily portions of fruit and vegetables, no matter how much she drinks. That's because other goodies in the flesh are not included in juice, and digesting whole fruit and vegetables benefits her system.

✔ **Make sure that your child eats breakfast.** Studies show that if your child eats breakfast, she's far less likely to become obese in later life. Skipping breakfast can cause blood-sugar problems and make your child's metabolism sluggish, which is bad for the digestive system. Most experts say that breakfast's the most important meal of the day: Breakfast eaters are less likely to contract diabetes or have high cholesterol, which is a known risk factor for heart disease.

✔ **Maintain your own healthy diet.** You're important too! Eating healthy food yourself is one of the best ways of getting your child into good habits, so make sure that you tuck in to your greens. Studies also show that children who have regular family mealtimes are more likely to have healthier diets than those who don't. Snacking in front of the telly is a definite no-no.

✔ **Offer as much unprocessed food as possible, and get into the habit of reading labels on the foods you serve.** Check for things such as hidden fats, sugars, additives, and salt. Foods with lots of preservatives and added flavourings are often deficient in essential nutrients and high in unhealthy (and unnecessary) chemicals. Salt's a particular danger – it can cause health problems, including high blood pressure and heart conditions. And sugar (and sugar substitutes), additives, and colourings have been linked with everything from behavioural problems to physical ailments.

✔ **Get your child to drink six to eight glasses of water a day.** Drinking enough fluids is vital. Water's the best drink by far – try to keep sugary drinks and juices to a minimum, and don't serve them at all between meals because they are lethal to tiny teeth. The British medical profession has been telling us for many years that most children aren't drinking enough. Dehydration leads to many short-term and long-term health problems: Lack of water can cause headaches, constipation, and poor concentration, to name but a few things.

A good way to tell whether your child's dehydrated is to check the colour of her urine. Her urine should be a pale straw colour: If it's dark yellow, she may well be dehydrated. A sunken fontanelle (the soft spot on a baby's head) can also indicate dehydration.

For more on healthy eating habits, head to Chapter 9.

A moving story

Exercise is vital for everyone – especially your child. Whether your child's dancing around the living room or entering a swimming gala, getting active is all good stuff. Exercise boosts circulation and helps infection-fighting lymphatic fluid to move throughout the body. Exercise is great for your child's emotional health too: When your child exercises, her brain releases chemicals called endorphins, the body's natural feel-good chemicals. Your active child develops stronger muscles and bones, is less likely to become overweight, has a reduced risk of developing type 2 diabetes, and has lower blood pressure and cholesterol levels compared with inactive children. For more details on the benefits of exercise and for suggestions for keeping your child active, check out Chapter 10.

Breathing easy

In the UK, around 17,000 children under the age of 5 years are admitted to hospital every year with illnesses related to passive smoking. Not smoking around your child is a crucial way of safeguarding her health. Scientists have shown that passive smoking has a lasting impact on the long-term health and respiratory system of children. Inhaling cigarette smoke increases the risk of asthma and other acute respiratory conditions and contributes to many childhood illnesses, including bronchitis, pneumonia, asthma, middle-ear infections, cot death, and possibly even autism. If your child inhales cigarette smoke, she's also at increased risk of developing certain kinds of cancer, including lung cancer. Research has even found a link between lower IQ levels and exposure to cigarette smoke.

Going outside the house to smoke doesn't fully protect your child – although of course outside is far better than smoking indoors. Research shows that poisonous chemicals from cigarette smoke cling to your clothes and hair and are released back into the air – and then inhaled by your child. When researchers measured toxic chemicals in the blood of children whose parents smoked outdoors, they found the levels of chemicals to be far higher than in children whose parents never smoked at all, inside or out.

Giving up the smokes

Giving up smoking is one of the best things you can do for your own body and your child's. The risk of premature death in smokers is double that in non-smokers. By stopping smoking, you reduce your risk of lots of diseases. You can buy aids to help you to stop smoking: Try nicotine gum, skin patches, hypnosis, or acupressure bands, all available over the counter in your local pharmacy. Go and see your GP or practice nurse if you feel you need more support, particularly if you'd like to attend a smoking-cessation clinic or self-help group funded by the NHS. Or try calling Quitline, run by an independent charity, on 0800-00-22-00.

Getting good sleep

Lack of sleep is the number-one cause of problems for all parents of young children. Sleep's particularly important for your child's health because it stimulates the hormones that make her grow. Sleep's also the time when your child's body does all its repair work, replenishing damaged tissues and cells and building a healthy immune system. Getting your child into good sleep habits can have a positive impact on her health and development. The best way of doing this is to establish a bedtime routine and make sure that your child is able to go to sleep by herself. Read more about bedtime routines in Chapter 11.

Staying safe

More than half of all accidents that happen to children under the age of 5 years occur in the home. The peak age for accident-prone behaviour is around 2 years, but babies enter the danger zone at around 9 months when they become mobile. In the early days, your baby needs complete protection. You need to develop a watchful caring eye, but safety equipment gives you extra peace of mind by protecting your little one in potentially dangerous areas such as the kitchen. Chapter 22 covers the basics.

The most important thing you ever buy your child is likely to be a child car seat. When you buy your car seat, ask a qualified shop assistant to check that the seat is suitable for your car and is fitted correctly. Research shows that up to 80 per cent of child car seats are not fitted properly, leaving many children extremely vulnerable.

All protected

Many doctors agree that vaccinating your child against dangerous diseases is the single most important thing you can do to protect her health. Before the use of vaccines, many children died from diseases such as whooping cough and polio. Immunisations have now all but eradicated many serious diseases in the UK, but illnesses such as polio can still be brought back from trips abroad and caught by children (and adults) in the UK who haven't been immunised. If your child hasn't been vaccinated and is exposed to germs, her body may not be strong enough to fight the infection. To find out more about the pros and cons of vaccinating your child, head to Chapter 3.

All you need is . . .

. . . love! To thrive, your child needs lots of cuddles and human contact, particularly with her main carers. Studies show that lack of love and affection is as damaging to children as food deprivation: Adequately nourished babies deprived of human relationships become impeded in their development in both mind and body.

We cannot overemphasise the importance of touch – human contact is critical for development and well-being. Babies who are held cry less than those who aren't, and those who're cuddled and massaged frequently tend to have better immune systems and handle stress more efficiently than those who aren't. The need for touch continues into childhood and beyond. One study showed that when children were massaged regularly for a month, blood glucose levels dropped dramatically in diabetic children and the children were able to reduce their medication, while asthmatic children had fewer asthma attacks. Massage also reduced the symptoms in children with autism, severe burns, cancer, and arthritis.

Spotting the Signs That Something's Wrong

Even if you do everything right, your child'll get ill – and probably quite frequently. This isn't a bad thing: Your child's body needs to come into contact with bacteria and viruses in order to build up a good resistance to the germs. In fact, some research shows that the more illnesses your child gets in the first few years of life, the healthier she's likely to be later.

Of course, you won't welcome every cold and tummy bug your child falls victim to. After all, caring for an ill child can be extremely worrying, especially when you can't quite work out what's wrong. Try to keep things in perspective: All children get ill, and in the vast majority of cases the illnesses aren't serious and don't pose any threat to your child's long-term health. However, if you're at all concerned about your child, get her checked out by a doctor. And try to be aware of the signs of diseases such as meningitis, which need urgent medical treatment (skip to Chapter 13).

The person who can tell better than anyone else whether your child is ill is *you*. Follow your instincts: You're likely to be able to spot when something's not quite right. Signs that your child has a bug include the following:

- ✔ **A fever:** The presence of a fever almost always means an infection. Fever itself is not dangerous – it's the body's normal reaction to the presence of foreign organisms – but you need to bring down your child's temperature to avoid overheating, which can cause a febrile convulsion.

- ✔ **Irritability or lethargy:** Your child's behaviour may be influenced by a fever. The raised temperature may make her irritable, drowsy, or lethargic.

- ✔ **Coughing:** This is a common sign that your child has an infection.

- ✔ **Vomiting and diarrhoea:** Symptoms like these are usually associated with problems directly involving the tummy or bowel, such as gastroenteritis or food poisoning, although sometimes they occur for other reasons. Some children vomit if they have a high temperature; others vomit if they're emotionally upset.

Yes, diarrhoea really can be a cause for celebration! If your child is suffering from diarrhoea as well as vomiting, she probably has a tummy bug, which usually settles on its own with no ill effects (you can find out more in Chapters 14 and 17). Vomiting without diarrhoea, especially if accompanied by fever, may have a different cause such as a urine infection. If you're in doubt, ring NHS Direct (0845-4647) or speak to your GP or health visitor.

- ✔ **A rash:** Rashes often suggests a viral infection. The presence of a rash doesn't usually make the illness any more serious – in fact, it can help your doctor diagnose illnesses such as German measles and chickenpox. But if your child has a rash, ask your doctor to check it out to ensure that she's not displayinga symptom of meningitis or another dangerous illness.

The easiest way to test for meningitis is the 'glass test'. Press the bottom of a glass on to your child's rash. If the rash fades or disappears, it is almost certainly not meningitis; if the rash remains, your child may have meningococcal septicaemia (blood poisoning) – so call an ambulance immediately.

The list above is a very general description of a few of the most common childhood symptoms. More detailed info on what to look out for appears elsewhere in the book. If you're caring for an infant, head to Chapters 7 and 8, which are devoted to infant healthcare. For older children, go to Chapter 14.

Knowing When to Call a Doctor

You may find it hard not to worry about the slightest sniffle your little darling gets, but more often than not it's nothing serious. However, you do need to call a doctor if:

- Your baby under 3 months old has a fever – this must always be regarded as potentially serious.
- Your child's listless or miserable even after you've brought down her fever.
- Your child's breathing is rapid or laboured.
- Your child's colour changes from pink or red to mauve or blue.
- Your child has a convulsion (fit).
- Your child loses consciousness.
- Your child has blood in her urine, vomit, or stools.

Keep in mind that young children can develop dangerous symptoms quite rapidly. If your child's poorly, keep a close eye on her and call your doctor if you're in any doubt.

Who You Gonna Call?

For most of us, the local doctor's surgery is our first port of call for health problems. Your GP can make a diagnosis, prescribe medication, and refer your child to other health services if necessary. But you don't always need to see a doctor if your child's under the weather. No one wants to go to the doctor unless they really have to – there may be a DIY solution, but if not, you need to decide whether a visit to the doctor or A&E is necessary.

Trying a bit of DIY

- A well-stocked medicine cabinet helps you treat many everyday illness and minor ailments at home. A small supply of infant paracetamol or ibuprofen syrup goes a long way and can help a whole array of problems, from coughs and fevers to toothache. Keep stocked up on infant paracetamol – fevers and other symptoms are more common at night, and the last thing you need at 3 a.m. is to discover that the medicine cabinet is bare. Chapter 18 tells you what you need to know about medications. Have a look at the Cheat Sheet at the front of the book for a list of basic first aid supplies.

✔ Your local pharmacist's a good source of help. She's an expert on medicines and how they work and can offer advice on common childhood complaints. Your pharmacist can recommend over-the-counter remedies for your child and give advice on whether you should take your child to the doctor. Chapter 4 gives info on pharmacists and other healthcare professionals.

✔ NHS Direct (0845-4647) is a nationwide service providing health advice over the phoneNurses and professional advisors staff the lines. The NHS Direct service is a good place to start if you need non-emergency medical help outside normal surgery hours. NHS Direct is open every day of the year, 24 hours a day.

✔ There are nearly 70 NHS walk-in centres throughout the UK. They offer free, fast, convenient access to healthcare advice and treatment for minor illnesses and injuries and can be a good alternative to A&E. Most of the walk-in centres open seven days a week, from early morning to late evening, and are run by experienced nurses. You don't need an appointment. To find out about your nearest walk-in clinic, check out www.nhs.co.uk.

Going to your doctor or casualty

Working out whether you to take your child to the doctor or straight to A&E depends on the severity of the problem. If the problem's not urgent, you should be able to get an appointment at your local surgery within a day or two – but remember to cancel it if your child's symptoms subside. Most GPs' surgeries fit you in if you just turn up with your child, although you may have to wait a while. Your doctor likely has an emergency out-of-hours service for urgent medical problems that can't wait until the next day. Most surgeries have an answering-machine message giving an out-of-hours telephone number or referring you to NHS Direct. Go to Chapter 17 to find out what to expect if your child needs to take a trip to hospital.

Many people go to A&E, but they can be treated just as professionally – and often more quickly – at a minor-injuries unit. Minor injuries units, which are usually located near major hospitals, cater for patients with less serious injuries and ailments, such as sprains, cuts, bites, stings, and eye or head injuries. The waiting times at minor injuries units are usually much shorter than those in A&E. You don't need an appointment. If you aren't sure if your child's injury can be treated at a minor injuries unit, call NHS Direct on 0845-4647, which can advise you and direct you to the most appropriate place.

Call 999 or take your child straight to A&E if the situation is critical or life-threatening – for example, if she's losing a lot of blood, is unconscious, is having difficulty breathing, or has been poisoned by something.

Chapter 2

Your Child's Body and Development

In This Chapter

▶ Discovering how your child's body works

▶ Watching your child grow

▶ Assessing your child's health

A really fulfilling aspect of parenthood is watching your child develop and grow and helping him to learn new skills. The four main areas of development are physical, intellectual, social, and emotional. Your child's development is influenced by the genes both parents pass on, the nurture you give him, and the environment in which you bring him up. Play, stimulation, affection, and a good diet all play important roles in your child's development.

Your child grows and develops most rapidly during the first five years of life. But remember that no two children develop at the same rate, even in the same family. This chapter outlines your child's development, from infancy to adolescence.

Meeting Developmental Milestones

How do you know whether your baby's developing normally? Doctors now agree that a child passes a number of physical milestones on his way to maturity. Newborns follow a sequence of events. The rate of development is influenced by factors such as temperament, environment, past medical history, and genetics. Having a basic understanding of these milestones helps you to know that your child's developing normally.

Your baby's development can be divided into three main areas:

- Movement and handling skills
- Language skills
- Social skills

Children usually develop movement skills in sequence, from top to bottom and from the middle of the body to the fingers and toes. Children gain control of large muscles before smaller muscles. With thinking skills, children grasp concrete concepts ('Mummy is here because I can feel her cuddling me') before abstract concepts ('I may not be able to see Mummy at the moment, but that doesn't mean she's gone for ever'). Social development and gaining confidence and skills are gradual, so give your child lots of opportunities to interact with others and to explore his environment.

Table 2-1 gives a rough idea of the age ranges for developing certain skills. All children are different and develop at different ages, so use this table only as a guideline. This chapter discusses these developmental milestones in more detail and gives you an age-by-age breakdown of what to expect and when.

Your baby's development is not a race! All babies develop different skills at different rates, and there's several weeks (or sometimes months) of leeway before any problems with development are diagnosed. If you have any concerns about your child's development, your health visitor will always be happy to answer queries.

Table 2-1	Age-related Skills
Age	*Developmental milestone*
Birth to 1 month	He has primitive reflexes – for example, if you touch his cheek, he turns his cheek towards you or give a little jolt if he hears a loud noise (the 'startle reflex')
	He sucks objects placed near his mouth and grasps hold of things. This is reflexive – he doesn't have fine motor skills yet
	He can hear and responds to sound by turning his head
	He can see objects 20–30 cm in front of him and follows your face with his eyes
	He recognises people around him and begins to show a preference for his mother
	He moves his head to the side when placed on his stomach
	By 3 weeks, he can move forward – so don't leave him alone on a bed or sofa

Age	Developmental milestone
2 months	He smiles spontaneously at a face he recognises with increasing frequency over the next few weeks
	He starts to make cooing sounds
	The grasping reflex gives way to purposeful reaching and slapping with his whole hand at objects in his vision (fine motor skills – being able to use the fingers – come later)
	He follows objects with his eyes
	He's aware of colours, explores objects visually and orally exploration, controls his eye muscles, and lift his head when lying on his tummy
3 months	He smiles when spoken to
	His eyes follow moving objects and search for sounds
	He holds objects placed in his hand
	He rolls from front to back
	When lying on his tummy, he lifts his head and keeps it there for a short time
4 months	He grasps for and holds objects and may not want to let them go
	He controls his head and arm movements
	He puts everything into his mouth (and we mean everything!)
	He laughs
	He rolls over and kicks his legs
	He may be able to see across the room
5 months	He loves being tickled
	His head doesn't lag if you pull him up to a sitting position from lying down
	He plays with his hands and fingers
	He rolls from front to back, and vice versa
6 months	He sits up with your help
	He babbles to his toys
	He passes objects from one hand to another

(continued)

Table 2-1 *(continued)*

Age	Developmental milestone
	He makes most vowel sounds and about half the consonant sounds
	He will drink from a cup held for him
7 months	He's aware of food and hunger
	He bangs the table repeatedly with a toy or spoon – much to your annoyance
	He pivots around in a circle when placed on his tummy
	He recognises Mum and Dad as important and cries out when a 'stranger' approaches
	He makes all vowel sounds
	He finger-feeds, using a pincer movement to grasp things with his index finger and thumb
8 months	He makes simple consonant sounds (da, ba, ka)
	He crawls (some babies crawl backwards before they crawl forwards, and some are 'bottom shufflers' who never crawl, but go straight from moving in a sitting position to walking)
9 months	He sits up, unsupported
	He may pull himself up to standing and maintain this position with support
	He may become more anxious about being separated from his Mum and Dad
	He waves goodbye
10–12 months	He walks without the help of furniture by holding on to you with his hands
	He recognises and responds to his name
	He stands on his own two feet for the first time
	Despite his new independence, he may still be clingy and afraid of strangers
	He uses his fingers to feed himself and drink from his cup, and he helps you dress him by holding out his arms and legs
	He can say 'Mama' and 'Dada' and other meaningful words

Age	Developmental milestone
13–15 months	He crawls up stairs – so make sure you have a safety gate in place!
	He imitates words – so don't swear in front of him!
	He shows a range of human emotion and squeals to get your attention
	He holds his cup and drinks from it without help
16–18 months	He likes to run
	His vocabulary has grown to double figures
	He wants things his own way and may be possessive over his toys
	Temper tantrums are common
	He manages the stairs by holding on to your hand (of course, he may not realise that he needs to hold on to your hand, so never leave him anywhere near stairs without a stairgate!)
	He feeds himself using a spoon and fork
19–24 months	He's much steadier, falls over less, and walks up and down the stairs one at a time
	He likes kicking and throwing a ball
	He follows you around and copies you
	Mealtimes are a bit tidier as he gains control of muscle movement, fine motor skills, and hand–eye coordination
	With help, he undresses himself at bedtime and turns the pages in books
	He may be able to say up to 50 words and string phrases together such as 'I love Mummy' – but his sentences aren't complete at this point
3 years	He rides a tricycle
	He builds a tower block of ten cubes, indicating good hand–eye coordination and balance
	His hands are steadier
	He knows his age and sex
	He wants to dress himself without your help, indicating independence

(continued)

Table 2-1 *(continued)*

Age	Developmental milestone
	He can talk in sentences and talk clearly enough to be understood by strangers
	He can chant rhymes or songs and loves to repeat them
	He may have an imaginary playmate, which shows imagination and independence, sharing, a 'we' mentality, and curiosity about other children; if the imaginary friend is of the same sex as him, he has awareness of his own sex
4 years	He throws a ball
	He climbs independently to explore his environment
	He draws a person in parts
	He tells a basic story or monologue
	He goes to the toilet alone
	He likes playing with other children
	He may be able to write his name (unless it's Rumpelstiltskin!)
5 years	He dresses and undresses himself easily
	He likes domestic role-play, such as playing house and pretend cooking
	He counts and names colours
6 years	He starts to lose his teeth, replacing around four a year
	His muscular strength, coordination, and stamina increase
	He performs complex tasks such as dancing and playing the piano
	He has reading and writing skills and likes to play organised sports

Understanding Physical Development

From the moment he's born, your baby starts to develop and is longing to learn. Your newborn uses all his senses – he can see, hear, feel, taste, and smell. At age 2 weeks, your baby follows movements, recognises faces, and begins to smile. He recognises the voices of you and your partner and reacts to loud noises.

Development's rapid and continuous, but your baby will pick up some skills more quickly than others. The development of his body depends on the maturity of his muscles and nervous system: He won't be able to walk or talk until these are functional. Your baby develops from head to toe, so he won't be able to sit until he can control his head and he won't be able to stand until he can sit down.

To gain complete control of his body, your child needs to master the following three types of skill:

- **Gross motor skills:** These control the larger muscles needed for balance and movement – for example, to walk. Your child develops body control from the top down, starting with his head and shoulders and moving down to the arms and then the legs.

- **Fine motor skills:** These control the smaller muscles, such as those in the hands and fingers. Your child learns how to use his arms, then his hands, and then his fingers. At age 3 months, your child plays with his hands and fingers. At 6 months, he grasps using his whole hand; by 9 months, he has an inferior pincer grasp (holding things with his first finger and thumb); and at 1 year, he has a primitive tripod grasp (using the thumb and first two fingers). By 15 months, your child uses his whole hand to pick things up. By age 2 years, your child is more dextrous and can hold a pencil and draw.

- **Sensory skills:** These control your child's ability to perceive the world through his senses – taste, touch, vision, smell, and hearing. Your child engages all five senses to learn as much as possible about his new environment.

Encourage your child's physical development by playing indoor games to help his fine motor skills. Outdoor play is also very important because it allows him to burn off excess energy.

From birth to 24 months

Children develop and grow at different rates. Progress is usually measured in 'milestones' indicating the skills most children have acquired by a certain age.

Movement begins with head control. Your baby won't be able to sit, crawl, or stand until he can control the position of his head. At 2–3 months, his neck muscles strengthen and you notice less head lag, although you still need to support his head when you lift him. He can hold his head steady for a while when you hold him. He can hold his head up when he's lying on his tummy. He is captivated by and plays with his fingers. Try propping up your child with a cushion so he sits upright, helping him to be more aware of what's going on around him.

After he gains some control over his neck muscles and his head, your baby starts to support himself with his hands, wrists, and arms. He also begins to bend his knees. These are the first movements of crawling. Although he may not move anywhere, he's developing strength and coordination.

At 4–5 months, your baby can control his head and move it from side to side. He supports himself on his arms and has good upper-body strength. He branches out into new and exciting endeavours, such as rolling over. His first rolling feat will probably be from his tummy on to his back, followed shortly by rolling from his back to his tummy.

Although you should never leave your baby unattended when not in his cot, at the half-year stage you need to double your attention. Even if you think your baby's first rollover was a fluke, keep in mind that if this 'fluke' happened once, it'll happen again.

At 6–7 months, your baby can lift his head and chest off the floor using his arms. He can sit up for a while if you support him with a cushion. He may roll from back to front and may try to crawl. He likes putting things into his mouth at this age, so don't leave anything unsuitable lying around. He grabs his toys using his whole hand and moves things from one hand to the other.

At 8–9 months, your baby wants to stand. He tries to crawl by rocking back and forth, and he may pull himself to standing if he uses his knees first. He can now sit on his own for longer periods. He may try to crawl upstairs, so make sure you have a stair gate in place. He uses his thumb and first finger to pick up small things and search for his toys if he drops them.

Your baby loves to stand, even before he can do so unaided. Help him develop leg strength by letting him stand on your lap while you hold him around the tummy. You may consider buying a bouncy chair for your baby. You put your child in the chair and he can sit, stand, or bounce to his heart's content. Some of these chairs swivel so that your baby can change direction. Some have an attached tray of toys.

At 8 months, your baby's muscles have developed to the point where he can sit for 10 minutes without tiring and crawl – probably backwards. His brain hasn't grasped the right muscle use for front and back movement. Different babies crawl in different ways: Your baby may shuffle on his bottom or move sideways like a crab – whatever he does, encourage him as he's learning how to control his body. Try holding a toy above his head and encourage him to reach for it. Some babies don't crawl at all but still develop normally.

At 9–10 months, your baby has good balance and good flexibility to swivel and twist his body to get what he wants.

At 10–11 months, your baby stands and tries to walk by holding on to furniture. Encourage him to walk by holding his hand as he moves along. By 12 months, he should be able to walk independently. At this point, your baby uses his thumb and first finger to pick things up precisely, such as raisins. He can also put small toys into a box – although he may prefer to throw them around!

From 2 to 3 years

From the age of 2 years, your child walks up and down stairs with two feet to a step. He loves climbing on the furniture and enjoys more challenging toys such as Lego and building blocks: these toys encourage his fine-motor skills. Your child can run by this age and kick a stationary ball.

He can turn the pages of a book individually, so read him plenty of stories to encourage him to do this. He may be able to hold a pencil to draw. At this age, your child has fairly good hand–eye coordination and should be able to recognise you and his family in photos: Encourage this by having plenty of photos and drawings around the house.

By 3 years, your child can run and walk, both normally and on his tiptoes. He will probably be able to kick, throw, and catch a big ball between his arms. He walks upstairs with one foot per step, eats with a spoon, washes and dries his hands on his own, and puts on and takes off his coat. Encourage your child's independence by playing ball games, giving him safe cutlery to eat with, and getting him to wash his hands unaided before mealtimes.

From 4 to 5 years

By now, your child runs up and down the stairs and balances on one foot. Help him develop further by encouraging him to ride a bike – he should be able to pedal well. He's now more skilled at ball games and activities such as climbing, skipping, and swinging. He can do jigsaws and colour in pictures well. By this age, your child's hearing and vision are pretty much developed to adult level.

Considering Cognitive Development

Cognitive development is the development of your child's ability to use his mind, imagination, creativity, and problem-solving skills, allowing him to organise his ideas and thoughts and make sense of the world around him. He begins to develop an understanding of concepts – shapes, colours, time – through different methods, including playing, talking, listening to you, asking questions, and imitating. He also learns by using his senses – watching, touching, tasting, smelling, and listening.

Your baby needs stimulation. Support his cognitive development by encouraging regular play activities and showing him repeatedly how to do things. He learns by copying you. Let him go at his own pace and give him plenty of encouragement and praise when he gets it right.

The age at which your child acquires knowledge and understanding depends on his genetic pattern of development and how much play and stimulating activity he takes part in. However, you can look out for some milestones, which we describe in the next three sections.

From birth to 24 months

From the moment he's born, your child discovers the relationship between his body and environment. He relies on his senses – seeing, touching, feeling, and sucking – to learn. By experimenting, he starts to develop an awareness of himself as being separate from his environment. He begins to realise that he can move things with his hands. A major breakthrough comes at around 4 months, when your baby discovers that objects are permanent and don't disappear just because he can't see them. After your child grasps this concept, he starts experimenting to see what happens: He may pull a pillow towards him when a toy is sat on it, or squash a teddy so that he can push it through the bars of his cot. Help your child's development by playing games such as peek-a-boo, making him realise that you don't disappear behind a pair of hands. Try doing the same with his toys: put Teddy behind your back and then reproduce him with a flourish.

From 2 to 4 years

At this age, your child's speech is egocentric, relating everything to himself – for example, 'My toy'. Don't worry – he's supposed to think that he's the centre of the universe at this stage! Your child has a hard time understanding the world from any perspective other than his own – hence the temper tantrums and the 'Me! Me! Me!' attitude. He begins to use symbols, words, and language, but he's not really thinking logically at this stage. By 3 years, your child's much better at communicating and tries to use words to understand his world. He's very imaginative and responsive at this stage.

Foster your child's intellectual development by giving him lots of picture books and reading to him regularly. Games that encourage thinking skills are a good idea – try paints, crayons, alphabet games, and jigsaws. Encourage his imagination by letting him dress up in different costumes and play in different environments such as water and sand.

From 4 to 7 years

From age 4 years, your child's speech is more social and less egocentric. He understands logical concepts but still focuses attention on one aspect and ignores other parts of an object. He responds to your dos and don'ts and is capable of problem-solving, such as basic sums.

By 4 years, your child forms complete sentences and has a vocabulary of around 1,540 words. He's very inquisitive, questioning, and imaginative. Books, jigsaws, construction sets such as Lego, and dressing-up boxes are great ways of helping him to express himself.

By 5 years, his vocabulary has grown to around 2,070 words and he can tell longer stories. He reads his own name, counts up to 20, and knows his colours and textures. He begins to question the meaning of words and understands the difference between what's real and what's not. He reasons, based on his experiences. Visits to museums and zoos encourage him to explore his environment at this age.

From 7 years, your child reasons logically and organises his thoughts. He can still only think about physical objects though, and he isn't capable of abstract reasoning. He starts to lose his egocentric thinking pattern at this age. He can now do multiple tasks, for example arithmetic – encourage this by setting him sums, giving him an abacus, and choosing games and cards that encourage numerical awareness.

 Keep on top of the teaching methods his school uses (such as using a phonetic alphabet), and be consistent when you're helping your child at home. There's quite enough for him to take in at this stage, without the added confusion of different learning styles!

Looking at Social Development

Developing social skills is an important part of your child's growth. He needs to learn how to share his things, consider others, communicate well, and have a positive self-image in order to grow into a mature, emotionally balanced adult. Your child also needs to learn how to feed, wash, and dress himself and go to the toilet.

You can do lots of things to aid your child's progress. Get him to socialise with other children, expose him to new environments on holidays and at playgroups, give him lots of love and affection, and praise and encourage him. All of these help him develop confidence, sociability, and independence.

From birth to 24 months

For the first month, your baby's totally dependent on you. He communicates through touch, his eyes, crying, and smiling. He learns how to interact with you by watching your facial expressions.

By 3 months, your baby expresses his happiness and discomfort through different facial expressions. He enjoys touching and being held by you.

At 5 months, he may be a little clingy and anxious about being separated from you or having to deal with strangers. He may play alongside other children, but not necessarily with them – this is known as *parallel play*.

By 6 months, your baby may be more accepting of other children.

At 9 months, your baby's familiar with his family and may still be wary of strangers.

At 1 year, he's affectionate towards you and enjoys playing with you. He may demand his own way.

At 15 months, he's keen to get out into the world and explore his environment – as long as you're close by! He begins to use single words to communicate and points to express his meaning. He starts to develop a sense of himself as a person. He knows that he needs the toilet, but he isn't yet able to control his bladder.

By 18 months, your child's vocabulary has increased and he communicates more easily. He may express stronger emotions such as fear or anger. He signals that he needs to go to the toilet, and he can undress himself.

From 2 to 4 years

At 2–3 years, your child's a lot more independent and able to feed himself with a fork and spoon, use the toilet, and wash and dress himself without your help. He may be prone to temper tantrums. He likes to *pretend play* – act out ideas and copy what you do – and *parallel play* – play alongside, but not with, other children.

At 3 years, your child is more aware of other children and more likely to interact with them – known as *cooperative play* – by sharing roles and activities. He may have a special friend and be less egocentric.

By age 4, your child forms longer-lasting bonds and friendships. He may have friends of the same sex. He can wash his hands and face and clean his teeth. By age 5, he can tie his shoelaces.

From 5 to 7 years

By school age, your child has more awareness of a special or 'best' friend and knows who he likes to play with – although this may change from day to day. He begins to be more social, as he's now interacting with teachers, other children, and other adults. As a result, he start to develop values and becomes aware of what is and isn't socially acceptable. He gains independence and confidence. Play time becomes more complex and competitive, with games such as hide-and-seek and school sports. Being popular with his peers is very important and has a huge impact on his self-esteem. This is an important and scary time in your child's life, so talk to him regularly about school, his friends, and his feelings.

Watching Your Child Grow

Physical growth refers to the increase in your child's height and weight and other body changes, such as hair growth and teething dramas. These are all part of the growth process.

Your baby is genetically programmed to reach a certain size and height. You and your partner's heights influence your baby's weight and height in later life. Genetics also determines your baby's metabolism and shape. Other factors include your ethnic group and nutritional input – but genetics is the main influence.

To reassure you that your child's developing normally, you may find it helpful to know about general growth patterns for children, why growth spurts occur and when to expect them, and why your doctor charts your baby's growth. Your health visitor or doctor checks your baby and compares him with national average weight and height charts from birth. But don't get too hung up on this – each child is an individual when it comes to growth.

Monitor your child's growth by recording his height on his bedroom wall or a height chart. Involve him in this – he'll be excited to know that he's getting bigger. The Child Growth Foundation (CGF) recommends measuring your child every six months from 18 months.

What's normal growth?

During the first year of life, your baby grows rapidly. Following this huge spurt, you may then be surprised when your child stops growing at such a speed. From day one, your health visitor keeps track of your baby's weight, length, and head size because growth is a good indicator of general health. The following is a guide to your child's growth from birth to puberty.

Children grow at different rates, and some are taller or shorter than others. If your child is big or small, avoid comparing him with his siblings or other children – this will make him feel self-conscious of his size.

Newborns

Most babies born full-term (37–40 weeks) weigh between 6 pounds, 2 ounces (2.75 kilograms) and 9 pounds, 2 ounces (4.5 kilograms). The average length is 19–21 inches (48–53 centimetres).

Various factors affect your baby's size at birth, including the height of you and your partner, and whether your baby was born early or late.

Most newborns are born with extra fluid, so they lose a few ounces as they lose this fluid. A healthy baby regains the lost weight within two weeks. During the first month, newborns gain around 5 ounces (142 grams) a week and grow around 1–1.5 inches (2.5–4 centimetres) in the first month. There may be a rapid period of growth from 7 to 10 days old and again from 3 to 6 weeks.

Between 1 year and puberty

In the first year, your baby grows rapidly – by his first birthday, he gains an average of 10 inches (25 centimetres) in length and triples his birth weight. However, he doesn't continue growing at such a rapid weight. After a year, your child's growth slows down, and by age 2 years his growth hits a fairly constant rate of 2–2½ inches (5–6 centimetres) a year until he reaches puberty.

By age 2 years, the growth in height continues at a steady rate of 2½ inches (6 centimetres) per year until adolescence. This isn't a 'perfect' rate – your child will have periods of growth spurts followed by periods of slower growth.

Puberty

Your child has a major growth spurt at puberty, between 8 and 13 years in girls and between 10 and 15 years in boys. Puberty usually lasts for two to five years. This growth is linked to sexual development: Your child grows body hair on the sex organs and under the arms, and girls begin to menstruate. By the age of 16–17 years, most boys and girls have reached physical maturity.

Growth spurts and growing pains

If your child wakes up with throbbing legs, you may wonder if you should take him to the doctor. The best thing is to reassure him and explain what's happening – the skeleton's being formed. These *growing pains* are completely normal. The most likely causes are aches and discomfort caused by physical activity during the day. The pains are concentrated in the muscles rather than the joints.

Growth spurts are linked to sexual development, so puberty brings pubic and underarm hair, fully developed sexual organs, and periods for girls.

Because your child's limbs grow at different rates, he may sometimes feel clumsy, weak, and uncoordinated. This is because his nervous system is trying to adjust to the rapid period of growth. His ligaments and tendons get tighter and he may get pains in his knees during exercise. Therefore, teach you child the importance of stretching properly before and after exercise.

Check how your child responds to touch when he's in pain. Children with serious medical conditions may not like to be touched, as touch intensifies the pain. But a child with growing pains feels better when he's massaged, touched, and held.

The following may help your child with growing pains:

- Offer him lots of cuddles and reassurance
- Massage the painful area
- Manually stretch your child's legs
- Put a heated pad on the painful area
- Paracetamol or ibuprofen in the appropriate dose for his age may help
- Explain what's happening to him and why it hurts sometimes

Growth spurts

All children have *growth spurts* – growth at a quicker rate than normal. These growth spurts are linked to important developmental changes. The most significant are between 3 and 5 years and between 8 and 12 years. This usually happens in spring as a result of lots of fresh air and exercise.

Playing your role in your child's growth

You can do lots of things to ensure that your child develops normally:

- **Make sure he gets enough sleep.** Most children need around 10–12 hours a night. Proper rest helps your child grow.
- **Feed him nourishing meals.** Ensure he gets a balanced diet full of essential vitamins and minerals. See Chapter 9 for more info on good nutrition.
- **Encourage him to exercise.** Child obesity in the UK gets a lot of press, so to avoid being another statistic make sure your child exercises regularly. Cycling, walking, swimming, and team sports all motivate him and keep him fit. Chapter 10 offers lots of tips on getting active.

Checking Out Growth, Height, and Weight Charts

Growth charts are an important way to monitor your child's growth and development and to check he's growing normally. The charts are available on the Internet so you can use them at home. Doctors use growth charts and body mass index (BMI) charts to compare your child's growth with other children in the same age range. These checks form a standard part of your child's medical check ups.

Growth charts are measured out in 'centiles', which compare the height, weight, or head circumference of an average spread of 100 children at the same age. If your child was born on the 10th centile, that means that he is bigger than 10 per cent of other children and smaller than 90 per cent. These lines give an indication of the rate at which height or weight increase over time for each of these centiles. So if your child is on the 10th centile, he will not only be smaller than a baby on the 90th centile, he'll grow at a slower rate, too. As long as your child is growing along about the same centile line, there's no need for concern. If his weight drops down from one centile line to another (and especially if it drops down by two centile lines) your health visitor may recommend that you get him checked out by the GP (you can find out more about this in the section on examining growth disturbance later in this chapter). But don't worry – even children whose weight tails off usually catch up, and turn out to have nothing wrong with them.

Contact the Child Growth Foundation (020-8995-0257; `www.childgrowth foundation.org`) for growth charts and instructions on how to use them.

Growth charts can be a bit complicated to use because of the detailed information they contain, so here are basic guidelines:

- ✔ Use the correct chart for your child's age and sex. You'll find two sets of charts: One for infants (age 0–36 months) and one for children and adolescents (age 2–20 years). Boys and girls use different charts, because they have different growth rates.

- ✔ Find your child's age on the bottom of the chart and draw a vertical line from that point on the growth chart.

- ✔ Find your child's weight on the right-hand side of the chart and draw a horizontal line from that point on the growth chart.

- ✔ Find the point where the two lines meet. Then find the curve closest to that spot, and follow the curve until you find the number that matches your child's statistics.

Growth charts are valuable tools, but don't focus on one reading. The charts are best used over a longer period to find a growth pattern. The growth of children aged between 6 and 18 months tends to fluctuate, but older children tend to follow the growth curve more closely.

Measuring body mass index (BMI)

Body mass index (BMI) is a calculation that uses your child's height and weight to estimate how much body fat he has. Your doctor uses BMI to determine whether your child is the appropriate weight for his age and height.

From the age of 2 years, a BMI check forms part of your child's regular check-ups. The doctor checks your child's BMI against other children and then puts the measurements on a standard child growth chart. There are separate charts for boys and girls to account for growth and body fat differences. After several checks, a pattern emerges and your doctor can track your child's growth.

BMI can be a helpful measurement if your child's at risk of becoming overweight as he gets older. In older children, there's a strong link between BMI and body fat. A child with higher BMI readings will probably have weight problems when he's older. If your child has high BMI readings, take steps to change his diet and exercise habits (see Chapters 9 and 10).

BMI isn't a perfect measurement. Children gain weight quickly – for example, during puberty – and a high BMI may be due to a high muscle mass. Monitor BMI as a trend rather than individual numbers.

Grappling with growth disturbances

Growth disturbances are departures from normal growth patterns. 'Normal' is hard to define, as no two children develop at the same rate. After birth, your baby should gain about 5 ounces (142 grams) per week from the second week to around 3 months. By 5 months, his birth weight should have doubled. If your child doesn't grow as expected, your doctor may look into whether he has a growth disturbance.

Children differ in size genetically, so your child's growth rate can't be based on just one examination. Monitor your child's growth over a period of time.

Your child will have regular professional health examinations by a health visitor or doctor. These check-ups may take place at school or during medical checks for other concerns.

If you're concerned about your child's growth, your health visitor or GP will measure and weigh your child and draw some growth curves for your child. Your doctor takes into consideration you and your partner's height and weight in childhood, adulthood, and puberty. Your doctor may ask questions about your child's diet, appetite, and exercise habits. The doctor may then examine your child – he make take an X-ray of your child's hand and wrist to examine the development of the bones. If the doctor thinks there may be a problem, he'll refer your child to a paediatrician for treatment.

Growth is determined mainly by genetics and environmental factors, particularly diet and exercise. Poor nutrition is one cause of growth disturbance. The other two leading causes of growth disturbance are the endocrine disorders *growth hormone deficiency* (GHD) and *thyroid deficiency* (which we talk about in the following sections).

Most children have no growth or developmental problems, but if you're concerned about your child ask your doctor or health visitor. You aren't being a pest – and it's their job to reassure you as a parent!

Growth hormone deficiency

GHD occurs when the pituitary gland doesn't produce sufficient growth hormone to help your child grow. From the age of 2 years, your child's growth pattern slows down if he has GHD. Doctors don't know why this happens, but the disease may be hereditary – 3 per cent of children with GHD have a brother or sister with the same disorder. GHD is three times more common in boys than girls.

A child with GHD may:

- ✔ Be small, but with normal skeletal proportions, facial appearance, and intellect
- ✔ Possibly be overweight
- ✔ Have a younger 'bone age' than normal (the bones aren't as developed as they should be)

If you suspect your child has GHD, ask your doctor to perform the relevant tests. The diagnosis is confirmed by measuring the level of growth hormone produced in response to a stimulation test – this usually involves a day trip to hospital.

With treatment, your child's outlook is excellent, provided treatment starts before age 6 years. Catch-up growth occurs following initial treatment and normal growth follows.

Thyroid deficiency

The thyroid is a small gland that lies beneath the skin and neck muscles. In the teenage years, the thyroid has a very important function – it makes the hormones that regulate metabolism and growth. If the thyroid is ineffective, it can interfere with physical development and cause further health problems.

If the thyroid is overactive (hyperthyroidism), too much thyroid hormone is released into the bloodstream and the body uses energy too quickly. Symptoms of hyperthyroidism include:

- ✔ Sweating excessively
- ✔ Unable to withstand heat
- ✔ Tiredness or sleeping problems
- ✔ Fast heartbeat
- ✔ Irregular menstrual periods
- ✔ Weight loss

Your GP can diagnose overactive thyroid problems. If your child has such a problem, the doctor may prescribe anti-thyroid tablets for your child. Once the hormone levels are corrected, your child should feel fine again.

If the thyroid is underactive (hypothyroidism), the body produces too little thyroid hormone and the body uses energy more slowly. Symptoms of hypothyroidism include:

- ✔ Depression
- ✔ Feeling sluggish
- ✔ Weight gain
- ✔ Growing at a slow rate physically and sexually
- ✔ Irregular menstrual periods
- ✔ Poor memory and concentration

Your GP can diagnose thyroid problems and suggest suitable treatment.

Chapter 3

The Immune System and Immunisation

*T*he immune system is the body's suit of armour, its unsung hero. The body can't survive without a heart to pump blood around it, or lungs to breathe oxygen, but how many of us give a thought to the intricate network that comprises the immune system? There it is, working around the clock without a single moment's rest, and it rarely gets a credit in the list of life's essentials. But without the immune system, we wouldn't be here: It provides our defence against the millions of bacteria, viruses, toxins, and parasites that are just itching to take over our bodies given half the chance.

The only time any of us becomes aware of this amazing piece of engineering is when the immune system goes wrong. Being poorly is a sign that the immune system has temporarily been unable to kill off an invading nasty. It can take a while for the body to fight and overpower the invader, but in most cases the body eventually wins – and that's all down to the power of the immune system.

Finding Out How Your Child Fights Infections

Keeping bacteria, viruses, and any other potential invaders at bay is a complex operation involving the efforts of several essential organs, blood cells, glands, and hormones. The immune system is often compared to an army because it comprises many different forces that work together to protect the body from unwanted bugs.

Do not enter: keeping the invaders out

The most visible part of the immune system is the skin. Supplying our first line of defence, it provides a primary boundary between germs and the body. Part of the skin's job is to act as a barrier in much the same way as you use cling film to protect food. Healthy skin is tough and impermeable to bacteria and viruses, not only because it seals the body's organs but also because it contains special cells that secrete antibacterial substances, such as the salt found in sweat, to kill off invaders.

The nose, mouth, and eyes are obvious entry points for germs. They too contain germ-fighting chemicals: Tears, nasal mucus, and saliva contain enzymes that destroy the cells of many kinds of bacteria. And since the nasal passage and lungs are coated in mucus, many germs that aren't killed immediately are trapped in the mucus, swallowed, and then destroyed by stomach acid.

Looking for troublemakers

If harmful germs do manage to get inside the body, the immune system needs to deal with them in order to stop them overrunning the body. It has to detect and eliminate the invaders before they can make themselves at home and reproduce – which they can do rapidly. If this mission is accomplished, then the viruses or bacteria are killed off before they cause feelings of illness; if the mission fails, however, the germs temporarily get the better of the immune system and illness ensues, continuing until the system has tackled and destroyed the invaders.

The main defenders of the immune system are white blood cells. They travel through the bloodstream and the lymphatic system, and are programmed to recognise troublemakers, whether bacteria, viruses, or other infecting agents, so that they can mount an organised attack against them.

Taking a systematic approach

The lymph system is a pivotal part of the immune system. It consists of an internal network of vessels throughout the body that are saturated with a special clear liquid called lymph, which contains white blood cells and carries them around the body. The whole body is soaked in lymph, although you rarely see it. Unlike blood, which is pumped around the body by the heart, lymph relies on exercise and muscular activity in order to circulate.

TECHNICAL STUFF

The amazing white blood cell

There are many types of white blood cell, each with its own specific job in keeping the body infection-free. White blood cells work together to detect, neutralise, and destroy invading bacteria and viruses. They do so in many ways; for example, some neutralise the invaders or make them more easily devoured by larger, so-called 'scavenger' cells. Other white blood cells ingest the invaders or release enzymes and chemical agents such as histamine to attack the invaders.

White blood cells are not like other cells in the body: They act like living single-cell organisms and are able to move and capture things on their own. Many white blood cells cannot divide and reproduce on their own – instead, they are made by the body's bone marrow. Unlike red blood cells, white blood cells have the ability to move on their own and are able to pass through cell walls, allowing them to assemble rapidly at the site of infection or injury.

Lymph also carries away waste products, which are filtered out by the lymph nodes located all over the body. Within the lymph nodes, harmful micro-organisms are trapped, attacked, and destroyed by white blood cells. This is one of the body's most efficient lines of defence. Lymph nodes are storage sites for cells – they're the 'swollen glands' often present during an infection. The tonsils, adenoids, and appendix are all important parts of the lymph system. If any of them is swollen, your child's body is probably fighting an infection.

Antibodies are manufactured in the lymph system. They are protective substances that the body produces in response to invasion by a hostile organism or the presence of a foreign substance. Antibodies counteract a number of the invading bacteria and viruses by inactivating them and making them powerless.

Like an elephant, the immune system never forgets

One of the remarkable things about the immune system is its ability to remember and recognise past invaders, allowing the body to respond quickly to a second attack. Disease-causing viruses and bacteria invade and reproduce rapidly in their millions, with an ability to respond quickly that is extremely important. Immunity is the body's ability to resist an invasion of disease-causing bacteria and viruses. Once antibodies have been made to fight a certain type of micro-organism, that micro-organism usually no longer poses a threat to the body, which is why one attack of a disease often prevents its recurrence later down the road.

This 'memory' is the basis of immunisation. Hundreds of years ago, forward-thinking scientists realised that having one infection not only allowed us to fight off that same disease if we came across it again, but also would be resistant to related diseases. Three hundred years ago, Edward Jenner worked out that milkmaids who had been infected in the course of their work with a relatively mild disease called cowpox never caught the infinitely more serious smallpox. He 'innoculated' his first patient by exposing them to material taken from a cowpox blister – sure enough, they, like the milkmaids, became immune to smallpox.

Living Examples: Seeing the Immune System in Action

In order to understand how the immune system works, you need to see it in operation. Here are a few examples of how the system does such an amazing job:

- ✔ **Cuts and grazes:** If your child cuts herself, all sorts of germs enter her body through the break in the skin. Her immune system responds by producing white blood cells to eliminate the invaders while the skin heals itself. In rare cases, the cut is infected: Then the area becomes inflamed because germ-fighting cells collect at the site of an infection, or the cut fills with pus, which is made up of millions of dead cells from the immune system that have tried to deal with the infection.

- ✔ **Insect bites:** If an insect nibbles your child's skin, your child gets a red itchy bump – a sign that the immune system's doing its job. The bump consists of a collection of millions of fighter cells that have gathered to protect the invading substance entering the bloodstream.

- ✔ **Colds and 'flu:** Each day your child inhales thousands of bacteria and viruses that are floating in the air. The immune system normally deals with these without a problem, but occasionally a germ gets past the first lines of defence and your child catches a cold or another bug. This is a visible sign that her immune system failed to stop the invading germ. Cells from the immune system rush to the mucus membranes in the nose and upper airways, killing off the germs before they get a hold deeper in the body, such as in the lungs. The fact that not every cold develops into pneumonia or life-threatening blood poisoning shows just how well your child's immune system is working each and every day. In time, the immune system kills off all the germs causing symptoms, and your child recovers completely. Getting over the illness is a visible sign that your child's immune system is working. In some cases, a bug is so virulent that antibiotics or other medication are needed to help your child's body fight the invaders.

✔ **Tummy upsets:** Every day, your child swallows hundreds of germs, most of which die in her saliva or the acid in the stomach. Occasionally, however, a germ gets through and causes food poisoning, with obvious visible effects – vomiting and diarrhoea are two of the most common symptoms. Again, the immune system can usually prevent these germs from taking over the whole body, so their effects tend to be local to the gut and digestive system (hence the copious quantities being produced at both ends!). Within a few days your child's immune system fights them off completely.

A helping hand: antibiotics

Sometimes the immune system can't respond quickly enough to outpace the reproductive rate of the invading bacteria, or the bacteria produce toxins so quickly that the toxins cause damage before the immune system can get to work. When this happens, antibiotics help the body kill off the bacteria without affecting the body's own cells. Different antibiotics work on different bacteria. But antibiotics do *not* work on viruses.

If your child is prescribed an antibiotic, the drug should kill off all the target bacteria over 5–10 days. Your child will feel better within just a day or two because the antibiotic kills the majority of the bacteria extremely quickly. Even though she feels better, however, your child should finish the course in order to prevent the illness recurring.

Although antibiotics can be real lifesavers, overuse of these drugs is a growing problem. Sometimes bacteria *mutate* (change the way they're made) and are able to survive the antibiotic. These bacteria then reproduce, the disease changes, and the antibiotic becomes totally ineffective in fighting that disease in everyone. This process is known as *antibiotic resistance*, and it has become a large concern among doctors, who are now much more measured in their prescriptions.

If an antibiotic worked the first time for an infection your child contracted, but not the second, the reason is not that your child has become resistant to the effects of the antibiotic. The germ, not the child, mutates! That also means that just because an antibiotic hasn't worked for your child in the past doesn't mean it won't work in the future.

Many infections are *self-limiting* – your child's immune system fights them off on its own within a few days. If the cause is a virus infection, the antibiotics won't do any good, but you may assume that they have because your child recovers.

Looking at disorders of the immune system

Many human ailments are caused by the immune system working in an unexpected or incorrect way. Allergies, for example, are a sign that the immune system is overreacting to certain stimuli that other people don't react to. Diabetes is caused by the immune system inappropriately attacking and destroying cells in the pancreas. Both allergies and diabetes are becoming more common in children.

Boosting Your Child's Immune System

So what can you do to protect your child from the endless array of germs that she's exposed to every day? Unfortunately, for a child, getting sick is simply part of the job description. The immune system is built up only by coming into contact with bacteria, viruses, and other organisms: The system is actually strengthened by battling with germs. Many experts consider six to eight colds, 'flu-like illnesses, and ear infections per year in the first five years to be normal – and even more (sometimes up to 12 or 15) if your child is in close contact with other children, such as older siblings or nursery playmates.

Turbo-charging your child's defences

Despite the fact that your child is bound to get ill sometimes, you can adopt the following healthy habits to give your child's immune system a boost.

✔ **Breastfeed your baby.** Breast milk contains turbo-charged immunity-enhancing antibodies and white blood cells. It guards against myriad health hazards, including ear infections, allergies, diarrhoea, pneumonia, meningitis, urinary tract infections, and sudden infant death syndrome (SIDS). Read more about SIDS in Chapter 11. Studies show that breastfeeding may also enhance your baby's brainpower and protect her against insulin-dependent diabetes, Crohn's disease, colitis, and certain forms of cancer later in life. Colostrum, the thin yellow pre-milk that flows from the breast during the first few days after birth, is especially rich in disease-fighting antibodies. For maximum benefit, experts recommend breastfeeding for a year and exclusively for the first 6 months.

Even if you manage to breastfeed for only a short while, every single bout of breastfeeding makes a difference to your child. Many mums give up breastfeeding because they find it difficult or painful. But breastfeeding should be neither: The key is to get as much support as possible, so ask your midwife, health visitor, or breastfeeding counsellor for help. See Chapter 6 for the how-tos and whys of breastfeeding.

✔ **Serve more fruit and veg.** All fruit and vegetables contain immunity-boosting phytonutrients such as vitamin C and carotenoids. Phytonutrients are believed to increase the body's production of infection-fighting white blood cells and interferon, an antibody that coats cell surfaces to block out viruses. Studies show that a diet rich in phytonutrients can also protect against diseases such as cancer and heart disease in adulthood. Try to get your child to eat five servings of fruit and veg a day: A serving's about two tablespoons for toddlers, or a piece of medium fruit (apple, orange), or two pieces of smaller fruit (plums, satsumas), or a 4-ounce portion of berries or veg for older children. Munch your way through Chapter 9 for all sorts of info on your child's nutrition.

✔ **Boost sleep time.** Studies of adults show that sleep deprivation can make you more susceptible to illness by reducing *natural killer cells*, immune-system weapons that attack microbes and cancer cells. The same holds true for children. Go to Chapter 11 for tips and advice on how to ensure that your child gets enough sleep.

✔ **Exercise as a family.** Research shows that exercise increases the number of natural disease-fighting cells in adults – and regular activity can benefit children in the same way. The lymphatic system is dependent on exercise to circulate efficiently, and so movement and exercise really are crucial to health. To get your children into a lifelong fitness habit, be a good role model. Check out Chapter 10 for practical tips on getting the whole family active.

✔ **Guard against germ spread.** Fighting germs doesn't technically boost immunity, but is a great way to reduce stress on your child's immune system. Make sure that your child washes her hands frequently – with soap. Pay particular attention to your child's hygiene before and after meals and after playing outside, handling pets, blowing her nose, using the toilet, and arriving home after being at school, in the garden, and on public transport. When you're out, carry disposable wipes for quick cleanups.

Here's another key germ-busting strategy: If your child gets ill, throw out her toothbrush straight away. Your child can't catch the same virus twice, but the virus can hop from toothbrush to toothbrush, infecting other family members. If your child has a bacterial infection, such as tonsillitis, then she can actually re-infect herself with the same germs that made her sick in the first place.

✔ **Banish second-hand smoke.** If you or your partner smokes, quit. Cigarette smoke contains more than 4,000 toxins, most of which can irritate or kill cells in the body. Your child's more susceptible than you to the harmful effects of second-hand smoke because she breathes at a faster rate and her natural detoxification system is less well developed. Breathing second-hand smoke increases your child's risk of SIDS, bronchitis, ear infections, and asthma. It may also affect intelligence and neurological development. If you absolutely can't stop smoking, then reduce your child's health risks considerably by smoking only outside the house.

✔ **Don't overdo antibiotics.** Urging your doctor for a prescription for antibiotics whenever your child has a cold or sore throat is a bad idea. Antibiotics treat only illnesses caused by bacteria, but the majority of childhood illnesses are caused by viruses.

Appreciating the role of nutrition

Making sure that your child gets the right vitamins and minerals can increase the number of white blood cells she produces, boosting her immunity and helping her to function better. Vitamins and minerals can also help to eliminate toxins.

Most children in the UK, unless they're extremely fussy eaters, can get plenty of vitamins through their diet alone and do not need vitamin supplements.

Nutrients that are particularly good for boosting immunity include the following:

✔ **Vitamin C:** Many experts consider that high levels of vitamin C increase the production of white blood cells and antibodies, including interferon, which protects cells from viruses. Vitamin C may also protect the heart and lower blood pressure. Studies suggest a link between high vitamin C consumption and lower rates of cancer. Children under the age of 6 years benefit from an intake of vitamin C of around 250 milligrams per day, while older children and adults can take 500 milligrams per day. If your child eats at least five servings of fruit and veg a day, she'll be getting the right amount of vitamin C. Foods that contain vitamin C include oranges, kiwi, papaya, and strawberries.

✔ **Vitamin E:** An important *antioxidant*, which means it can counteract the damaging effects of toxins, stimulates the production of antibodies and natural killer cells, which seek and destroy germs and cancer. Vitamin E also protects the heart. Foods high in vitamin E include seeds, vegetable oils, and grains.

✔ **Carotenoids, such as beta carotene:** They also increase the number of infection-fighting and killer cells and are good antioxidants. Beta carotene is converted by the body into vitamin A, which has immune-boosting functions. Foods rich in carotenoids include carrots, yellow peppers, and sweetcorn.

✔ **Zinc:** An invaluable mineral that increases the production of white blood cells and stimulates the release of antibodies. Sources of zinc include fortified cereals, beans, dark turkey meat, and beef.

A word about garlic and echinacea

Garlic is known as nature's antibiotic, a powerful immune booster that stimulates the multiplication of infection-fighting white cells. Garlic is also an antioxidant. Raw garlic is more powerful than the cooked stuff.

Echinacea is a popular healing herb known for its infection-fighting and immunity-boosting properties. It can be taken in pill or liquid form, and a number of herbal teas are also infused with it. Unlike antibiotics, which kill bacteria directly, echinacea works indirectly by strengthening the body's immune system to kill off invading bacteria. Although echinacea is still being researched, evidence suggests that it can stimulate the body to produce more infection-fighting white blood cells and killer cells. Echinacea also has a marginal effect on the recovery time from the common cold.

✔ **Selenium:** A *trace element* (a natural product present in tiny quantities) that is essential for the production of antibodies. The best sources of selenium are tuna, whole grains, brown rice, egg yolks, and cottage cheese.

✔ **Omega-3 fatty acids:** These are great immune boosters because they increase the activity of the white blood cells that eat up bacteria. Foods high in omega-3 fatty acids include oily fish, nuts, and seeds.

✔ **Probiotics:** Also known as acidophilus. Probiotics are healthy bacteria that live in our intestines and help our immune system. For most children, they don't make a big difference to the digestive system, which works very effectively on its own. However, if your child has digestive problems such as chronic diarrhoea, your doctor may advise of probiotics such as lactobacillus and bifidobacteria, which are available in in certain 'probiotic' foods in supermarkets or in liquid, powder, and capsule forms.

Certain foods are known to weaken the immune system. Sugar, for example, has an immune-suppressing effect. In fact, studies have shown that eating or drinking as little as 100 grams (eight tablespoons) of sugar – the equivalent of a can of fizzy drink – can reduce the ability of white blood cells to kill germs. Too much fat can also lead to a depressed immune system because it can affect the ability of white blood cells to multiply. A diet consisting mainly of highly processed and synthetic foods can deplete the body's stores of nutrients, leaving the body more vulnerable to infection. Therefore, a healthy diet with lots of fresh foods helps your child stay in tip-top condition.

Pricking the Surface: The Low-Down on Vaccinations

The vast majority of medical experts agree that one of the best ways to protect your child against harmful diseases is to make sure that she has her vaccinations. In fact, most doctors have no doubt that vaccinating your child is the single most important step you can take to protect your child's health, because it offers her protection against a range of potentially life-threatening or disabling infectious illnesses. Indeed, over the last couple of centuries, immunisation has done more to improve infant survival rates in the UK than any other advance apart from, perhaps, clean water supplies. Since vaccination against smallpox began on a large scale at the start of the nineteenth century, the number of children dying from common infectious diseases has plummeted.

Diseases such as diphtheria, polio, and whooping cough used to be common in the UK and posed a very real threat to children's lives. These diseases can only be kept at bay if the vast majority of the population is immunised against them. Known as *herd immunity* (no, your child is not a cow, but kids do spend a lot of time in close contact with each other!), herd immunity means that at least 90 or 95 per cent of the children that an infected child comes into contact with are resistant because of immunisation, and the germ can't spread far enough to become an epidemic. So, immunisation protects not only your child but the rest of the population too. Studies have shown that when the number of children being vaccinated drops, the number of cases of the illness in question increases.

Even though many diseases are now rare in the UK, the diseases can be brought back from trips abroad and caught by children (and adults) who have not been immunised. Vaccinations are not compulsory in the UK, and as a parent you have a choice. However, diseases such as polio and meningitis aren't the only ones that kill or permanently damage children; measles, mumps, and pneumonia can also have a devastating effect (see Chapter 14). You may worry that you're doing your child harm if you get her vaccinated, but immunisation rates for certain diseases in the UK are well below the levels needed to prevent epidemics. So bear in mind that statistically, you're much more likely to harm your child by not having her immunised. Make sure that your choice is an informed one, so read as much as you can (not relying on media headlines!) before making your decision about whether to have your child immunised.

Available vaccines and the vaccination schedule

It may seem that your child is offered an awful lot of immunisations in the first year or two of life. However, that's because an awful lot of nasty germs are out there, and kids need protection! Many of these infections cause far worse complications if they are contracted in the first year of life than they do if they're caught later on, so delaying immunisation carries its own risks. However, before you decide to have your child immunised, discover as much as possible about the issue, so you can decide whether you are doing the best for your child. Hopefully this book answers your queries, but don't hesitate to ask your health visitor, GP, or practice nurse about any further concerns.

The diseases your child is offered vaccination against are so rare in the UK – and have been for some time, because of the use of vaccines – that you may have never known anyone who's had the diseases. So here's a brief refresher course on the nasties that your child can be immunised against:

- ✔ **Diphtheria:** A disease spread by droplets from the nose and mouth. It causes fever, sore throat, and severe difficulty in swallowing. If complications set in, diphtheria can cause breathing difficulties and damage to the heart, respiratory system, and nervous system. Diphtheria can be fatal.

- ✔ **Tetanus:** Sometimes called lockjaw, this disease is transmitted in soil. Germs enter the body through cuts or burns, causing muscular and breathing problems, which can be fatal. The symptoms of tetanus are painful spasms of muscle contraction and it kills about 1 in 30 people who get it. Tetanus can have a *incubation period* of 4–21 days (which means it can live in the body without showing symptoms). The organism that causes tetanus is found in soil and animal saliva.

- ✔ **Pertussis:** Commonly known as whooping cough, this causes long painful bouts of coughing and can lead to vomiting and choking. This highly infectious disease is transmitted by droplets from the nose or mouth. The incubation period is 7–10 days. Whooping cough starts in the same way as a cold, but as the disease progresses the coughing spasms become more and more severe. The 'whoop' occurs as the child draws breath between bouts of coughing. These distressing symptoms can go on for more than 10 weeks. Severe cases may be complicated by pneumonia (which affects about 1 in 5 infants who get pertussis under 6 months of age), vomiting, weight loss and, more rarely, brain damage and death. Young babies are most at risk (it kills about 1 in 40 babies who get it under one month and 1 in 300 infants who get it under 1 year old).

✔ **Polio:** The polio virus attacks nerve tissue in the brain and spinal cord and can cause paralysis. Polio is still very common in a few developing countries, but cases are rare in the UK. The disease is spread by contact with the faeces, mucus, or saliva of an infected person. The incubation period varies between 3–21 days.

✔ *Haemophilus influenzae B (HIB):* Infection with this organism has 'flu-like symptoms but complications such as meningitis, *septicaemia* (blood poisoning), and pneumonia can follow, which is why the vaccine was introduced.

✔ **Meningitis C:** Meningococcus is a bacterium that causes meningitis and septicaemia. The bacterium has several strains and this vaccination is against one of the most common strains – C. Meningitis is a serious illness that can be fatal or cause long-term damage to the brain and nerves. The illness is spread through droplets from the nose and mouth.

✔ **Measles:** This highly infectious disease used to be the most common childhood illness. It was all but eradicated in the UK when the MMR vaccine was introduced, but since immunisation levels have dropped (see the sidebar 'The MMR debate' later in this chapter), cases have risen again. It has an incubation period of 10 days. Infection is spread by droplets from the mouth and nose. Measles may start like a bad cold, with catarrh and a high temperature. The rash generally appears two days after the first symptoms. Common complications include diarrhoea, ear infections, and the chest infections pneumonia and bronchitis. One in 1,000 children with measles develops meningitis or encephalitis (inflammation of the brain).

✔ **Mumps:** A viral illness usually causing considerable swelling around the cheeks and neck. The incubation period is 14–21 days. Complications include meningitis or encephalitis, which between them affect 1 in 300–400 children who get mumps; deafness (in up to 1 in 25 cases); and inflammation of the testes in boys, which may permanently damage fertility.

✔ **Rubella (German measles):** This is generally a mild illness in children, causing fever, rash, and swollen glands. Complications are rare in children. However, if a pregnant woman contracts rubella in the first 8–10 weeks of pregnancy, the effects on her unborn baby can be serious: Her baby may be born with deafness, blindness, heart problems, and/or brain damage. Rubella has an incubation period of 14–21 days.

If you've already had a child, you should have had a blood test in your first pregnancy to check that you're immune to rubella. If you weren't immune, you should have been offered a vaccination after your baby was born, with a blood test to check that it worked in boosting your immunity. However, if you're pregnant and come into contact with a possible case of rubella, you must contact your GP as soon as possible to check you are immune.

✔ **Tuberculosis (TB):** In areas in the UK that are at high risk for TB, a disease that affects the lungs, your child may be offered the BCG vaccination (Bacillus of Calmette and Guerin) to protect against TB soon after birth. Your baby will probably get a small sore at the injection site after this vaccination, but it heals gradually.

Table 3-1	Typical Vaccinations at Different Ages
Age in months	*Vaccine*
2	DTaP/IPV/Hib + pneumococcal vaccine
3	DTaP/IPV/Hib + Men C vaccine
4	DTaP/IPV/Hib + Men C + pneumococcal vaccine
12	Hib/Men C
13	MMR + pneumococcal vaccine
4–4½ years (pre-school booster)	DT/IPV

Key: D: Immunisation against diphtheria; Ta: Immunisation against tetanus; P: Immunisation against whooping cough (pertussis); IPV: An *inactivated* ('not live' – see the section 'Explaining how jabs work') immunisation against polio; Hib: Immunisation against Haemophilus influenzae type B; Men C: Immunisation against meningitis C; MMR: Immunisation against measles, mumps, and rubella (German measles); Pneumococcal: Immunisation against pneumococcal infection.

Explaining how jabs work

Immunity from a disease occurs naturally when, for example, your child catches an infectious disease such as chicken pox. Your child's immune system launches an assault on the virus by forming antibodies against it. After the immune system has destroyed the infection, the symptoms of the disease disappear, leaving the antibodies to guard the body to prevent further invasion by the same enemy.

Immunisation works by introducing a particular virus or bacterium (or part of it) artificially, so that your child's body develops antibodies against it without actually developing the illness. A vaccine contains a version of the virus or bacterium and tricks the immune system into reacting as though it had met the real thing. White blood cells then make antibodies to the germs and remain in the body, ready to annihilate the real germs should they ever arrive. Your child won't actually develop the infection when she's immunised because the virus or bacterium has been pre-treated to make it harmless.

A number of vaccines, such as the pneumococcal vaccine, are made from an inactivated version of the germ. The pertussis (whooping cough) vaccine is made from proteins from the skin of the virus. When the body develops immunity to these proteins it protects it against the whole germ if it comes into contact with it. Still others, such as diphtheria and tetanus vaccines, are made from small doses of the toxins that these germs produce.

Others, known as *live vaccines*, such as measles, mumps, and rubella, contain a weakened strain of the disease-causing bacterium itself.

What to expect on the day

You will probably be sent a reminder when your baby's jabs are due. In the UK, the vaccination programme starts at age 2 months, with further doses at 3, and 4 months of age (see Table 3-1 in this chapter). Three vaccine doses are given to ensure that your child's body makes a good immune response to the diseases. The first dose of the vaccine may not provide lasting protection, and a protective immune response may not develop fully until the second or even third dose. Injections are usually given by a general practice nurse or health visitor, often in the thigh or the top of the arm. You'll be asked to hold your baby close to you on your lap as she has her injections.

Breastfeeding (or bottle feeding) is a powerful painkiller. If you're worried about the jabs hurting your baby, try feeding her while the nurse vaccinates her. Some doctors suggest giving infant paracetamol before or just after the vaccination, just in case your child's prone to running a temperature after an immunisation (see the next section for more on the side effects of vaccinations).

Your baby may cry briefly while she's being vaccinated, but cuddles and reassurance will soon calm her. You may want to take along a favourite toy or blanket or offer her a feed after she's had the vaccine. The doctor or nurse may ask you to stay in the surgery for 10 minutes or so to check that your baby doesn't have an adverse reaction to the vaccine.

Dealing with side effects

Minor side effects after immunisations are relatively common, but they're usually short-lived. Your child may get redness and swelling at the site of the injection, have a fever, feel unwell, or seem generally out of sorts. A slight rash, particularly after the MMR jab, is common. You can usually relieve such side effects by giving your child the recommended dose of infant paracetamol or ibuprofen, before or after the jab.

Serious side effects after vaccination are rare, but seek medical advice if your child has any of the following after immunisation:

✔ A convulsion (fit)

✔ Persistent fever over 39.5°C

✔ Extreme reaction, such as continual and painful swelling, at the site of the injection

✔ Breathing difficulties, large weals on the skin, or loss of consciousness, which can be symptoms of a relatively rare allergic reaction called anaphylaxis (described fully in Chapter 15). If you suspect your child is suffering from anaphylaxis, take her to your nearest accident and emergency department immediately.

Serious side effects are rare, but they do happen. But bear in mind that all the immunisations offered in the UK are far less likely to cause complications than getting the disease. For instance, meningitis or encephalitis affects fewer than one in a million infants receiving the MMR vaccine, but 1 in 300–400 children who contract mumps.

Seek advice from your GP or health visitor before immunisation if your child:

✔ Has an acute illness accompanied by fever. Your GP is likely to advise you to delay vaccination until the illness has settled. (This does not include mild coughs, colds, and earaches.)

✔ Has had a bad reaction to a previous immunisation. This significantly increases the chance of a bad reaction to later similar immunisations.

✔ Has an allergy to eggs (the MMR vaccine is prepared in eggs. While the amount of egg contained in the vaccine is so small that it probably won't cause a problem even if your child has a severe allergy, your GP may recommend that your child has the vaccination carried out under close supervision at the hospital).

✔ Has ever had a convulsion (fit).

✔ Has any illness that affects her immune system, for example HIV or AIDS. (A child whose immune system is not working properly should not have live vaccines.)

✔ Is taking any medicines that affect her immune system, for example immunosuppressants following organ transplant, high-dose steroids, or chemotherapy.

Answering commonly asked questions

Vaccinations are a hot topic among parents. While everyone wants to protect their baby from serious illnesses, parents naturally want to be absolutely sure that the jabs their baby receives are absolutely safe. Parents quite rightly ask questions about safety, including the following:

✔ **Why does my baby need to be vaccinated so early in life?**

Doctors like to vaccinate from as young as 8 weeks to ensure that your baby is not left vulnerable in the early months of life. An 8-week-old baby who hasn't been immunised is open to infection by the germs that cause meningitis C, whooping cough, and HIB, which can be killers in this age group. Many parents worry that their baby's immune system won't be able to cope with the vaccine, but most doctors regard these fears are unfounded. Apart from anything else, your baby is exposed to thousands of germs every day – far more than they encounter in any number of immunisations.

✔ **Are vaccines safe?**

Before a vaccine is licensed, its safety and effectiveness are tested thoroughly. After a vaccine has been licensed, its safety continues to be monitored. Any side effects that are discovered, no matter how rare, can then be assessed further. All medicines cause side effects, but vaccines are believed to be among the safest of drugs.

✔ **Is it possible to overload the immune system by giving too many vaccines?**

From birth, your baby's immune system protects her from the germs that surround her. Without this protection, your baby would not be able to cope with the tens of thousands of bacteria and viruses that cover her skin, nose, throat, and intestines. Vaccines are designed to strengthen your baby's immune system and protect her from extremely serious diseases. Most doctors believe that there is no evidence that any vaccine programme overloads a child's immune system. In the USA, where more vaccines are given in a single GP visit than in the UK, a study found no difference in hospital admission in children who had had multiple immunisations compared with children who had had only polio vaccine. Immunising against several diseases at once was just as safe as immunising against one.

The MMR debate

Some parents have decided against the combined MMR vaccine for their children, choosing either for their child to have no vaccinations at all against measles, mumps and rubella or to have single jabs instead. Their decision follows adverse media publicity, which began after a paper was published in the *Lancet* reporting a study that suggested a link between the combined MMR vaccination, autism, and bowel disease. The research has since been discredited, and none of the many studies looking for a link between MMR, autism, and bowel disease, have shown any evidence of a link. Examples of the most compelling evidence against any link between MMR and autism include:

Because of a problem with the mumps element of their vaccine, routine use of the MMR vaccine was stopped in Japan for several years. Halting the immunisation programme made absolutely no difference to the number of cases or autism that were diagnosed.

Finland has carried out the biggest study ever done of the MMR vaccination. Over a 14-year period, scientists monitored 1.8 million children for side effects including autism and inflammatory bowel disease. No evidence of any link was found.

A Swedish study looked at the incidence of autism over a 10-year period, before and after the introduction of the MMR vaccine into the national vaccination programme. The incidence of autism was not affected by the introduction of the MMR vaccine.

For more information about vaccinations and the diseases they are designed to prevent, visit www.immunisation.org.uk

Considering alternatives to vaccinations

With more and more childhood vaccinations and boosters being introduced every year, many parents, concerned about possible side effects, are looking for alternatives.

Homeopathy is one of the most commonly considered alternatives to vaccinations. Sadly, no evidence shows that homeopathic alternatives offer protection against any of the diseases mentioned in this chapter, and the Faculty of Homeopathy does not recommend homeopathy as an alternative to standard immunisation. However, you can consult a homeopath about using homeopathic remedies in conjunction with routine immunisation. See Chapter 18 for more about homeopathy.

Chapter 4

Who's Who? The Roles of Healthcare Professionals

In This Chapter

▶ Making the most of your doctor and health visitor

▶ Getting to know your local pharmacist

▶ Taking your child to the dentist

• •

*E*very parent needs advice, support, and help from time to time, especially soon after birth. This help comes from a variety of sources, depending on the nature of the problem and how your local healthcare system's organised. If you've recently given birth, for example, your main contacts are your community midwife and your family doctor. If your child's ill you seek help from your GP, and if your little one needs medication you visit your pharmacist.

This chapter outlines the roles of the healthcare professionals you'll probably come into contact with so you know what to expect.

Getting to Know Your Child's Doctor

You'll probably visit your doctor if your child's ill or you're worried about his health and development. For example, you may be concerned that your child isn't growing properly, or he has a rash, or he's sleeping all the time.

Your child's doctor can:

✔ Show you how to monitor your child's health.

✔ Explain your child's growth and development and what you can expect at the next stage.

✔ Diagnose minor and serious illnesses in your child.

> ✔ Refer your child to other specialists for help with specific conditions.

> ✔ Help you with other concerns about your child, such as exercise, nutrition and weight issues, and behavioural and emotional problems.

The key to a decent relationship with your doctor is good communication and realistic expectations. Doctors are under pressure to see more patients in less time these days, so you'll probably take a lot of responsibility for your child's health and development. You can help by being specific when you take your child to the doctor – make a note of your child's temperature, for example, or how many times he vomited. Also write down any questions or concerns you have before you go to the surgery.

Finding a doctor

Choosing a doctor for your child is an important decision. You must find a doctor that you feel comfortable with, as you'll likely see a lot of him after your child's born. If you don't have a good rapport with your current GP, find a new one. Your local library or Citizens' Advice Bureau has a list of GPs and their contact details. Many health authorities and primary care trusts also have Web sites where you can find out about doctors in your area.

A paediatrician is a doctor who specialises in child illnesses and is up to date with trends in child healthcare. Paediatricians focus on preventive healthcare and help you with problems that require specialist treatment. Many paediatricians are based in hospitals, but community paediatricians work with schools. In the UK, you cannot book an appointment directly with a paediatrician – you need to be referred by your GP.

Here are some pointers and questions to ask when choosing a GP for your child:

> ✔ Ask friends, colleagues, and family members for recommendations.

> ✔ Does your child have any special healthcare needs? If you want a doctor who specialises in children's health, look for a GP with 'DCH' after his name, which means he has a diploma in child health.

> ✔ What are the opening hours of the surgery? Do patients always see the same doctor? Does the surgery accept after-hours phone calls or e-mails?

> ✔ Does the doctor support your approach to childcare? Is he open to discussing complementary therapies if you value an holistic approach?

> ✔ Does the surgery have a baby clinic or a paediatric nurse?

✔ Is the surgery relaxed, efficient, and friendly? Take a look around several surgeries before making a decision.

✔ What hospital is the surgery attached to? Does the hospital have paediatric care and 24-hour nurses? If not, you may want to find a different one.

✔ Is the surgery large or small? A larger surgery may have longer opening hours but may be less intimate than a smaller place.

✔ What is the surgery's policy on seeing children? Are children prioritised? Can you get a same-day appointment? What are the usual waiting times?

Scheduling standard doctor visits

Your doctor and health visitor (see the later section 'Getting the Most Out of Your Health Visitor') see your child from birth to the age of 5 years a number of times as part of the NHS child-surveillance programme. These sessions help to pre-empt development problems before they occur. Appointments are normally at ages 6–8 weeks, 6–9 months, 18–24 months, 3–3½ years, and 4½–5½ years (when your child starts school). Your doctor or health visitor can tell you when the next visit's due.

If you're concerned about your child's health in any way, don't wait for your next scheduled appointment. Always seek help when you need it.

If your child needs more specialist help, your doctor may refer him to a consultant community paediatrician, with special skills in developmental problems, a physiotherapist, a speech therapist, an ophthalmologist (sight specialist), or an audiologist (hearing specialist), depending on your child's problem.

Getting the Most Out of Your Health Visitor

Your health visitor is a qualified nurse, usually linked to your doctor's surgery, with specialist training in childcare. A month after you've given birth, your health visitor visits you and takes on some responsibility for your child's health and development up to the age of 5 years. Health visitors often see families at home, but they also run regular clinics based in local general practices, where you and your partner can take your child. Theclinics offer a good chance for you to voice any worries you have about your child's health and development, such as feeding, weight gain, teething, sleeping, and immunisations.

Your health visitor's also a source of information about your local area and childcare amenities. He'll be able to tell you about your local parent-and-baby groups, play care, nurseries, and childminders.

Your health visitor is likely to contact you in the last month of your pregnancy, depending on the healthcare policies where you live. He then visits you at home about 10 days after the birth of your baby to check on you both and answer any questions you have. However, you can see your health visitor at the local clinic (usually your GP's surgery) at any other time if you need to.

The length of each appointment with your health visitor depends on the age of your child and the questions you need to discuss. But on average a new birth visit lasts about an hour and subsequent visits half an hour.

To make the most of your health visitor, follow these suggestions:

- **Be prepared.** Make a list of any questions or niggles you have in order of priority. And keep your notes handy – for example, jot down your child's weight or height measurements if you need to discuss them, or a diary of events if your baby's been ill.

- **Bring in a babysitter.** Ask your partner or a friend to be in the house and look after your child while the health visitor's there so you can talk without being too distracted.

- **Say what's on your mind.** Your health visitor's there to help you, so don't be afraid of asking obvious or silly questions.

- **Make plenty of time for the visit.** And try to relax and enjoy it.

- **Keep your own medical history to hand.** Your health visitor can advise you on your own health and well-being issues, such as dealing with postnatal depression, employment and benefit rights, and where to look for childcare.

- **Ask your partner to be there.** Your health visitor can advise new mums *and* dads on their roles.

- **Find out about between-visit hours.** Ask whether you can call your health visitor between visits or whether he runs a pop-in clinic at your GP surgery.

Making Friends with Your Pharmacist

Your pharmacist is a trained expert who issues medicines prescribed by doctors. He also dispenses over-the-counter medicines without prescription. To get the best from your pharmacist when buying medications, always describe your child's symptoms and how long he's had them, mention any other medications he's taking, and tell the pharmacist if your child suffers from any allergies.

If your child's feeling a little under the weather, your pharmacy's a good place to start. You don't need an appointment to see your pharmacist, so this can be quicker than waiting to see your doctor. Your pharmacist can advise you on the best medicines for your child and whether you need to take your child to the doctor.

Your pharmacist also provides the following services for you and your child:

- ✔ **Getting the low-down on your child's medications.** If you're uncertain about a prescription your doctor has prescribed for your child, ask your pharmacist.

- ✔ **Making sure that you give the right dose.** If your child needs to take different medicines at different times of the day, ask your pharmacist for a dosette box (for a minimal fee) to help you organise the medicines.

- ✔ **Treating minor illnesses.** If your child has a minor illness, your pharmacist may be able to recommend a suitable treatment. Most pharmacists are happy to help with the following:

    • Infections, coughs, colds, and sore throats

    • Skin problems, spots, and minor skin infections

    • Stomach problems such as diarrhoea, nausea, constipation, and indigestion

    • Minor injuries such as cuts, bruises, and sprains

    • Allergies such as hay fever and dermatitis

    • Pain such as headache, toothache, and muscle pain

  • Common babyhood problems such as teething, colic, head lice, and nappy rash.

- ✔ **Recording your child's medication history.** Your pharmacist keeps a record of all medicines issued to you and your child. That way, your pharmacist is aware straight away if your doctor prescribes your child two drugs that he mustn't take together. This record of the medicines your child's taken can be helpful later if he becomes ill due to the drugs or to track what has and hasn't worked.

- ✔ **Delivering to your door.** Some pharmacists offer home delivery services, which is useful if you can't make it to the pharmacy during the day or need emergency help.

- ✔ **Disposing of old medications.** Your pharmacist can dispose of your out-of-date medicines – after all, you don't want medicines lying around the house or in the dustbin, just in case your child finds them.

Dealing with the Dentist

Like it or not, children need regular dental check-ups. For this reason, your dentist's likely to be one of the healthcare providers you see most regularly. For a list of dentists in your area, contact your local health authority (look in Yellow Pages) or check out the British Dental Association's 'Find a Dentist' service at www.bda-findadentist.org.uk. Before signing up with a dentist, check that he treats children, whether he provides NHS treatment, his surgery opening times, and whether he offers any other services, such as a hygienist, who works to prevent decay by scaling and cleaning teeth.

Chapter 4 covers keeping your child's teeth clean.

Understanding what the dentist does

Your child should go for a dental check-up every six months. At each check-up, the dentist does the following:

✔ Checks your child's teeth and gums are in good shape.

✔ Gets rid of any *plaque* (a film of bacteria on teeth), which contributes to cavities and gum disease.

✔ Looks out for early signs of serious oral health problems, such as dental caries.

✔ Shows your child how to floss and look after his teeth and gums properly.

Overcoming fear of the dentist

Your child is probably anxious at the thought of a stranger prodding and pulling his teeth with strange implements. The following tips may be helpful:

✔ Talk to your dentist and express your concerns.

✔ Stay with your child during his treatment.

✔ Encourage your child to ask questions about what may happen – this helps him feel in control.

✔ Explore relaxation techniques, hypnosis, psychotherapy, and acupuncture if your child develops a phobia about visiting the dentist. Check out the British Dental Health Foundation at www.dentalhealth.org.uk for more info.

Considering complementary medical professionals

Complementary medicine generally includes healing practices that aren't part of regular medical treatment – that is, any practice that isn't taught widely in medical schools.

In complementary medicine, the therapist treats the whole person rather than just the illness.

Chapter 18 gives some info on homeopathy, herbal medicine, osteopathy, chiropractic, and aromatherapy. We also cover how to find the best complementary medical professionals.

A Final Word and a Gentle Reminder

Dealing with your child's health – especially when your child's ill or hurt – can be frightening, and manoeuvring your way through the healthcare industry can be intimidating. Try to remember that you have lots of medical resources at your disposal and seek advice from healthcare professionals when you need it. Make full use of the resources in your community. Don't worry about being a pest or that your questions aren't important. Keep the following tips in mind:

✔ Look at medical examinations as a way of learning more about your child's health and development.

✔ Turn a trip to the doctor into play time. Most surgeries have some toys and a play area. Let your child understand he's allowed to play to make him less scared of the experience. Your child will probably recover from the experience faster than you do!

✔ Have confidence in yourself as a parent and get involved in local child-care groups. Seek parent-to-parent advice and support if you need to.

Part II
The First Year of Life

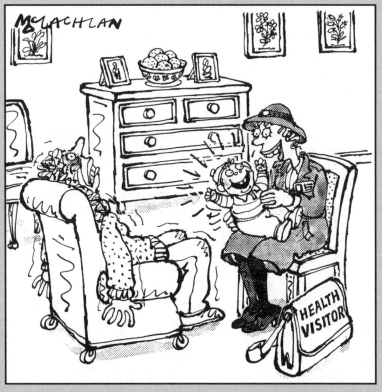

"Well, Mrs. Frimling, your baby's <u>very</u> happy, <u>very</u> lively & <u>very</u> healthy – you should be <u>very</u> proud."

In this part . . .

*I*f you're finding the first year of your baby's life daunting you're not alone. How do you really know if your
child is eating properly, developing at the right pace, and
generally thriving? How do you hold and clean your baby
properly?

Put your mind at rest – in this part you'll discover the
answers. We explain the health checks you can expect for
your baby – when they happen and what they tell you –
and how and when to wean your baby. We also explain
common newborn health blips such as jaundice, nappy
rash, and milia. Chapter 7 covers the signs that something
a bit more serious is wrong, such as infections, allergies,
and tummy bugs.

Chapter 5

Is My Baby Okay? Health and Development Checks in the First Year

. . . .

In This Chapter

▶ Making sure your baby's healthy at birth

▶ Recognising possible causes for concern

▶ Knowing all about your baby's weight

▶ Attending follow-up checks

. . . .

*F*rom the moment your baby's born, your GP and health visitor will examine her regularly to ensure she's healthy and developing well. They'll ask you to take your baby for regular check-ups and weigh-ins and more formal appointments that concentrate on how she's developing. It's a good idea to attend these because it gives your health visitor a chance to make sure all's well and pick up any potential problems regarding her growth and development. Many parents find these sessions invaluable because you can discuss any concerns you have about your baby, no matter how trivial they may seem. Your midwife or health visitor will keep you informed about your baby's appointments: you don't need to arrange anything – just turn up at the clinic when you're due.

These vital checks should reassure you that everything's okay and give you a great chance to ask questions and talk to your GP or health visitor about yourself and your baby.

Your baby will grow rapidly during her first year, and you're bound to have lots of questions. Before your appointments with your health visitor or GP, make a list of things you're worried about and any questions you want to ask. The appointments are there to help you as well as your baby.

Checking the Basics

In the first year after your baby's born, you may feel as if you live in your local surgery. The first check your baby has is usually done at the hospital, unless you've had a home delivery. Your midwife then visits regularly for the first 10 days of your baby's life to check up on you and your baby and to answer your queries. After that, most of the checks are carried out at your GP's surgery. If your baby's healthy, you'll see a health visitor or your GP rather than a paediatrician. Most GPs' practices have one or more health visitors who run clinics in the surgery. If your GP doesn't offer this service, you'll probably attend a community clinic close to where you live. At these appointments, the health visitor checks your baby's weight and sometimes the head circumference and length. At some appointments, your GP gives your baby a physical check-up. Table 5-1 gives the low-down on what to expect at which appointments.

Table 5-1	Typical Infant Check-up Schedule	
Check-up	*With whom*	*What they look at*
Weekly until 6 weeks	Health visitor	Weight, length, head circumference
6–8 weeks	GP and health visitor	Feeding and sleeping habits, vision and hearing
Every 2–4 weeks until 7–8 months	Health clinic	Weight, length, head circumference
7–8 months	Health visitor and GP	Development, hearing, physical examination

Making the Most of Your Clinic Appointments

Although your GP and health visitor look at some specific things during your baby's health checks, you can also take the opportunity to ask questions. Here are a few tips for making the most of your appointments:

✔ Don't hesitate to ask questions. Your doctor and health visitor are only too aware that babies don't come with a 'how to' manual and that all babies are different. No matter how trivial or silly you think your question is, if it's troubling you it's worth asking. And even if you're embarrassed, your healthcare professionals won't be – they're bound to have heard similar questions before.

✔ Keep a notebook, where you can write down any questions you have and observations that you make. Take the notebook with you to your appointments and jot down anything you need to remember during the visit.

✔ If you're not sure of the person to whom you should direct your query, ask your health visitor when you take your baby for a routine health check. If your health visitor thinks you need to talk to your GP, she can arrange this for you.

✔ Ask your health visitor for her phone number. She'll be more than happy to talk to you between your routine appointments about any queries that arise.

✔ Your midwife or health visitor will give you a health record – your baby's 'little red book' – that keeps together all your baby's vital info. Take the book with you whenever you go for an appointment.

✔ At the end of your current visit, check with your health visitor to see when you need to come again.

Finding Out About Your New Baby

Every baby's unique. But whatever yours looks like when she makes her first appearance, you're bound to be surprised. Perhaps she's smaller, bigger, hairier, or wrinklier than you'd imagined; shrivelled prunes may not have held much appeal before, but now you've given birth to one your feelings may have changed. Don't despair if your baby doesn't have the perfect peachy skin you'd imagined: She's been steeped in amniotic fluid for the past 9 months – that's one long bath – and it can take a while to adapt to life in the open air.

Testing, testing: Checks at birth

Straight after birth and then 5 or 10 minutes later, the midwife does five short tests – collectively known as the *Apgar test* – to assess your baby's overall health. These tests help the healthcare professionals to decide whether your baby needs immediate medical attention. You may not notice the tests being carried out: Experienced midwives can do them by assessing your baby as you hold her. The Apgar test looks at the following:

✔ **Respiration:** Breathing shows the lungs are healthy.

✔ **Muscle tone:** Limb movement signals strong muscles.

✔ **Heart rate:** A strong regular heartbeat shows that your baby is acclimatising well to her new surroundings.

✔ **Skin colour:** A healthy skin tone shows that that your baby's lungs are taking in oxygen efficiently.

✔ **Grimace:** Facial responses are a sign that that your baby's responding to stimuli.

Each test is given a score of 0, 1, or 2. A total of 7 or more shows that your baby's in good condition. A score below 4 means your baby needs help: The doctor may have to clear her airways and give resuscitation.

Most low-scoring babies score highly when they're retested a few minutes later. Few babies score a perfect 10 on the Apgar test. Even if your baby has a low score, it may simply mean that her nostrils are blocked or she needs a kick-start to get her breathing. The Apgar test gives no prediction of your baby's future health: It simply lets the doctors know whether your newborn needs some assistance at the beginning of life outside the womb.

Your baby's first full examination

A paediatrician (or a GP if you had a home birth or were discharged from hospital soon after delivery) carries out your newborn baby's first detailed check-up within 36 hours of birth. The doctor records your baby's weight and head circumference, feels her tummy to check the internal organs, makes sure her limbs match in length and her feet are aligned, and checks her spine. The doctor may also feel the inside of your baby's mouth to make sure the top of the mouth is formed.

The following sections detail the various health checks that the doctor carries out on your newborn baby.

Going head to toe

When your baby has her first detailed check, the doctor looks at her head, her toes, and everything in between. One of the things the doctor checks on your baby's head is the fontanelle – the 'soft spot'. This normal opening (well, two actually – one on top of the skull in the middle and one just behind it) between the bones of the skull feels soft because there's no bone under the scalp. If the soft spot bulges, it can indicate raised pressure inside the skull, an uncommon condition called *hydrocephalus*. The doctor will investigate this – and your baby may require an operation. If the soft spot is sunken, your baby may be dehydrated – although this is more common later in the first year of life, especially if your baby has diarrhoea and vomiting or is unwell for some other reason (see Chapters 7 and 8 for more on illnesses in the first year).

You probably won't be able to resist counting your baby's ten tiny fingers and ten tiny toes – and even when they're all accounted for, it can be hard to stop looking at them. But the doctor has other things on his mind; he will be more interested in your baby's feet and will check for club foot or *talipes*. Positional talipes is a mild condition due not to a physical problem but to the way the baby holds her feet. Positional talipes is most common in babies who are breech before delivery. It usually settles on its own, although the doctor may show you how to straighten out your baby's foot to stop problems developing.

If the club foot is caused by a physical abnormality, the doctor will refer your baby to a paediatric orthopaedic surgeon, who deals with bones and joints.

Listening to the heart and lungs

The doctor listens to your baby's chest to make sure that air is going into both lungs when your baby breathes in. Problems with the lungs are very rare if a baby's Apgar scores were reasonable (usually 7 and over).

When the doctor checks your baby's heart, she may hear a *heart murmur* – a sound in addition to the normal heartbeat. Heart murmurs are very common in newborns: While your baby was in the womb, she had an extra blood vessel leading from her heart to her lungs to provide the lungs with blood. As your baby starts to breathe air, the extra blood vessel shuts down, but this can take a few days. If your baby has a heart murmur but she's feeding well and isn't breathless, the doctor probably won't examine her heart again until the 6–8-week check-up.

If the murmur is still present at the next check-up or your doctor is worried about your baby, the doctor may refer your baby for some tests, including an electrocardiogram (ECG). An ECG is not painful or uncomfortable for your baby. The doctor may also do a blood test to measure your baby's oxygen levels.

If the tests reveal any problems, the doctor will refer your baby to a paediatric heart specialist.

Most of the time, heart murmurs are normal and do not indicate that there is anything wrong with the heart. However, sometimes they may result from a hole in the heart or a narrowed valve. Even if your baby is diagnosed with a heart defect, she's unlikely to need treatment. Around 70 per cent clear up unaided within a few months or years. Your child will be monitored regularly while the murmur persists. If your child does need treatment, it will probably entail drugs rather than an operation.

Examining the eyes and mouth

The doctor will look at your baby's eyes through a special instrument with a light called an ophthalmoscope to look for something called the *red reflex*. This is a red light caused by a reflection from the back of your baby's eyes. If the red reflex isn't there – and it nearly always is – there may a problem called *congenital cataracts*, where the lens at the front of the eye has clouded over. To put this into perspective, I've never seen a case of congenital cataracts in 19 years of practice.

The doctor will also check that your baby's eyes aren't sticky. If the eyes are sticky, the doctor will do a test to see whether your baby has an infection called chlamydial conjunctivitis. Congenital chlamydial conjunctivitis, which your baby can catch from you, is uncommon and completely treatable with antibiotic eye drops.

Lots of babies develop sticky eyes in the first few months of life – and only rarely because of a chlamydial infection. As long as your baby doesn't have sticky eyes from a few days after birth, and as long as the whites of her eyes aren't red, just bathe her eyes in cooled, boiled water every few hours. If this doesn't work, your doctor can give you some antibiotic eyedrops to treat your baby's sticky eyes.

The doctor will check your baby's tongue to make sure she doesn't have *tongue tie*, where the band of tissue under the tongue is too short and restricts tongue movement. Tongue tie usually doesn't cause many problems, but occasionally it leads to feeding difficulties and speech problems. If your baby has severe tongue tie, she may need a minor operation to clip or divide the tissue under the tongue to free it up. This is usually carried out under a general anaesthetic, but your baby probably won't need to stay in hospital. The operation completely clears up the problem.

The doctor will also check for a condition called *cleft lip* or *cleft palate*, where there is a split in the lip or the palate, or both. A cleft lip is obvious from the outside, but a cleft palate can only be felt by gently popping a finger into your baby's mouth. Cleft lip and cleft palate may cause problems with feeding. Both can be treated with surgery – usually between the ages of 3 months and 1 year – under general anaesthetic.

Hunting for hernias

Hernias are gaps in the tissue under the skin that keep your baby's insides inside. The two most common hernias, which the doctor will check for, are inguinal and umbilical hernias.

- ✔ **Inguinal hernia:** This is a gap in the tissues under the skin around your baby's groin. In boys, it can cause a swelling that goes down into the scrotum, where the testicles sit. An inguinal hernia can cause problems if a bit of your baby's intestine pushes through the hole and gets stuck. The doctor will probably recommend a simple operation to repair your baby's inguinal hernia.

- ✔ **Umbilical hernia:** This is a gap in the tissue around the tummy button. If your baby has an umbilical hernia, her tummy will have a bulge under the skin around the tummy button. This kind of hernia is not dangerous because nothing gets stuck. Over time, the hernia stays the same size or gets smaller as your baby grows, becoming much less noticeable and probably disappearing completely. Therefore, you don't need to do anything about this sort of hernia.

Making sure the genitals are normal

About 1 in 25 boys is born with *undescended testes*, in which the testes are still in the abdomen. Undescended testes usually descend naturally by the age of 6 months, but if not your baby boy may need a routine operation at the age of about 18 months.

The doctor will check for *hypospadias* in boys, in which the opening of the urethra (the hole through which your baby passes urine) is in the wrong place. Most boys with hypospadias have no problem passing urine, but some develop a condition known as *phimosis*, where the foreskin balloons out during urination. Your baby may need surgery to allow him to pass urine normally.

Checking the legs and hip joints

The doctor checks your baby's hips by gently rotating her legs, looking for a condition called clicky hips or congenital dislocation of the hip (CDH). In *CDH*, the hip joint is not formed correctly and dislocates easily. One or both hips may be affected. If the doctor suspects CDH, he will refer your baby for an ultrasound scan. Treatment starts as soon as possible so that the hip joint can develop normally. If CDH is relatively minor, your baby may be fitted with a lightweight removable splint to hold her legs apart and encourage correct growth of the hip joint. If CDH is more severe, your baby will need stronger splints or a plaster cast for several months. More rarely, your baby may need a short period of traction or an operation to correct the problem.

The sooner CDH is spotted, the easier it is to correct successfully. If CDH is not picked up until later, your child may need surgery to correct it. Most children with CDH go on to lead normal active lives. Even if no problems are picked up at the newborn stage, your GP or health visitor will check your baby's hips again during routine developmental checks. In the meantime, if you have any concerns about your baby's hips, talk to your health visitor or GP.

Ensuring the anus is open

The doctor will ask you whether your baby has passed her first poo, which should be a greenish-black sticky substance known as *meconium*. Bowel movements show that your baby's bowels aren't blocked.

Testing the reflexes

The doctor will test some of your baby's reflexes to make sure that her central nervous system is functioning well. The main tests are these:

- **Blinking:** Your baby should blink if a flash of light or puff of air is directed at her eyes.

- **Rooting:** Your baby should turn automatically towards you if you stroke her cheek. Her mouth should be open, searching for something to suck.

- **Sucking:** Your baby should start sucking automatically if a clean finger or teat is put in her mouth.

✔ **Moro or 'startle':** Supporting your baby with the back of her hand, the doctor will let your baby's head drop back slightly. This will startle her and she should spread her arms, legs, and fingers in surprise before slowly curling back up.

Catching Up with Your Baby at 6–8 Weeks

Your baby's come a long way in 6–8 weeks, and it's time to get her checked out again. This check-up focuses on all areas of your baby's development, including her general well-being and alertness. The doctor or health visitor will ask you about your baby's feeding and whether she's smiling yet. Smiling is an important developmental milepost, as it shows that your baby's responding to you well.

The health visitor will usually see your baby first to weigh and measure her, ask questions about her development, and answer your queries. After that, your GP will give your baby a physical examination, checking her heart, lungs, genitals, ears, eyes, mouth, hips, and legs again. We explain these checks in the earlier section 'Your baby's first full examination'.

Your baby's checks are thorough, but your GP or health visitor might not spot all potential problems. Let your GP or health visitor know if you have any worries yourself about your baby's progress.

Looking at what your baby can do at 6–8 weeks

At your baby's 6–8-week check, your health visitor will check that your baby's developing normally. The following are signs that all is well:

✔ Your baby's closed fists are more open and readily grasp a rattle if you touch it to her palm.

✔ Your baby has a stronger neck and more head control, although you still need to support her head when you're holding her.

✔ Your baby may be able to hold a toy in her fist, although she won't look at it – at 6–8 weeks your baby won't have made the connection between the toy she's holding and what she's doing with her hands.

- ✔ Your baby listens intently when you talk. She may even turn to the sound of your voice, watch your face, and smile.
- ✔ Your baby starts to make 'ooh' and 'aah' noises – her very first attempts at verbal communication.

Muscling in or flopping out

The health visitor may hold your baby under her tummy and chest in horizontal suspension to see whether her muscles have developed enough for her head to keep in line with her body and to partially bend her hips.

Some mildly 'floppy' infants have simply not had enough opportunity to move around and strengthen their muscles. This may be the case with babies who are frequently left in their car seats. Try to give your baby plenty of opportunity to move around and kick her arms and legs to help develop muscle tone.

If your health visitor thinks your baby is 'floppy', she may refer your baby for tests, and teach you some exercises to do with your baby to improve muscle tone.

Most 'floppy' babies just take a bit more time than usual to develop muscle tone.

Helping your baby make sense of the world at 6–8 weeks

You can do lots of things to help your baby's healthy development, even at this tender age. Cuddling and talking to her will help her learn vital communication skills and show her that you love her and that her needs are important. Although your baby will develop at her own sweet pace, you can maximise healthy development by interacting with her as much as you can. Try some of the following:

- ✔ Carry your baby around and show her shapes, colours, and lights: Everything's fascinating the first few times she sees it.
- ✔ Make conversation whenever you have the chance, and particularly when your baby makes noises or looks your way.
- ✔ Talk to your baby as you do everyday things: 'Where's daddy?' 'Here's your blue rattle!'
- ✔ Share a book, ideally with simple black-and-white pictures. Even your young baby will find images stimulating and enjoy listening to your voice.

That's Progress! Check-ups at 7–8 Months

The first few months of your baby's life are filled with regular visits to the clinic to be checked and weighed. Your baby will have a more thorough developmental check at around 7–8 months or so. The timings and range of tests done vary between health authorities: Your health visitor will explain the normal procedure for your area. Your GP or health visitor may check your baby's hips one last time, although many health authorities are phasing this out because the check is unlikely to be helpful if your baby has had her hips checked straight after birth and at 8 weeks.

The health visitor may formally test your baby, or she may simply watch your baby play and ask questions about her development. The health visitor uses a variety of tools, including wooden bricks (to see if your baby can pass them from hand to hand or bang them together), raisins (to see how your baby picks up small objects), and a pot (to see whether your baby can get a raisin out of the pot).

During this check-up, your health visitor may do some or all of the following:

✔ Test your baby's hearing.

✔ Carry out an overall assessment of your baby's physical development.

✔ Assess your baby's social skills.

✔ Check your baby's hand–eye coordination.

✔ Test your baby's cognitive skills (ability to understand).

The 7–8-month check is not the first hurdle in your child's path to adult success, and there's no need to 'cram' her beforehand by rehearsing the tasks the health visitor will be giving her. All babies vary in the speed at which they develop different skills. The check-up is just a general guide to how your baby is developing. Even if your baby doesn't carry out all the tasks perfectly, she's unlikely to have a problem in her overall development.

My (Sarah's) son didn't start walking until he was 16 months old, and I was terrified that there was something wrong with him. My health visitor was very kind, gently reminding me that different skills develop at different rates and that failure to walk independently was unlikely to indicate brain damage when his vocabulary was already 50 words.

Looking at what your baby can do at 7–8 months

During this developmental check, your health visitor will be looking to see whether your baby has reached certain milestones. For example, between 6 and 9 months, most babies can sit up unsupported – but remember to stay close for the first couple of weeks of her doing this to prevent her nose-diving out of her precarious new position. Many (but by no means all) babies make their first attempts to crawl at this stage. A significant minority of babies never crawl, preferring to bottom-shuffle their way across the floor.

Here's a rough idea of what you can expect over the next few months, but remember – this is only an approximate guide. Babies reach their milestones when they feel like it, not when the books say so.

- ✔ By around 9 months, your baby will begin to pull herself up to standing, using whatever's handy at the time – perhaps the sofa or your legs. She'll probably just stand until she bumps down again, but this great new vantage point will increase her urgency to get on the move to check out all those exciting places she can see.

- ✔ Your baby may be able to stretch out with one hand to grasp small toys, pass them from hand to hand, let go with the first hand as the fingers of the other hand close around the toy, and examine the toy with concentrated interest.

- ✔ Your baby will be able to poke at small things with her index finger and begin to point. She'll also be able to use the pincer grip – holding with the finger and thumb – to pick up small objects.

- ✔ Your baby will love experimenting with sounds and will babble away in her cot or pram. She'll turn to your voice or a quiet noise from across the room unless she's distracted.

- ✔ Your baby may be able to shout now – and she'll let you know it! She may also sing a few notes of a familiar nursery rhyme.

Helping your baby develop at 7–8 months

At this age, most games should be just that – games. You'll reduce the fun for both of you if you limit play to educational stuff. Most babies learn from everything they do. Singing nursery rhymes, for instance, will teach your baby about sounds and how to use her voice. Playing peek-a-boo will show your baby that things don't stop existing just because she can't see them. Looking at picture books together will help your baby to associate objects with names. Here are a few more suggestions:

- ✔ Play 'this little piggy' and 'round and round the garden'. Your baby'll love the actions and the songs.
- ✔ Talk about the objects around you so that your baby can match up things with their names.
- ✔ Use your baby's name whenever you talk to her: 'Where's Emma's hat?'

Weighing It Up: The Big Picture

Your baby's weight can give a very good general indication of her overall physical health and vitality. Steady weight gain indicates that your baby's food intake is sufficient and that her food is being absorbed by her body. Persistent weight loss may be a sign that something isn't right. Baby weight is one of the biggest causes of anxiety among new parents: Every ounce gained tends to be greeted with the kind of pride usually reserved for winning an Olympic medal, and every ounce lost sends parents into sheer panic.

Healthy babies come in all shapes and sizes. A petite baby weighing 3 kg can be as vigorous and sound as a baby who weighs a strapping 4 kg. Steady weight gain can be reassuring, but beware of falling into the trap of comparing your baby with others. As long as your baby's healthy and feeding well, the number of grams she has or hasn't gained is unlikely to be an issue.

In the first couple of weeks after birth, your baby will likely lose several ounces – a drop of 5 per cent of her birthweight is perfectly normal, as her body and digestive system need time to acclimatise to life outside the womb. By 2 or 3 weeks, after you've established feeding, she'll likely reach her birthweight again – and possibly more.

Monitoring your baby's weight

For the first few months, your health visitor will advise you to attend your local baby clinic every week or so to have your baby checked and weighed. The health visitor will record your baby's weight using graphs in your baby's 'little red book'. These graphs, called *centile* or *percentile charts*, show *centile curves* based on the measurements of average babies. If your baby's weight is on the 25th centile curve, this means that 25 per cent of babies are lighter and 75 per cent are heavier than your baby.

Perfect miniatures

If you and your partner are both under 5 foot 3 inches tall, don't expect your baby to be on the 95th centile. Many babies are on the lower centiles for weight but grow steadily along that centile line and develop normally in every other respect. For decades babies have tended to grow up taller than their parents, but on the whole your baby's likely to follow the same trends in height as you and/or your partner. If you're both fairly short, your baby will probably be both short and light compared with other babies of the same age.

Whatever line your little bundle of joy sits on, your health visitor will be most interested in checking whether your baby is consistent, follows her own curve, and doesn't drop too far below her curve. By following your baby's centile measurements, your health visitor can check that your baby's developing normally.

Centile charts are just guidelines, and a single divergence from your baby's percentile line is not cause for concern. What matters is the pattern over several months. Also, the rate at which your baby gains weight will change – for example, her weight gain may slow down once she becomes mobile.

'Light' babies

Many babies fail to put on weight steadily, or even lose weight for short periods when they're ill or if they don't take easily to weaning. A lengthy failure to gain weight or continued weight loss over several weeks or months with no apparent cause can be a cause for concern and is known as *failure to thrive*. If your baby has failure to thrive, the doctor will need to assess her carefully so that she can be treated. Symptoms of failure to thrive include a drop in weight over 3 months or more, refusing to feed or poor feeding, listlessness, and unhappiness. True failure to thrive is unusual – fewer than one in 100 babies investigated for failure to thrive have a serious problem. There are many causes of failure to thrive, and your baby will be treated on an individual basis. See Chapter 7 for more on failure to thrive.

'Heavy' babies

Even if your baby comes in on the 95th percentile, she isn't necessarily overweight – it just means that 95 per cent of children her age weigh less. If your baby's long or heavy-framed, she's bound to weigh more. Excess weight gain before weaning is rare. If you're breastfeeding, your baby's very unlikely to be overweight, because your milk's tailored perfectly to suit her individual needs. However, it is possible to overfeed a bottle-fed baby, so ask your health visitor for advice if you're concerned.

Focusing on Your Baby's Eye Checks: Squints

The doctor or health visitor will check your baby's eyes at birth and regularly during the first year. In the early weeks, you may notice that your baby's eyes veer off in different directions. This is perfectly normal, because your baby may take some time to gain control of her eye muscles. If your baby still shows signs of this after 12 weeks or so, she may have a *squint*, which means that one of her eyes is weak. A squint, also known as a 'lazy eye', affects around 3 per cent of babies. Your baby won't be able to tell you if she has symptoms of squint such as poor, blurred, or double vision, but she may give you a clue by covering or closing the affected eye.

A squint won't disappear on its own, so seek a diagnosis and treatment as quickly as possible to prevent the sight in your baby's affected eye worsening. Squints can run in families, so if you have an older child with a squint, ask your doctor to check your baby.

If the doctor suspects a squint, she'll refer your baby to a specialist for further investigation. Treatment may include patching the normal eye to encourage the weaker eye to work harder and glasses if your baby is old enough to wear them without constantly pulling them off. Sometimes, an operation is necessary to tighten the muscles around the affected eye. During the operation, only the muscles attached to the outside are moved, so there's no significant risk of damage to your child's sight.

From about the age of 4 months, you can check for a squint by holding a toy about 20 cm from your baby's face and moving the toy from side to side. Your baby should follow the toy with both eyes. If one of her eyes drifts, she might have a squint.

Many parents think their baby has a squint, only to be reassured otherwise by a doctor. Your baby may simply look as if she's squinting if the fold of skin between her eyes is broad. If you have any concerns about your baby's vision, see your GP.

Listening In: Your Baby's Hearing Tests

Most health authorities test hearing within 24 hours of birth. The doctor tests your baby's hearing by inserting into her ear a probe that looks like a thermometer and can detect tiny echoes from the eardrum to show that the ear is functioning normally.

If the first test does not show a strong enough response, the doctor will refer your baby for a second screening. This does not necessarily mean that hearing loss is suspected: Conditions at the time of the first test may simply not have been right.

A small proportion of babies are referred for an auditory brainstem response (ABR) test, which can give better information about the hearing. The *ABR* test is usually carried out at an audiology (hearing) clinic in your local hospital. Sounds are played through earphones placed on your baby's head, usually when she's asleep. A computer records how your baby's ears respond to the sounds. If the ABR responds strongly, your baby's unlikely to have a hearing loss.

If the test results are abnormal, the doctor will refer your baby for further testing and possibly treatment for conditions such as glue ear (which we discuss in Chapter 13). If your baby has deafness, she may be fitted with a hearing aid. If the hearing loss is profound and permanent, she may be assessed for cochlear implants, which can be very effective in helping her to hear.

Making Exceptions: Your Premature Baby

If your baby was born prematurely – before 36 weeks' gestation – she'll probably be very small. Missing out on time in the womb means missing out on growing time and some getting-ready-for-independent-life time. The more weeks inside the womb your baby misses, the more difficulties she's likely to face. A baby born after 37 weeks' gestation will probably need only a little extra help – being kept in an incubator with extra warmth, extra oxygen, and tiny feeds of breast milk at frequent intervals. A baby born earlier than 37 weeks' gestation may need more help, as she may not have developed the capacity for independent life. She may be fed by a tube passed down her nose into her stomach if she cannot suck or swallow and she may have a respirator to breathe for her.

As your baby develops, you will need to allow for her prematurity. As an example, take a baby who was born at 34 weeks – in other words, 6 weeks early. Although her birthday is the day she was born, and therefore 6 weeks later she is 6 weeks old, she will not be comparable with full-term 6-week-old babies until 6 weeks after her expected rather than actual date of delivery. Your health visitor will keep your preterm baby's gestational, or corrected, age in mind right through the first 2 years of life, although the significance of this age will gradually diminish: There's an enormous difference between a 3-month-old baby and a prematurely born 3-month-old baby whose corrected aged is only 3 weeks. But the difference between the two babies will be much less noticeable by the time they reach their second birthdays.

Chapter 6

Feeding Your Baby

● ●

In This Chapter

▶ Looking at the benefits of breastfeeding

▶ Considering bottle-feeding

▶ Working out when to wean

▶ Troubleshooting: When food and your baby don't agree

● ●

During your baby's first year, little is likely to preoccupy you more than the subject of feeding. You'll spend many of your waking moments either thinking about it or doing it. By the time your bundle of joy's blowing out the candle on his first birthday cake, you'll be the world's number-one expert on feeding. But it isn't only about making sure your baby gets the right vitamins and minerals to grow. Feeding's also an integral part of the bond between you and your baby – you'll soon tune in to his needs and his likes and dislikes, and in turn he'll learn to trust you as the person who provides the comfort and security of food. Being sensitive to your baby's nutritional needs also provides a firm foundation for healthy eating habits as he grows older.

 Your baby has a brand-new digestive system that needs a considerable amount of breaking in. To cut a long story short, babies are sick. A lot. Whether they're breastfed or bottle-fed, new babies are likely to bring up a fair amount of milk after a feed. This is called possetting and is nothing to worry about.

Choosing to Breastfeed

Unless you've been living on Mars for some time, you're probably already aware that breast milk is by far the healthiest food for your baby. The World Health Organization recommends breastfeeding exclusively for at least the first 6 months. But although breastfeeding is often hailed as the most natural thing in the world, it can be hard work. The decision whether to breastfeed isn't simply a medical one: Issues of convenience, aesthetics, and body image all play a part. Deciding whether to breastfeed is personal, and you shouldn't feel pressurised into doing so if your heart's not in it. But without a doubt-, if you can breastfeed, it's the best thing you can do for your baby.

If the jury's still out, try to arm yourself with the facts about breastfeeding and bottle-feeding before you start.

Spouting on about the health benefits of breast milk

As well as being free (other than the cost of a healthy diet for yourself), easy (once you get the hang of it), and convenient (you won't leave home without your milk and you don't need to heat it up), breast milk gives your baby a tailor-made formula for good nutrition. The makeup of your breast milk changes constantly according to your baby's needs throughout the day and adapts as he grows, so he's always got exactly the right nutrients on tap. Best of all, breast milk has a whole host of health benefits that money just can't buy. For example, breastfeeding:

- **Protects against infection.** Breast milk contains germ-fighting antibodies that help protect your baby from infection until his own immune system matures. So your breastfed baby is less likely to suffer from a whole host of nasties, including ear infections, pneumonia, botulism, bronchitis, meningitis, and German measles, to name but a few.

- **Reduces the likelihood of your baby developing allergies, eczema, and wheeziness.** This is particularly important if allergies run in the family: studies show that the longer a baby is breastfed, the better his immune system is going to develop. The opinion of experts is that allergies are caused by early exposure to allergens, so the longer you put off introducing other foods, the better.

- **Protects against cot death.** Although all sorts of factors contribute to cot death (we talk about safe sleeping in chapter 11), research shows that for each month of breastfeeding the chance of cot death is halved compared with that in formula-fed babies.

- **Lowers your baby's risk of obesity.** Babies who are fed exclusively on breast milk for the first few months have been found to be up to four times less likely than those fed on formula to become obese in later childhood.

- **May help to prevent childhood cancer.** Incidences of diseases such as leukaemia are lower among breastfed babies – for example, US researchers discovered that babies who were breastfed for at least 1 month were significantly less likely to develop leukaemia than formula-fed babies.

- **Reduces the likelihood of tummy troubles such as constipation, food poisoning, diarrhoea, and colic.** This is because breast milk is completely tailored to meet your baby's needs; it has exactly the right nutrients and fluids necessary to keep his digestive system healthy. There's also less chance of unwittingly introducing harmful bacteria to your baby's digestive system: just one bottle or teat that hasn't been properly sterilised can wreak havoc on his digestion. And to cap it all, breastfed babies' bowel movements don't smell nearly as bad as bottle-fed babies'!

✔ **Provides the perfect brain food.** Breast milk not only is ideal for your baby's physical development but also boosts brain power. One study found that premature babies who were breastfed scored, at the age of 7 years, up to ten points higher in IQ tests than those who are bottle fed. This may be due to the fact that breast milk contains certain biological chemicals, called long chain fatty acids, which are vital for the development of the brain, eyes, and nervous system.

✔ **Is good for you, too.** Breastfeeding reduces your risk of developing hip fractures and early breast or ovarian cancer. It can also help you get your body back more quickly after your baby is born, as it burns up lots of calories. Breastfeeding also offers limited contraceptive effect (but it should not be relied upon – 10 per cent of women who breastfeed start ovulating after 10 weeks, and 50 per cent by 25 weeks).

Even if you breastfeed for only the first few days of your baby's life, he will still get some benefit. Infection-fighting antibodies are especially plentiful in your *colostrum* – the yellowish watery-looking milk you produce in the first few days after delivery. Colostrum is also choc-full of essential vitamins and proteins.

Getting started

You've done the classes and read the books, but when it comes to breastfeeding for real it can feel a bit daunting. Breastfeeding your baby as soon as you can after delivery is a good idea, as his sucking reflex is at its strongest then.

Breast milk is produced on a supply and demand basis: The more you feed, the more you'll produce. Feed your baby on demand to ensure you produce as much as he needs.

Here's what you do:

1. **Make sure you're relaxed and comfy.** Use pillows to support your back and arms.

2. **Hold your baby close, with his head and body in a horizontal line and your nipple pointing towards his nose.** Then touch his top lip with your nipple. He'll instinctively open his mouth and turn towards your nipple.

3. **When your baby's mouth is wide open, move him towards your breast (don't do it the other way round unless you want stretched nipples!), aiming your nipple towards the roof of your baby's mouth.**

His bottom lip and chin should touch your breast first. With his mouth open, he should take in all of your nipple and part of the *areola* (the dark area surrounding the nipple). His bottom lip should be curled back towards his chin.

Once he's latched on, he'll settle into a rhythm of drinking. You will very soon feel your *let-down reflex* kick in, which gets the milk flowing. You should be able to see more of your areola above your baby's mouth than below it.

If you hear a slurping or clicking sound as your baby feeds, he's probably not latched on properly. This can result in sore cracked nipples. Unlatch him by sliding a (clean) finger into the corner of his mouth and follow Steps 1–3 again.

4. **Feed your baby for as long as he wants on one side.** For the first few minutes, he will be getting *foremilk*, which is watery, to quench his thirst. After a while, the *hind milk* starts to flow, which is more calorific and satisfies his hunger. For this reason, keep feeding on one side for a good few minutes before swapping breasts, otherwise he may only get foremilk and be hungry again very soon.

If you need to take him off, slip your finger into the corner of his mouth to break the suction.

Many new mums worry that their babies seem to need to feed constantly, day and night, without a break. New babies have tiny tummies that can hold only enough food to keep them going for short periods. They also have a lot of growing to do, so at first your baby may feed every hour or so. Later, he may go through growth spurts when he wants to feed more often than usual, but these usually last only a few days.

To increase your changes of successfully breastfeeding your baby, the most important thing you can do is get as much help as you can. Don't be afraid to ask – as many times as necessary, for as long as necessary. If you're still in hospital, a midwife can advise you and check that your baby is latching on correctly. You may find you need help with positioning and finding a comfortable position, too:

- ✔ Ask for the help of a breastfeeding counsellor. Most maternity units now provide qualified counsellors who can ensure your baby is latching on properly. This can take time and a lot of patience – a breastfeeding counsellor should have both of these.

- ✔ Go to antenatal classes, where you'll be taught the basics. A number of hospitals run in-depth courses, as do the National Childbirth Trust (0870-444-8708; www.nctpregnancyandbabycare.com) and La Leche League (0845-456-1855; www.laleche.org.uk).

✔ Watch someone breastfeeding to see how to do it. But choose someone you know!

✔ Find the phone numbers for a few breastfeeding support groups in advance, so you can get help quickly if you need it.

Expressing milk

You don't have to be permanently attached to your baby if you're breastfeeding. *Expressing* your milk to be bottle-fed to your baby later by your partner or babysitter, for example, means you can have the best of both worlds.

You can express breast milk by hand or by using a breast pump. If you want to express only occasionally, you may decide to try expressing by hand and save on the cost of a breast pump. To express manually, gently squeeze the area around your nipples, pushing your fingers back towards the chest. Some women find they simply have to massage their breasts to express, while for others it can take time and practice. Wash your hands before you start, and hold a sterilised container underneath your nipple to catch the milk. Try looking at your baby while you're doing this, or imagine feeding him, to help let down the milk. Expressing manually can be tiring. Massage towards your nipple to help the milk come out. You may find it easier to grasp your breast in one hand and massage the whole thing in a stroking movement towards the nipple.

If you plan to express breast milk regularly or don't have the stamina to do it by hand, a breast pump may be a good investment. Electric and manual pumps operate on the same principle as hand expressing. Manual ones usually involve you physically squeezing the pump to get the milk out. Electric ones are often faster and more efficient, even if you do start to feel a strange affinity with a dairy cow while you're using them. A suction cap extracts the milk, which sounds painful, but it shouldn't be. If it hurts, stop. You may need the help of a breastfeeding counsellor or health visitor. A good breast pump mimics the sucking action of a baby but should not hurt you.

Breast pumps come in all shapes and sizes, and prices vary hugely. New ones come onto the market all the time, claiming all sorts of scientific advances. But don't just rush out and buy the most expensive, unless you are going to use it frequently. Ask friends or your health visitor what they'd recommend before investing in one.

When you want to express milk, choose a time when you're feeling relaxed, warm, and comfortable, because expression can take as long as 45 minutes. Whether you express by hand or pump, you'll need to collect your expressed milk in a sterilised bottle, storage cup, or bag. You can keep expressed milk in this sealed container in the fridge for up to 48 hours – but don't keep the milk in the fridge door, as it's not as cool as the main compartment. You can freeze breast milk for up to 6 months at –5°C and then defrost it as and when you need it. Never refreeze breast milk.

After your baby is into a pattern and sleeping for a little longer at night (yes, you probably feel it's never going to happen, but trust us on this one!) you're likely to have more milk in the mornings. You may find it easiest to express a good amount of milk at this time, which can be useful to 'top up' your baby if he's been feeding all evening and you want to get him to settle at night.

Overcoming common breastfeeding problems

Breastfeeding is a knack and, despite poplar belief, this knack often takes some time to develop. In the meantime, problems such as soreness and engorgement can ensue. But the good news is that you can easily manage most breastfeeding problems. Breastfeeding counsellors are an excellent place to start if you have any problem of any kind. But here are a few tips to help you stave off some of the most common complaints.

Coping with cracked nipples

Sore, cracked nipples can have you climbing the walls in agony – and they're the number-one reason for new mums resorting to the milk bottle. Sore nipples are usually caused by your baby not latching on properly, so check your positioning when breastfeeding to make sure he's getting the whole of the nipple and most of the areola in his mouth. Ask for help from your health visitor or breastfeeding counsellor immediately if you're in any doubt about your positioning. Cracked nipples in themselves are painful, but not dangerous. If your breasts become red and tender, however, you may have mastitis (see the 'Managing mastitis' section later in this chapter).

If you find yourself with cracked nipples, take this advice:

- Keep the nipple dry with breastpads (change as soon as they become damp) or clean tissues and go topless whenever possible – the air helps heal the skin.

- Try applying a few drops of breast milk or dab on some lanolin, vitamin E ointment, olive oil, or petroleum jelly onto the nipple after feeding.

- Try to continue feeding from the sore nipple – it may be agony, but do it if you can bear it, even if only for a few minutes, to keep the nipple conditioned to feeding.

✔ Increase the number of feeds, and feed for a shorter period each time. That way, your baby may not be as hungry as usual and may not suck as hard.

✔ Express a little milk manually before you put your baby to the breast. This starts the milk flow, so your baby won't have to suck so hard to get the flow going.

Eradicating engorgement

If your breasts become over full, they'll feel hard and painful, making it difficult for your baby to latch on. To avoid engorgement, try the following techniques:

✔ Feed your baby regularly. Keeping your milk flowing regularly is important, so try not to miss feeds – many experts recommend waking your baby up if necessary in the early days. He shouldn't go more than six hours without a feed, day or night.

✔ If you have to miss a feed, express some milk. Check out the section 'Expressing milk' earlier in this chapter for some suggestions.

✔ If, despite your best efforts, your breasts become engorged, try gently expressing a little milk by hand or with a breast pump. Massage your breast with a warm flannel to ease the discomfort and stimulate the let-down reflex.

Beating blocked ducts

When a milk duct becomes blocked, you'll feel a hard red patch or lump on the outside of your breast. The best way to prevent this is by feeding often and encouraging your baby to empty your breast. If the baby won't do it, assume the chore yourself: Get expressing. If your ducts get blocked anyway, try these things to improve the situation:

✔ Check that your bra fits properly, because tight clothing can make the problem worse.

✔ Feed often. Offer your baby the affected breast first, massaging towards the nipple as you do so.

✔ Apply heat to the lump. A warm bath or shower can also work wonders.

✔ Most importantly, keep feeding.

Managing mastitis

Bacteria from your baby's mouth or a blocked duct that has not been treated can lead to mastitis, an acute infection that can make your breast swollen and painful, with red patches. Mastitis is often accompanied by fever (over 38°C), malaise, and general body aches, similar to having flu.

Asking for help

If you'd like to find out more about breastfeeding, plenty of people and organisations are available to give you advice, including the following:

- ✔ Your midwife, both before and after you leave hospital.

- ✔ Your health visitor, who gets in touch shortly after your midwife stops visiting.

- ✔ The breastfeeding counsellor at your local hospital.

- ✔ Friends and family members – but beware of conflicting advice from too many sources!

- ✔ *Breastfeeding For Dummies* by Sharon Perkins and Carol Vannais (Wiley) – a comprehensive book covering everything about breastfeeding, down to the smallest details.

- ✔ The National Childbirth Trust (0870-444-8708; www.nctpregnancyandbaby care.com).

- ✔ La Leche League (0845-456-1855; www.laleche.org.uk).

- ✔ Association of Breastfeeding Mothers (0870-401-771; www.abm.me.uk).

- ✔ The Breastfeeding Network (0870-900-8787; www.breastfeedingnetwork.org).

Soothe sore swollen breasts by placing a couple of chilled cabbage leaves on to the affected area. Really! Try it! You don't need to tell anyone what you've got down your bra . . .

If you suspect you've got mastitis, see your doctor as soon as possible, as you may need antibiotics to clear up the infection. Try to continue to breast-feed your baby, in order to avoid engorgement, which makes the condition more painful. Ibuprofen, paracetamol (both safe to take while breastfeeding), or warm compresses may help relieve the pain while you're waiting for antibiotics take effect (usually around 2 days).

If you see white spots on your breasts and in your baby's mouth, and your breasts feel itchy, you may have contracted thrush, a common fungal infection. Make an appointment to see your doctor immediately, as you and your baby are going to need treatment with antibiotics or anti-fungal creams. Seek immediate help; you and your baby need to be treated simultaneously to prevent re-infecting each other. Check out Chapter 8 for more on newborn niggles.

Considering Bottle-feeding

Women may opt for formula feeding for a number of reasons. Some are simply not comfortable with the idea of breastfeeding, while others may have had a bad previous experience and not want to go there again. Whatever your reasons, this is a personal decision, and only you can decide what is right for you. In addition, health issues may mean you opt to bottlefeed. They include the following:

✔ If you have a chronic infection such as human immunodeficiency virus (HIV), formula feeding helps ensure that you don't pass the infection to your baby via your breast milk. (Women who carry the hepatitis B virus can breastfeed as long as the baby has been vaccinated against hepatitis B.)

✔ If you have inverted nipples, breastfeeding can be extremely difficult. Inverted nipples are often confused with flat nipples, which can be 'coaxed out' using nipple shields or stretching exercises. A truly inverted nipple is still attached to the chest wall.

✔ If you have had previous surgery on your breasts, bottle-feeding may be your best bet as you may not be able to breastfeed. Sometimes, surgery means cutting the milk ducts from the nipple, which can make it physically impossible to breastfeed.

✔ If you take certain medications, bottle-feeding may be best. Certain medications can pass through the breast milk and affect the baby adversely. Drugs to be wary of include anti-cancer drugs such as cyclophosphamide, doxorubicin, methotrexate, and ciclosporin; bromocriptine; lithium; and some migraine treatments, particularly ergotamine. Ask your GP about any medications you take regularly before you start breastfeeding.

✔ You may simply find breastfeeding too painful or exhausting. You may also feel you're not producing enough milk – although this is a common misconception, as about 95 per cent of women produce the right amount of breast milk.

Even if you're planning to bottle-feed, you'll probably be encouraged to breastfeed in the very early days so that your baby can benefit from your colostrum, the antibody-rich pre-milk that your body produces before your milk comes in. I talk about breastfeeding in the section 'Choosing to Breastfeed' earlier in this chapter.

Finding out about formula

Although formula can't replicate breast milk exactly, you can rest assured that your baby is getting all the nutrients he needs from formula. Scientists have spent many years trying to make formula milk as chemically close to human milk as possible. Consider the following:

✔ Formula milk is generally made from specially treated cows' milk. To make the milk easier for babies to digest, manufacturers modify the carbohydrates, proteins, and fats, and add vitamins and minerals, including iron.

✔ The quality of traditional infant formula has improved tremendously over the years. One major discovery has been that breast milk contains long-chain polyunsaturated fatty acids (LCPs), which are essential for the healthy development of your baby's nervous system. A number of formula milks now contain versions (although not identical) of LCPs, which have been shown to benefit the development of intelligence and eyesight in bottle-fed babies.

Formula falls into two categories. First milks are suitable from birth to 6 months. Then you switch to follow-on formula, which contains more iron, vitamins, and minerals to meet your growing baby's needs. If the milk doesn't agree with your baby – for example, if he starts being sick more frequently, gets diarrhoea, appears to be in pain or bloated – discuss alternatives with your health visitor. She may suggest a different brand, or perhaps even a dairy-free alternative, but get advice from her before changing your baby's milk.

Don't give your baby normal cows' milk (except in cooked food) until he's 12 months old. Cows' milk is difficult to digest and won't meet your baby's nutritional needs.

Bottle-feeding the healthy way

Good hygiene is essential when you're bottle-feeding, as babies are at a high risk of contracting tummy infections such as gastroenteritis. To prepare a bottle, follow these steps:

1. **Sterilise equipment (until your baby is at least 6 months old) and wash your hands before preparing feeds.**

   You can sterilise by steaming, boiling, using sterilising tablets, or using your dishwasher. For a more in-depth look at ways of sterilising and food hygiene, have a look at Chapter 12.

2. **Fill the sterilised bottle with the right amount of cooled, boiled water and add the correct amount of milk powder.**

   Follow the instructions on the formula tin, using the scoop provided and levelling off any excess with a knife.

   Never add more than the recommended amount of formula to your baby's bottles: This can cause dehydration and is a common cause of constipation in young babies.

3. **Screw on the cap, shake the bottle until all the powder has dissolved, and replace the cap with a teat and lid.**

4. **If you prepare several feeds at once, store them in the fridge.**

   Be sure to put the prepared bottles in the body rather than the (warmer) door of the fridge, and don't keep them for longer than 24 hours.

Feeding baby

Although your baby may be happy to drink formula milk straight from the fridge, most babies prefer it slightly warmed. Stand the bottle in a jug of hot water, shaking the bottle occasionally to distribute the heat.

Never heat your baby's milk in a microwave, as this can cause hotspots that can burn him.

Test the temperature by shaking a few drops of milk on to the inside of your wrist. Then you're ready to go! Follow these steps:

1. **Sit comfortably in a supportive chair and use a pillow to raise your baby on your lap if necessary.**
2. **Tip the bottle before you offer it so the teat is filled with milk. Adjust the angle as your baby feeds to avoid him gulping air.**
3. **Wind your baby halfway through the feed by sitting him upright after he has finished on one side and gently stroking his back until he burps**
4. **Throw away any milk that's left after 30 minutes.**

   Formula that's been out of the fridge for more than 30 minutes is an ideal breeding ground for bacteria, which could make your baby ill.

As with breastfeeding, you can offer your baby a bottle whenever he seems hungry – he'll let you know how much he needs by crying for it!

Moving from breast to bottle

If you want to wean your baby off the breast and on to the bottle, give him (and yourself) a while to adapt to the change. If you're returning to work and need to have established bottle-feeding by a certain deadline, give your baby at least 2 weeks to acclimatise – don't wait until the day before he goes off to nursery. If you're fully breastfeeding, stopping immediately can be physical agony! You'll probably find that substituting one bottle feed for one breast feed in a day, and increasing the number of bottles by one every few days, reduces breast engorgement.

Starting to feed from a bottle with expressed milk makes the transition to bottled formula milk easier because at least this way he gets the same taste, even if the technique is different. Many babies take to the bottle without a hitch, but others don't like it at all and take a while to acclimatise to this new way of feeding. If your baby objects to bottle-feeding, try these tips:

- ✔ Leave the room and get someone else to offer the bottle, so that your baby can't smell your breast.

- ✔ Wait until your baby's hungry (but not starving, otherwise he'll just scream!) before offering him a bottle.

- ✔ If your baby's older than 6 months, you may find it easier to move straight from the breast to a spouted beaker, which is better for his teeth. This is particularly good if you want to introduce *mixed feeding* (part breast, part bottle), as it prevents nipple confusion.

Many experts believe that offering a bottle before breastfeeding is established properly can cause nipple confusion. Sucking from a bottle and a breast use different techniques, so your baby may struggle to latch on to your nipple if he gets used to drinking from a bottle teat. Remember, too, that replacing breastfeeds with bottles of formula reduces your milk supply, and you'll have difficulty starting breastfeeding again after you've stopped.

Working Out When to Wean

Where did your helpless newborn go? Only yesterday, your wriggling bundle of joy was interested in nothing more than a drop of warm milk and a snooze. Suddenly he's sitting up, gurgling away, and showing a sophisticated fascination in your Sunday roast with all the trimmings.

Weaning is a major milestone for every baby (and every parent). It's an exciting time – the beginnings of family meals, picnics in the park, and fun-filled party teas. But before any of that happens, you've got a great deal of mess to get through.

Fun it may be, but weaning is also stressful – and not just because your home's likely to get an interior makeover (puréed carrot can make interesting wallpaper). Deciding when to wean isn't always easy either. The World Health Organization recommends breastfeeding exclusively for the first 6 months to boost your baby's immunity and avoid allergies – and that means no solids. But some babies seem ready for weaning earlier, and many health professionals agree that babies can start solids as early as age 4 months.

Spotting the telltale signs that your baby's ready for solids

As a rule, the best guide to the right time to wean is by looking at your baby and seeing whether he displays any of the obvious symptoms, such as the following:

- ✔ He seems hungry again quite quickly after a big breast- or bottle-feed.
- ✔ He seems more restless than usual or starts waking at night even though he used to sleep through.
- ✔ He's interested in your food, makes chewing motions as he watches you eat, or even tries to help himself to what's on your plate.
- ✔ He's doubled his birthweight.

Don't start weaning earlier than 4 months, because your baby's digestive system can't cope with complex foods. Weaning too early can also increase the risk of allergies in later life. However, leaving weaning until much later than 6 months is also not advisable: At 6 months, milk alone does not provide your baby with enough nutrients, especially because the stores of iron he was born with are depleted.

Getting started

Put away the dinner plates – you only need to give a tiny spoonful or two to begin with. The idea is to get your baby used to the taste and texture of solids to begin with, not to fill him up on them. Before you start, take the edge off your baby's appetite by giving him a little of his usual milk. Sit him in a high-chair or on your lap and offer him a spoonful of the food you have chosen – puréed vegetable or fruit are good first foods – mixed with a little breast milk or formula – the food ought to be warm and runny. Put a tiny amount on the spoon and into your baby's mouth. It'll probably all come back out, but keep trying. As you do so, give him lots of eye contact, smile, chat, and tell him how tasty it is. If he turns his head away or gets upset, stop – he's had enough.

If your first attempts go badly, don't panic! Try again the next day, but be prepared to back off and leave it a week or so if your baby's really reluctant. There's no point in force-feeding him. For now, his usual milk is more than adequate to keep him full up and healthy.

Moving on up: step-by-step weaning

Weaning is a very gradual process, and for the first few weeks at least, your baby will probably take no more than a couple of spoons of food at each sitting. Take it slowly and stay relaxed and you'll both take to it like ducks to water.

Week 1: Puréed vegetable such as carrot is an ideal first food. Mix it to a runny consistency with breast milk or formula, and just give one or two spoonfuls once a day.

Even when weaning, your baby still needs plenty of breast milk or formula milk – milk is still his most important source of nutrition, so be sure to offer at least 600 ml of milk a day until he's 12 months old.

Week 2: Introduce smooth purées of single vegetables, such as carrot, swede, or potato, watered down with breast milk or formula. Stick to the same purée for a couple of days before introducing a new one, so your baby gets used to each flavour. If your baby is happy, aim for two small servings a day.

Make up quantities of puréed vegetables, and then freeze them in ice cube trays. This lets you prepare food in advance and increase the size of servings as your baby's appetite increases. Life's too short to cook a tablespoon of purée at a time!

Week 3: Add purées of fruit, such as banana, apple, or mango. You can also combine purées to make new flavours. Give two or three servings a day.

Week 4: If your baby's over 6 months of age, you can start to introduce more filling meals such as lentil and vegetable purée. You can also try small amounts of dairy products, such as unsweetened natural yoghurt or fromage frais, or mild cheddar cheese. If your baby's happy, he can now be having two quite substantial meals a day.

Week 5: You can now start to add thoroughly puréed meat and fish, or lentils, if your baby's over 6 months of age. All of them are rich in protein and great for your baby's growth. Give your baby two or three meals a day, with at least one protein-based serving.

Introducing lumps and textures

From between the ages of 7 and 9 months, you can start to introduce lumpier purées and finger foods, such as chunks of banana or well-cooked carrot sticks. You can also offer bread, pasta, and couscous.

As you introduce textures, let your baby feed himself with his fingers or a spoon if he likes – the more control he feels he has, the more he'll enjoy the experience.

When your baby has happily accepted lumps and finger foods, you can introduce chopped foods rather than purées. As a general rule, from around the age of 9 months your baby can eat small *unsalted* portions of your meals (see the section 'Avoiding foods that could be harmful' later in this chapter, for why you mustn't use salt). Encourage him to feed himself and sit at the table with the rest of the family.

Harnessing health hazards

You can keep your baby safe and healthy when weaning by doing the following:

- Wash your hands before handling and preparing bottles and food, and before feeding your baby.

- Wash all fruit and veg thoroughly. The UK government advises peeling fruit and veg if they're not organic, because farming chemicals can cause stomach cramps. Peel is also a choking hazard.

- Sterilise all bottles and feeding equipment until your baby is 12 months old.

- Remove potential choking hazards from your baby's food: Check fish and meat for bones, remove stones and pips from fruit, and cut up food into small pieces.

- Cook meat, fish, and poultry thoroughly to kill off parasites.

- Make sure your baby's food isn't too hot: Taste it before serving to check the temperature.

- Store food in the fridge in a sterile lidded container for up to 24 hours. Do not re-store food once your baby's spoon has been in it, as saliva can spread bacteria.

- Remember to defrost frozen food thoroughly before serving.

- Keep surfaces for raw meat separate: Don't prepare other foods on the same surface.

- Don't microwave your baby's food or milk, as it can develop hotspots that can burn your baby's mouth.

- Don't reheat food more than once. If you're using jars, heat up the amount you expect your baby to eat and refrigerate the rest.

- Never leave your baby unattended while he's eating, in case he chokes.

Weaning your baby on to solid foods is an important step in his healthy development and a huge learning curve for both you and your baby. Don't be afraid to ask for advice from your health visitor if you're not sure about something.

Avoiding foods that could be harmful

To begin with, stick to puréed fruit and veg, baby rice, and breast milk or formula. Your baby's digestive system not only needs time to get used to new stuff, but sticking to these foods makes him less likely to react badly or develop and allergy. Beyond the age of 6 months, many foods are considered safe, but some can cause allergies or illness or pose a choking risk. Here's what not to give:

- **Cows' and goats' milk:** These milks don't provide the right proportion of nutrients for young babies. Don't even use them to mix up your baby's cereal – use only breast milk or iron-fortified formula for the first 12 months, after which, go ahead and introduce your baby slowly to full-fat cows' milk. Don't be tempted to serve reduced-fat or skimmed milk to your child until he's at least 2 years old, as he needs the extra fat in whole milk to provide energy for his growing body.

- **Nuts:** All are a choking hazard.

- **Peanut and other nut products:** Avoid because they may cause allergies. If you have a family history of asthma, eczema, or allergies, avoid giving your baby peanut products until he's at least 36 months old.

- **Salt:** Babies under 1 year of age cannot process any salt. If you add salt to food, it can cause serious kidney damage. Gravy granules, stock cubes, and ready-made sauces are packed with salt, so don't go near them.

- **Honey:** Avoid honey for the first year of your baby's life, as it can contain spores that cause botulism poisoning in infants. Although rare, botulism poisoning can make your baby extremely ill.

- **Sugar and any foods containing sugar:** Avoid it altogether – it has no nutritional value and is bad for your baby's teeth.

- **Eggs:** A whole lot of nutrition is packed into a little egg. But wait until your baby's at least a year old before scrambling up eggs for him. If you feed eggs any sooner, you'll run the risk of causing an allergic reaction in your baby.

- **Tea, coffee, and fizzy drinks:** The caffeine in these prevents your baby's body from absorbing iron.

- **Low-fat foods:** These don't provide enough calories for your baby's growing needs.

Young children need fat in their diet because it provides instant energy, and allows them to metabolise essential vitamins. As long as your baby's weight gain is steady, don't concern yourself with cutting fat. We discuss this and other nutrition issues in more depth in Chapter 9.

✔ **Foods that may cause an allergic reaction, including chocolate, beans, corn, nuts, seafood, and citrus fruits and juices:** Avoid these foods for baby's first year, especially if you have a family history of allergies.

Making the transition from formula to cows' milk

Experts agree that babies should beat least 12 months old before they drink cows' milk, because of their immature digestive systems. Yoghurts and cheese are fine in small quantities, but use follow-on formula milk for drinking until your baby is 12 months old, by which time most babies' digestive systems can handle the proteins contained in dairy milk. When you do introduce cows' milk, use whole milk rather than skimmed varieties. Whole milk contains proteins, fats, vitamins, and minerals that are essential for your baby's growth and development.

For optimum health, it may be beneficial to wait even longer than 12 months before you introduce cows' milk. Children who switch to cows' milk at 12 months of age may be more at risk of iron deficiency: Formula is fortified with iron to meet your baby's needs, but cows' milk is naturally low in iron. When you feel that your child is eating a well-balanced diet with plenty of iron-rich foods, such as leafy green veg, pulses, and red meat, you can start him on cows' milk. Talk to your health visitor if you are concerned.

Introducing drinks with meals

When your baby has started to eat solid foods, he'll need to drink with his meals. Water is by far the best drink because it is thirst-quenching, and not harmful to your baby's teeth. Use cooled, boiled water for at least the first 6 months. Many babies don't take to the taste of water after drinking milk exclusively, as milk's naturally sweet. Persist by giving your baby regular little sips of water – he'll get used to the taste if you persevere. If your baby really hates the taste of water and starts to become dehydrated (constipation is a warning sign), try diluting a little fresh fruit juice with water. Avoid commercial baby juices because these are sweetened and bad for your baby's teeth. Infants under 1 year old shouldn't drink more than 6 fluid ounces of juice per day. Too much juice can displace the needed protein, fat, and vitamins in breast milk or formula. Give your baby diluted juice in a sipping cup rather than a bottle, as this can help prevent cavities forming in young teeth.

Troubleshooting: When Food and Your Baby Don't Agree

Introduce foods gradually to your baby's diet. That way, you'll find it easier to tell whether a particular food doesn't agree with him. Signs that a food is a problem can include a whole series of symptoms, including abdominal swelling, diarrhoea, and agitated behaviour. Such symptoms can be an indication that your baby has a food allergy or intolerance.

A lot of confusion exists between the terms 'intolerance' and 'allergy'. Many people assume that they're different words for the same problem, but they actually refer to very different conditions. A *food allergy* is a reaction of the immune system to a substance it perceives, mistakenly, as harmful. A *food intolerance* usually involves a reaction within the digestive tract. Either way, both are problems for babies.

The foods that most commonly cause allergies and intolerances are eggs, cows' milk, wheat, gluten (found in wheat, rye, barley, and sometimes oats), fish, shellfish, citrus fruits, tomatoes, sesame seeds, and soya.

If you baby vomits several times a day, gags, chokes, or refuses to feed, call a doctor. Reflux disease is caused by acid from the stomach refluxing back into the oesophagus (gullet). Symptoms include vomiting several times a day, pain when vomiting, irritability, inconsolable crying, gagging, choking, or refusal to feed. For more information about reflux disease, head to Chapter 12.

Diagnosing food reactions in babies

A true food allergy usually causes an immediate reaction after the baby eats a particular food. The most common symptoms of a food allergy are itchy skin, itchy or swollen tongue and lips, sneezing, a runny nose, shortness of breath, vomiting, and coughing.

The symptoms of food intolerance are more likely to be tummy pain or colic (you may see him pulling his knees up to his chest or arching his back in pain) bloating, wind, diarrhoea, and sometimes vomiting. Agitated behaviour, and hot flushing may also be symptoms.

Never try to diagnose an allergy or intolerance yourself: If you suspect your baby is reacting to a food, seek a proper diagnosis from your doctor, so that your baby can get the correct medical treatment.

The most severe from of allergy is called *anaphylaxis*, a potentially life-threatening reaction that needs emergency medical treatment. Symptoms may include itchy skin, swelling on the lips and tongue, tightening of the throat, difficulty breathing, and appearing to be losing consciousness. Your baby may look pale and clammy. Left untreated, anaphylaxis can cause loss of consciousness and in rare cases may be fatal. For more info on allergies, have a look at Chapter 15.

Getting geared up on gluten

A reaction to gluten, a protein found in wheat, rye, barley, and sometimes oats, is common in babies. Gluten sensitivity causes damage to the upper intestine, leaving the body unable to absorb nutrients properly and causing digestive problems, which usually appear gradually. Symptoms can include a swollen-looking stomach, vomiting and diarrhoea, porridgy-looking poo, constipation, appetite loss, and slow weight gain or weight loss.

Breastfeeding and delaying feeding your baby foods with gluten in until he is 7 months old or more can reduce the likelihood of your baby having a gluten reaction. Therefore, try to avoid foods such as baby porridge and rusks, which are usually made with wheat flour, until your baby is about 8 months old. Most babies grow out of gluten intolerance, but occasionally gluten intolerance indicates coeliac disease, a lifelong condition that means your child must avoid glutinous foods permanently. If you suspect that your baby has a gluten intolerance, see your health visitor or doctor, who may refer him to hospital for blood, urine, and faeces tests.

The truth about milk intolerance

A reaction to cows' milk and dairy produce is one of the most common food intolerances in babies. The technical name is *functional lactase deficiency*, a temporary form of intolerance to lactose, which is a protein found in cows' milk and other dairy products. True lactose intolerance is rare in babies. A reaction to cows' milk in the early months is more likely to be down to your baby's immature digestive system, which may still be lacking the appropriate enzymes to metabolise lactose.

If your breastfeeding baby seems to be having a reaction – for example, if he's continually bloated or has diarrhoea – you may need to cut dairy products from your diet, as the proteins that cause the reaction can be passed on to your baby via your milk. However, don't cut out dairy products without first getting advice from your health visitor or GP.

If your formula-fed baby seems to be reacting to milk, you may want to switch to a soya-based formula – but never do so without first getting advice from your GP or health visitor. Bear in mind, however, that up to 30 per cent of babies who have a problem with dairy foods are also likely to react to soya milk, so this may not be the answer. Rice milk is sometimes recommended in severe cases, but always see your health visitor or GP before changing your baby's diet.

Chapter 7

Spotting the Signs that Something's Wrong

*I*f you find yourself worrying that your baby can't tell you when something's wrong, fear not. She *will* tell you – and loudly. The difficult bit is trying to work out exactly why she's doing it. Is she hungry, tired, teething? Does she have a tummy upset? Does she need a doctor? The trick is to look for other signs to see what's causing her distress. This chapter aims to help you a little with the detective work, but sometimes it takes trial and error or even a visit to the doctor before you can be sure just what's bugging your little treasure.

Finding Out Why Your Baby's Crying

One thing's for sure: crying certainly gets you sitting up and paying attention. Studies show that people's stress levels rise when they hear the sound of a crying baby, and you may find yourself responding to crying instinctively – even if it's only to join in the wailing. Having a crying baby can be frustrating, but remember that crying is your baby's only way of communicating with you and letting you know she needs something, so she's likely to do it rather a lot.

The most disturbing thing about having a crying baby is not knowing what on earth's wrong. Working out why your baby's crying usually involves a bit of trial and error, but after a few weeks of getting to know your baby you'll start to differentiate between her cries and be able to respond to her needs more easily. Here are the most common reasons for crying:

- **Hunger.** Your baby's tummy is tiny and can't hold much milk, so in the early days she'll need frequent top-ups, especially if you're breastfeeding her (babies digest breast milk more quickly than formula).

- **A dirty nappy.** How would you like to be left in one? Enough said. To avoid the soreness of nappy rash and infection, change your baby's nappy as soon as it's dirty and every three hours if it's wet.

- **Tiredness.** A newborn needs around 17 hours sleep a day. Just like you, your baby can become fretful and irritable if she's overtired. Try rocking her in your arms or taking her for a ride in the buggy or car to help her nod off.

- **Boredom.** Getting plenty of attention and having things to look at helps stimulate your baby. She'll love to look at you and listen to you, so hold her facing you while you chat or sing to her.

- **Over stimulation.** Too much noise and activity can make your baby fractious, so try laying her in her cot or Moses basket while you get on with things nearby.

- **Discomfort.** Check that your baby's clothes aren't too tight and that she's not too hot or cold. If her tummy feels hot and clammy, remove a layer of clothing or blankets. If she's cold, add another blanket and check that she's not in a draught. The ideal room temperature for a baby is around 18°C/65°F.

- **Loneliness.** Apart from food, your baby needs love and cuddles more than anything else. Many babies cry if they're put down or left alone even for short periods. If holding your baby is preventing you from getting anything done, try putting her in a sling so that you can carry her around but still have your hands free.

- **Anxiety.** Remember that your baby is very sensitive to your moods, so she may cry if you're feeling anxious, irritable, or stressed. To help you unwind, ask your partner or a relative or friend to look after her for a couple of hours to give you a break.

If your baby is crying and you don't know why, go through the preceding list to check that she's not suffering from any of the most obvious and common causes. If you're confident that your baby's crying is not for any of these reasons, it may be a sign that she is ill or in pain.

Reading the signs that your baby's in pain

Until relatively recently, doctors believed that babies didn't feel pain in the same way as older children and adults. However, more recent research proves that babies feel pain as much as anyone else – in fact, they may be even more sensitive than adults to pain. You may find it hard to tell whether, and where, your baby is hurting, but here are a few signs that you can learn to read:

✔ **Listen to her cries.** Your baby's pain cry is likely different from her other cries. Pain cries are often loud, high-pitched, urgent, and continuous. If you find it difficult to understand what the cries mean, work it out systematically by eliminating other causes of discomfort, such as those listed in the preceding section. If none of these things seems to be the problem, she may be trying to tell you that she's hurting.

✔ **Check her body language.** As well as crying, your baby will give you clues about how she's feeling by the way she moves her body. If she writhes around in an agitated manner, making involuntary movements with her arms and feet or pulling her legs up to her tummy, then she may be feeling pain. An older baby may touch the area that's hurting or withdraw when you try to touch the painful area.

✔ **Watch her face.** Certain facial signs may suggest that your baby is crying because she's in pain. Look out for her frowning and squeezing her eyes together and creating a bulge of flesh between the eyebrows, shutting her eyes tightly, or pulling her mouth taut, horizontally and vertically, causing deep creases running down from the nostril edges to the mouth.

If your baby's crying because she's ill, she'll likely display other symptoms as well, such as fever (temperature over 37.5°C/99.5°F), diarrhoea, rapid shallow breathing, and vomiting. She may also show behavioural changes, such as fretfulness, clinginess, or refusing food.

If you're at all concerned about your baby's health, call your GP, especially if your baby:

✔ Doesn't want to move or be moved by you

✔ Has blood in her poo or urine

✔ Vomits or has diarrhoea for more than 24 hours

✔ Is floppy and listless

✔ Has a bulging or sunken fontanelle (the soft spot on the top of her head)

✔ Has a fever (temperature over 37.5°C/99.5°F) and/or a rash, or has a temperature but his hands and feet are cold

✔ Has mottled skin

Give your doctor as much information as possible about your baby's symptoms, as this makes it easier for the doctor to make a diagnosis.

Most GP surgeries no longer look after their patients out of hours. But you can phone NHS Direct (0845-4647) 24 hours a day for advice.

Comforting your crying baby

The best way to soothe your baby depends on the cause of her pain, but here are a few tried and tested ways that may help her feel better:

- ✔ **Hold her.** If you cradle your baby gently, containing her limbs, she'll feel less panicky. Swaddling your baby may also be really effective in calming her: Hold her with her hands together on her chest and her fingers near her mouth, and then wrap her firmly in a small cotton sheet.

- ✔ **Rock her.** Many parents instinctively rock their babies to comfort them. A rocking motion is thought to stimulate a reaction in your baby's inner ear, which can have a calming effect on her.

- ✔ **Let her suck.** The movement of your baby's mouth muscles when she sucks may stimulate the release of endorphins – the body's natural feel-good chemicals – in her brain. Sucking on her thumb, a dummy, a teat, or a nipple can help her relax and block the pain. Sucking also offers a distraction from the pain and can be a very effective way to soothe her.

If your baby's really screaming, you may find that the measures suggested above make her more agitated and distressed. If so, try letting her lie quietly, as any kind of stimulation may be stressful for her. Do see a doctor or call NHS Direct if you are at all worried about your baby.

Coping with persistent crying

If nothing seems to calm your baby but she's not displaying signs of illness, she may have colic (read more about about colic in Chapter 8). If you're struggling to cope with persistent crying, try the following:

- ✔ Put your baby in her cot and leave the room for ten minutes to give yourself a chance to take a breather and calm down.

- ✔ Phone a friend or your health visitor – simply talking to someone can help.

- ✔ Contact Cry-sis (08451-228669; www.cry-sis.org.uk).

Getting to the Bottom of Tummy Troubles

All young babies bring up tiny amounts of milk, known as possetting. Stomach upsets are also common in babies, so sick-stained T-shirts are definitely in fashion if you're a new parent. In addition, you'll soon become an expert at dealing with exploding nappies.

Repeatedly bringing up large quantities of milk or food can be a symptom of illness, however. And severe vomiting and diarrhoea need prompt attention, as they can lead to dehydration, which can be serious in babies and young children.

Contact your doctor if your baby is under two months old and has vomiting and diarrhoea and any of the following symptoms:

- ✔ Dry mouth and tongue
- ✔ Sunken eyes and/or fontanelle
- ✔ Dark urine and/or nappies that stay dry for several hours
- ✔ Lethargy/listlessness
- ✔ Floppy muscle tone
- ✔ Lack of interest in feeds
- ✔ Racing heart rate

Contemplating causes of stomach complaints

Gastric problems in babies can be caused by a number of things, including viral infections, bacteria in food, and reactions to food. Breastfeeding your baby is the best way to avoid infection: Gastroenteritis is rare in breastfed babies because breast milk gives them extra immunity against infection.

Viral infections

A tummy bug, or gastroenteritis, is often caused by a virus passed from person to person via droplets in the air or unwashed hands touching food and toys. One of the most common viruses responsible is the rotavirus – fortunately a vaccine should soon be available to protect your child. Gastroenteritis generally causes sickness and diarrhoea for a few days, but your baby is likely to be completely better within a week. If you know someone who is suffering from a tummy bug, try to keep your baby away from them until the illness has passed – and if your baby has vomiting and diarrhoea, keep her away from other babies and children until she's better.

Monitoring milk

Bottles of milk are ideal breeding grounds for the germs that can cause tummy bugs, so remember the following tips:

✔ Keep prepared bottles in the main part of the fridge – not the door, which isn't cold enough – and discard any unused formula after 24 hours.

✔ If your baby feeds from a bottle, don't let her keep a bottle for more than two hours.

✔ Use cooled, boiled water in your baby's drinks and food until she's a year old. When you go out, take water and milk powder in separate containers, ready to mix up when she needs a feed.

For more feeding info, check out Chapter 6.

Green vomit is a common sign of gastroenteritis in older babies and toddlers, but in very young babies it can be a sign of a twisted bowel, which needs urgent medical attention.

Bacterial infections

Bacteria in food that hasn't been prepared or stored safely, or on bottles that haven't been cleaned properly, can make your baby extremely unwell. Your baby's immune system is still developing and she's particularly vulnerable to tummy upsets. You can help to avoid tummy upsets by taking care with hygiene. Wash your hands after using the loo and changing nappies and before preparing food. Clean your baby's bottles and feeding utensils thoroughly – and that means sterilising bottles until she's a year old.

Although maintaining basic hygiene is important, especially when preparing, storing, and clearing away food, if your baby never comes into contact with germs she won't build up any resistance to them. So take care with the essentials, but try not to worry about dusty surfaces and grubby toys, especially once your little one's crawling and cruising around.

Food intolerances and allergies

Some babies and toddlers have adverse reactions to certain foods, which may cause tummy upsets. When you're weaning your baby, try to introduce one new food at a time, so that you can see whether it disagrees with her; check out Chapter 6 for the low-down on weaning, and Chapter 15 for more on allergies. Occasionally, breastfeeding mums find that eating certain foods causes tummy upsets in their babies: If your baby has diarrhoea and seems otherwise well, take a close look at your own diet. If you're eating too many spicy foods, for example, it may be having an impact on your baby's bowels.

Other causes of vomiting

Vomiting can indicate the start of a range of illnesses, including ear infections, colds, and more serious problems, such as urine infection or meningitis. Keep an eye out for other symptoms, such as pain, rashes, and fever, and contact your doctor if necessary. Here are two more reasons why your baby may be vomiting:

✔ **Reflux.** Lots of young babies have reflux, whereby milk comes back up due to a leaky valve at the top of the stomach. The main symptom is bringing up significant amounts of milk, almost effortlessly, at the end of a feed. There are no other symptoms and your baby is otherwise well. The condition will resolve as your baby grows, although your doctor may prescribe a special feed thickener.

Never try to thicken your baby's food yourself, as doing so can lead quickly to dehydration.

✔ **Pyloric stenosis.** If your baby suffers from severe projectile vomiting – which can shoot up to several feet! – and seems very hungry, she may have pyloric stenosis, a condition where food cannot pass out of the stomach and is ejected forcefully the other way. Your baby may fail to put on weight, and seem hungry as soon as he's eaten and vomited. See your doctor if your baby regularly vomits like this. If your doctor suspects pyloric stenosis, your baby may need to have an ultrasound scan. The condition is treated with a simple operation carried out under local anaesthetic.

Pyloric stenosis is more common in first-born male babies and the symptoms usually start in the first four to six weeks of life. But babies don't always obey the rules, so if your baby gets symptoms that you think may be due to pyloric stenosis, see your GP.

Preventing dehydration

One of the most important things you need to do if your baby is vomiting or has diarrhoea is to make sure she doesn't become dehydrated. If your baby becomes dehydrated, she may need to be admitted to hospital to receive fluids via an intravenous drip. To keep your baby hydrated, try the following:

✔ If your baby is bottle-fed, do not give her milk. Instead, offer her frequent sips of cooled, boiled water. Keep encouraging her to drink, even if she can't keep anything down for very long.

✔ If your baby is breastfed, let her continue to feed normally. Try also offering cooled, boiled water between feeds.

✔ Your GP may prescribe rehydration drinks to help replace any vital fluids your baby has lost. Don't give rehydration drinks without first seeking advice from your GP.

Don't be too concerned if your baby loses weight while she has an upset stomach. You'll probably find that the weight goes back on quickly when she's better.

What's That in Her Nappy?

When you're learning to look after your brand-new baby, one of the first obstacles you'll encounter is a nappy full of sticky, tarry, dark-green poo – swiftly followed by bowel movements of a startling variety. Babies' stools vary enormously: The colour can range from lemon-yellow to green and the consistency from liquid to firm. Therefore, it can be hard to tell the good from the bad.

With wee, the story's a bit different. Instead of being fascinated by colour or consistency, most parents obsess about quantity: How much and how often?

Getting all blocked up about constipation

Constipation is relatively common in bottle-fed babies and babies who have been weaned on to solids. Although constipation is seldom a cause for concern, you must deal with it quickly, because waste matter that builds up in the rectum dries out quickly, making it more and more difficult – and painful – to pass.

Signs of constipation

The main concern is not the frequency but the consistency of your baby's poo. If she appears to be in distress during a bowel movement, and if her poo is hard and dry, then she's likely to be constipated. You may also notice that her tummy feels hard and she may have tummy ache – she may be difficult to comfort, pull up her legs to her chest in pain, and seem lethargic.

How often a baby should poo can be a worry for new parents. The answer is that there's no magic number. Some new babies can produce ten dirty nappies a day, while others, especially breastfed babies, can go for days without doing a poo. Breast milk is so well suited to your baby that there isn't much waste for her to get rid of. Try not to worry about quantity: If your baby seems well and comfortable and has plenty of wet nappies, then she's probably fine. If she's unhappy and seems to be in discomfort or pain, seek medical advice.

Don't delay in asking for help: The sooner constipation is dealt with, the easier it is to rectify. If your baby has any of the following, take her to a doctor:

- ✔ Cream- or white-coloured stools, which can sometimes indicate liver problems.
- ✔ Blood in the poo, which may be due to a slight tear (fissure) in the anus or the result of an inflamed bowel.

✔ Frequent watery poo, accompanied by lethargy, fever, or any other symptoms of illness.

✔ Hard, infrequent stools that cause discomfort and distress.

Treating constipation

A shortage of fluids in your baby's diet is one of the most common causes of constipation, although bugs and other illnesses can also trigger the problem. Once she's onto solids, a shortage of fibre can also be a cause. Your GP or health visitor is likely to suggest increasing your baby's fluid intake with cooled, boiled water. For babies on solid food, diluted juice or puréed fruit can help get things moving. If your bottle-fed baby has hard painful poos, check that you're adding the correct amount of formula to her bottles: Make sure you fill the scoops loosely and level them, as over-thick feeds are a common cause of constipation.

When you wash your baby's bottom, apply cream or petroleum jelly around the outside of the anus to help ease any soreness caused by constipation.

A warm bath can make your baby relax and help to open her bowels. Tummy massage is also a good way to get things going. With oil or moisturising cream on your fingers, start at the belly button and then massage outwards in circles in a clockwise direction. If your baby enjoys the massage and is comfortable and relaxed, continue. While she's lying on her back, hold her legs and turn them gently in a quick cycling motion. This makes the stomach muscles move and puts gentle pressure on the intestines, making them move.

Never put a thermometer or anything else inside your baby's anus to stimulate the bowel movement, because doing so may cause damage.

After you begin to offer your baby foods other than milk, you will notice changes in her poo. Until now, her digestive system has been used to only one type of food – milk. Your baby will react to new foods by producing more solid, smellier poos. You may find that pieces of food pass straight through, entirely undigested – a normal event that will happen less as your child's digestion matures.

When you've weaned your baby, give her lots of fresh fruit and vegetables to make sure her diet contains enough fibre. Dried fruits such as raisins, apricots, and figs help, as do peas, beans, sweetcorn, baked beans, and jacket potatoes.

Although you don't want your baby to be constipated, her digestive system isn't made to cope with a very high fibre diet. So while a good selection of puréed fruit and vegetable is invaluable, too much high-bran bread may do more harm than good.

Having a wee look at your baby's waterworks

A young baby can wee up to 30 times in 24 hours. Copious weeing is nothing to be concerned about. In fact, a dry nappy is more worrying. If your newborn's nappy stays dry for four to six hours, speak to your midwife, health visitor, or GP, because your baby may be unwell or dehydrated. If your baby's urine is yellow and concentrated , she needs more fluids. Offering plenty of drinks (cooled, boiled water for young babies) should solve the problem.

If you think your baby's urine contains blood, contact your doctor immediately. But bear in mind that certain foods and drinks, such as blackcurrant juice, can turn wee red. Also seek medical help if your baby's urine is very concentrated and smelly, because this may be a sign of a urine infection.

Weighing Things Up: Failure to Thrive

During the first year or so of life, most babies gain weight and grow rapidly. The pattern of this development can vary considerably, but the average term baby doubles her weight by four months and triples it at one year. However, some babies with underlying health problems don't meet these milestones and need extra help and possibly some closer attention to find out what's causing the problem.

If your baby is classified as 'failing to thrive', basically she isn't putting on weight or growing in the expected way. 'Failure to thrive' is a general term rather than a specific condition, but doctors take it seriously because failing to thrive is a sign that your baby's not getting the nourishment she needs. A baby who's failing to thrive may:

✔ Become disinterested in her surroundings and feeding

✔ Avoid eye contact

✔ Become irritable or withdrawn and whiny

✔ Not reach developmental milestones such as sitting up, walking, and talking at the 'usual' age

✔ Have faltering weight, which drops from an established growth curve for at least three months

✔ Have a skinny appearance, with thin arms and legs, but with a large stomach

✔ Have wispy hair and dark circles around the eyes.

Finding out what causes failure to thrive

Failure to thrive can result from a wide variety of underlying causes, such as the following:

- **Gastrointestinal problems:** Tummy troubles such as reflux or chronic diarrhoea can interfere with your baby's ability to hold on to the nutrients and calories from her milk or food.

- **Underlying illness:** Milk-protein intolerance and coeliac disease, a sensitivity to a protein found in wheat and certain other grains, can limit your baby's ability to absorb nutrients. Your baby may eat a lot, but her body can't absorb and retain enough food. Unless diagnosed, problems like these can cause failure to thrive.

- **Underlying infection:** A urinary tract infection, for example, can place great energy demands on your baby and force her body to use nutrients rapidly, sometimes causing short- or long-term failure to thrive. Underlying infection can also impair your baby's appetite. Other conditions that can lead to failure to thrive include heart, liver, and respiratory disorders.

- **Metabolic problem:** Metabolic disorders, such as gluten or lactose intolerance, limit your baby's ability to make the most of the calories consumed or make it difficult for your baby to break down, process, or derive energy from food. Other metabolic disorders can cause a build-up of toxins during the breakdown process, which can make your baby feed poorly or vomit.

- **Poor nutrition:** Some parents just don't feed their baby enough or lack the knowledge of how to feed their baby healthily. For example, they may restrict the calories they give their baby because they don't want a fat child. Other parents feed their baby according to their own limited diet. Make sure your baby is getting the nutrition she needs by giving her a varied diet.

- **Unknown cause:** In a few cases, doctors cannot pinpoint a specific cause.

Your baby may be slow to gain weight for a number of reasons. Genetics plays a big role in weight gain, so if you and your partner are slim your baby may not put on pounds quickly. Monitoring your baby's weight gain from home can be difficult, so attend regular weight and development checks with the health visitor.

Diagnosing and treating failure to thrive

Your baby's weight gain is likely to level out or even drop occasionally, but if she doesn't gain weight for three consecutive months during the first year of life for no obvious reason, your doctor will probably become concerned.

Failure to thrive is usually diagnosed by using standard growth charts, called *centile charts*, where your baby's weight, length, and head circumference are measured at each development check. Centile charts show the size of the whole 'normal' range of children at a given age. As a rule, your doctor will want to investigate your baby for possible failure to thrive if her weight gain slows down enough to drop down two 'centile lines'.

If your doctor finds that your baby is failing to thrive, she will take a thorough medical and feeding history and perform a detailed physical examination of your baby. Your doctor may carry out blood and urine tests on your baby if she suspects a particular disease to be the cause.

A baby with extreme failure to thrive may need to go to hospital so that she can be fed via a tube and monitored continuously. During this time, any possible underlying causes can be evaluated and treated appropriately. The length of treatment varies. Weight gain takes time, so several months may pass before your baby is back in the normal range for her age, although after she starts to gain weight satisfactorily, she will normally be allowed home.

If your baby's weight drops or she doesn't seem to have a normal appetite, get in touch with your health visitor, who can tell you if you need to see the doctor. Any major change in eating patterns warrants medical advice.

Teething Times: Nothing but the Tooth

Your baby was born with a set of 20 teeth hidden in her jaw, and at around six months of age she'll start to be painfully aware of them.

Looking after a baby who is cutting teeth can be a real nightmare. It's amazing how one little white thing poking through a gum can throw everything into chaos: Suddenly you've got a grizzly, dribbly little person who needs round-the-clock attention. Of course, teething isn't always troublesome – everyone knows someone whose baby cut her first teeth without so much as a whimper – but most babies go through a period of being uncomfortable and grumpy when they're cutting their pearly whites. The good news is that teething is usually relatively short-lived and you can do plenty to soothe the pain.

Spotting the signs of teething

Common signs of teething include irritability, drooling, chewing, crying, swollen red and bumpy gums, and seeing the whiteness of a tooth through the gum.

The whole tooth

The first white tip usually pops through at about age six months. Each baby is different, though: Some have teeth at three months old, others don't get any until they're almost 12 months old, and some are even born with a tooth or two. If your baby doesn't have a tooth by her first birthday, have a chat with your health visitor.

Babies' teeth don't necessarily appear in the same order. But the typical pattern is: lower central incisors at six months; upper central incisors at seven months; upper lateral incisors at eight months; lower lateral incisors at nine months; first molars at 12 months; canines at 18 months, and second molars at 24 months.

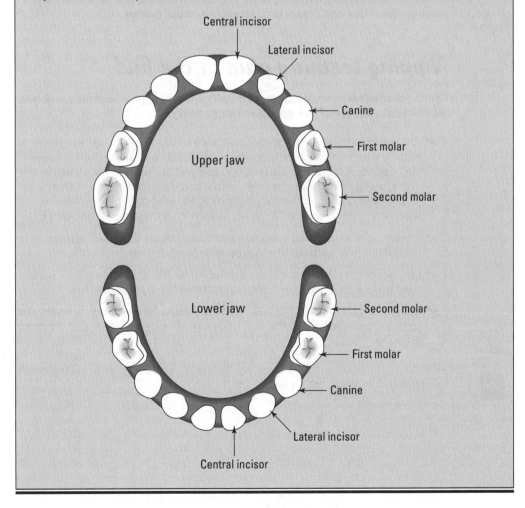

Central incisor
Lateral incisor
Canine
First molar
Second molar
Upper jaw
Lower jaw
Second molar
First molar
Canine
Lateral incisor
Central incisor

Talk to a group of parents, however, and the list of symptoms associated with teething is likely also to include red cheeks, fever, ear-pulling, going off food, diarrhoea, and nappy rash.

The experts aren't so sure. Although irritability, drooling, and chewing are certainly associated with teething, teething is unlikely to cause fever, ear-pulling, and diarrhoea.

Parents often blame teething for all sorts of symptoms that are actually more likely to be signs that your baby is ill. At six months of age, when the first tooth often comes through, your baby also starts to lose the immunity you passed on when you were pregnant and may come down with colds and tummy bugs more easily.

Beware of mistaking something more serious for teething. If your baby has a fever or diarrhoea and screams constantly, see the doctor.

Nipping teething pain in the bud

Finding the best way of soothing your baby's teething pain normally involves a bit of trial and error. Here are a few things to try:

- ✔ Give your baby something cool and hard to chew. Most babies love to chomp when they're teething, and something cold to chew on is especially good. A teething ring that you can put in the fridge is ideal – but don't put the ring in the freezer, as this can damage the gums. Or try giving your baby cold carrot sticks or apple rings to chew on – never leave your baby alone with these, however, as they pose a choking risk.

- ✔ If your baby's dribbling a lot, use a bib to soak up the drool and put petroleum jelly on her chin to stop it becoming sore.

- ✔ Distraction can take your baby's mind off teething. Take her for a walk, read her a story, and give her plenty of cuddles to reassure her.

- ✔ Your local pharmacist can help. Look for sugar-free teething biscuits and teething gels that numb the gum. You can also try homeopathic teething granules.

As soon as the first tooth appears, you'll need to start regular brushing every morning and bedtime with a baby toothbrush.

Chapter 8

Hello World! Common Newborn Health Niggles

. . . .

In This Chapter

▶ Finding out about your baby's body and skin

▶ Cleaning, carrying, and cooling your newborn

▶ Discovering jaundice and colic

▶ Tackling tender areas

. . . .

*N*ew babies have some distinct physical characteristics that can seem alarming to the untrained eye. But what may appear to be peculiarities or even defects are highly likely to be normal features that'll change as your baby matures. Don't be surprised, for example, if his head is an irregular shape: After all, it was a tight squeeze through the birth canal, as you can probably testify. If your baby was delivered using ventouse suction or forceps, his head may look pointed or flat on one side. In fact, looking like a Klingon is de rigueur among babies fresh out of the womb. Puffy eyelids and wrinkly skin are the norm – the result of all that water in utero – and swollen genitals are a side effect of hormones passed on from you. For the same reason, many newborn girls and boys appear to have 'breasts'. Rest assured that all these temporary special effects will soon disappear, and it won't be long before your little alien has transformed into a perfect, rounded little parcel.

When you're a new parent, there's no limit to the number of questions that pop into your head every day. Take full advantage of your midwife, health visitor, and GP – that's what they're there for.

Baby Basics: Holding, Bathing, and Keeping Warm

No matter how well prepared you think you are for your baby's arrival, the reality always seems to be different from the theory! If you're terrified you're going to drop, break, or otherwise harm your precious newborn, you're in good company – in fact, parents who don't worry are the exception! This section will boost your confidence.

This way up: Picking up your baby

The first few attempts at picking up a new baby can be nerve-wracking, but you'll soon be able to do it with your eyes shut (although we wouldn't recommend this!). You don't so much pick up as scoop a baby. Arrange your hands and arms around him while he's still supported by his mattress, and put one hand under his head. Once you've got him in your arms, the easiest way to carry a new baby is either against your chest in an upright position, or with his head in the crook of one of your arms and the rest of his body lying in the lower part of your arm.

Your baby won't break, honest! Vulnerable and fragile though he may look, he's actually a good deal more robust than you may think. Just remember the one golden rule: Never let his head flop. Your baby has no neck control at all at birth, and doesn't develop any for at least six weeks. Don't let his limbs dangle, either: Just like any of us, he'll feel insecure left hanging in limbo.

Making sure he's not too hot or cold

Your baby's body is not mature enough to regulate its own temperature very well. He can't sweat properly if he gets too hot, so you'll need to be extra sensitive to his body temperature. Being too hot can increase the risk of Sudden Infant Death Syndrome (SIDS, or cot death). These days, babies are much more likely to be too hot than too cold, but being very cold can cause problems with your baby's heart and circulation.

The best way of telling whether he's too hot or cold is to do it the way your granny used to: Feel the back of his neck or tummy. Don't feel his hands or feet: They won't give an accurate indication of his temperature, as they're usually cooler than the rest of his body.

As a rule, your baby will feel warm. If he's hot, damp, or sweaty, then he has too many clothes on – remove a layer of his blankets or clothing to help him cool down. If he feels cold to the touch or looks blue round the lips, then he's too cool – so add a layer.

Always strip off your baby's outdoor clothes and hat when you come in to a warm atmosphere from a cold one, even if you have to wake him up to do so: Overheating can be very dangerous to young babies.

Buy a room thermometer for your baby's bedroom. The ideal room temperature for a baby is around 18°C (65°F). This may feel a bit chilly to you, but if your baby's wearing a vest and body suit and has a sheet and a couple of blankets, then he'll be plenty warm enough. A room temperature between 16 and 20°C (60 to 68°F) is acceptable.

Keeping your baby clean

New babies don't get very dirty, so they don't need a lot of washing. Make the most of this stage! A daily bath for your newborn is unnecessary, because too much water can dry out your baby's skin. You'll be fine simply washing his face and bottom and any other bits, such as his hands and under his arms, that need sprucing up a little. For 'topping and tailing' all you need is a clean towel, a bowl of warm (never hot) water, and some cotton wool. Lay him on a changing table, a mat or a towel, or sit him on your lap. Keep your baby's head and body supported at all times unless he's lying on a mat or towel on the floor (your baby can't hold his head up yet).

Use a fresh piece of cotton wool for each body part, to avoid spreading any germs on the skin. Wash the genitals from front to back, to avoid spreading germs from the skin around the bottom.

If you're bathing your baby, wash his face before you put him in the baby bath by dipping a clean piece of cotton wool in warm water and wiping gently round his eyes, moving out from the nose. Never use soap on your baby's face. Also wash his bottom before you put him in the bath if he's produced anything more than wee!

Never use a cotton bud in your baby's ears – or yours for that matter! The lining of the ears is very sensitive, and putting anything into them can damage the lining and cause inflammation and ear infection.

Blotches, Spots, and All: Caring for Your Baby's Brand New Skin

Your baby's skin is his largest organ, a thin but tough barrier that protects him from the environment, helps regulate his temperature, and is full of nerve endings to make him responsive to touch. His skin is a living, breathing organ that has to acclimatise to life outside the womb. Acclimatisation takes some doing, so expect blotches and bumps, not peaches and cream, in the early weeks.

Chapter 14 covers rashes caused by common childhood infections.

Seeing spots

New babies often develop little yellow spots known as *milia* (refer to Image 1 in the colour section). They may look nasty, but panic not: They're usually harmless and clear up without treatment.

One of the most common forms of milia are yellow pinprick spots over the nose and forehead. Rather charmingly (not!) they're also known as neonatal acne. They are caused by an excess production of oil (*sebum*) stimulated by your hormones during pregnancy. As the effects of these hormones fade, so will the spots.

A light sprinkling of creamy-white spots on your baby's face or body may be tiny cysts containing a protein called *keratin*. As long as you leave them alone, the cysts will pop open and disappear within six weeks.

Apart from keeping your baby's skin clean with warm water and cotton wool, you don't need to do anything to treat these little blemishes. Never try to burst, pick, or pop spots, because this can cause nasty infections. The spots will fade gradually as your baby's skin settles down in its new environment.

Regarding rashes

Babies in baby magazines seem to have perfect skin but this has more to do with photographic techniques than nature – most babies have at least a few imperfections on their skins, and rashes of all sorts are very common. Fortunately, most rashes are nothing to worry about, and disappear on their own over time. As long as your baby is well in all other respects, doesn't have a fever, and is feeding normally, you don't need to rush for help. Get advice from your doctor or health visitor if the rash doesn't settle after a few days, or if your baby is unwell.

It's absolutely vital that you know how to recognise the rash caused by the *meningococcus* bacteria, which causes meningitis (thankfully, meningitis is very rare, despite all the media coverage). The rash of meningococcal infection usually causes a deep red, blotchy rash, associated with a very poorly baby. As a rule, any rash that fades when you press a glass against it is not the meningitis rash. If it doesn't fade, or if your baby is drowsy or generally unwell, get medical help immediately – a delay could be fatal. You can find out more in Chapter 14.

Erythema toxicum

Around half of all newborn babies develop *erythema toxicum*, a rash that appears in uneven red patches over the skin, especially on the back, chest, and stomach, in the first two or three days after birth. At the centre of each patch, you may notice a little blister, which may look sore or infected. The cause of this rash is not known – it's probably just your baby's skin adapting to its new environment – but it's harmless and will disappear on its own within a few days.

The best thing you can do is leave the rash alone. Creams and ointments may irritate your baby's skin, so steer clear unless your doctor advises you otherwise.

Cooling down heat rash

A bright red bumpy rash in the folds of your baby's skin or where his clothes fit tightly is probably a heat rash. This develops when your baby becomes so hot that his pores clog up, causing irritation. Although heat rash isn't serious, it's very itchy and a sign that your baby's too warm. Try the following to soothe your baby's heat rash:

- Give your baby a cool bath, place damp flannels over the irritated areas, and leave him naked for a while.

- Use calamine lotion to soothe your baby's itching skin, but avoid other lotions and ointments, as they can clog the pores even more.

- Don't let your baby get too hot. Stay in the shade on hot days and dress him in loose, light clothing. If he develops a high temperature (37.5°C/99.5°F), you can give him infant paracetamol, but always follow the instructions. If his temperature stays high, contact your GP. See Chapter 17 for more about dealing with fevers.

- If your baby's skin flares up, remove a layer of his clothes to help him cool down.

Focusing on birthmarks

Birthmarks are incredibly common: About one in three babies is born with a birthmark, but no one quite knows why. Birthmarks come in a huge assortment of sizes and colours, ranging from pale yellow to deep blue, but they rarely need medical attention: Only around one in 100 birthmarks needs treatment. Here are some of the most common birthmarks:

- **Stork bites.** About one in 40 babies is born with these small, pinkish marks, often on the back of the neck. The marks (also called salmon patches or angel kisses) usually disappear by the age of two years.

- **Strawberry naevi marks.** These bright red raised marks can change shape and size and can feel quite lumpy. They tend to appear around two to three weeks of age and grow rapidly up to the age of six to nine months. Strawberry naevi often appear on the face and neck, but they may also appear on the trunk and groin. Strawberry marks fade away untreated by the age of six or seven years. Rarely, if the mark is in a dangerous place, such as the throat or the eye, your doctor will want to treat it, perhaps with steroid treatments or surgery.

- **Port-wine stains.** These flat marks are purple-red in colour and often appear on the face. They are usually present at birth and can cover a large area of skin. Port-wine stains may grow with the child, but they don't alter radically in shape or size. The only treatment for port-wine stains is removal by laser. This usually starts before the age of two years. Up to six treatments, spread over three years, may be needed to remove the port-wine stain completely.

- **Mongolian spots.** These bluish-grey patches of skin, found on the lower back and buttocks, are particularly common in Afro-Caribbean, Asian, and Southern European babies. They are completely harmless and usually disappear in early childhood.

If you're worried about a birthmark, get medical advice. Your GP can tell you whether you need to worry, or whether you can let the mark disappear in its own good time.

Dealing with dry areas

Some babies, particularly those who are born late, have an outer layer of skin that looks shrivelled like a raisin and peels off unaided shortly after birth. Many parents worry that this dried skin is a sign of eczema, but this is rarely the case. Check out Chapter 15 for info on eczema.

On the whole, it's better not to use anything on this sort of dry skin unless your baby is irritated or troubled by it – dry areas usually settle down on their own. If you must use a moisturiser, make sure it's unperfumed.

Tackling cradle cap head-on

Cradle cap is characterised by thick scales of skin on the head (see Image 2 in the colour section). The scales may be yellowy-brown in colour or may just look like dead skin. Sometimes the whole head is covered, but cradle cap often affects only a small patch of the scalp. Many parents worry unnecessarily about cradle cap. Cradle cap may be unsightly, but it's not serious: It doesn't harm your baby and, contrary to popular opinion, isn't a sign that your baby has eczema. Cradle cap usually clears up on its own within a few days or weeks, although it may recur. When your baby's hair has grown and thickened, you'll probably no longer notice any of those scales.

Cradle cap is though to be caused by overproduction of sebum, an oily substance secreted by the *sebaceous glands* in the scalp that keeps the skin oiled and healthy. If cradle cap spreads beyond the scalp, it is known as *seborrhoeic dermatitis*.

You don't need to treat cradle cap, but if you want to try to remove it, the following can help:

✔ Soften the skin on your baby's head by gently rubbing olive oil or petroleum jelly into his scalp after his evening bath. Leave overnight to allow the dry skin to soften. In the morning, wash his hair with a gentle baby shampoo and rinse thoroughly: Shampoo will dry the skin if you leave any behind. Towel-dry your baby's hair and then brush or comb it with a soft brush or round-toothed comb, gently removing the scales of cradle cap. Repeat this treatment every day until all the scales have gone.

✔ A number of shampoos available from high-street pharmacies have been specially formulated for treating cradle cap. If you do try one of them, stop using it immediately if you notice your baby's skin becoming red or irritated.

Always leave the cradle-cap scales alone if they are stuck firmly to the scalp. Pulling them off may cause bleeding and infection.

See your GP if your baby's cradle cap is very stubborn and causing irritation, looks red, or appears to be infected. Best to seek medical attention as well if cradle cap spreads beyond your baby's scalp, for example to the face, cheeks, or skin folds under the arms or in the nappy area.

Jaundice, Colic, and Other Early Worries: Adapting to Life Outside the Womb

If you think that having a new baby in your life takes a lot of adjustment, imagine how your baby feels! After nine months comfortably wrapped up in your womb, he has to take in the sounds, sights, and even the air of the outside world. It's hardly surprising, then, that occasionally hiccups occur. But rest assured, most of the minor problems your baby will encounter will settle with no long-term consequences. You may age a decade in the process, but your baby won't know he's ill. As the old saying goes, 'They'll never remember, and you'll never forget!'

Making sense of newborn jaundice

During the first week of your baby's life, his skin may take on a yellowish-orange tinge. Think bad fake tan and you'll get the picture. This condition, known as *physiological jaundice of the newborn*, affects about a third of all new babies. If your baby is Afro-Caribbean, south Asian, or Chinese, he may have just a yellowing of the whites of his eyes, palms of the hands, and soles of the feet.

Newborn jaundice is caused by an excess of a substance called *bilirubin* in the blood, a natural by-product of your baby's red blood cells that is usually removed from the blood by the liver. Until your baby's body adapts to life outside the womb, your baby may produce more bilirubin than he needs and more than his immature liver can handle. As his liver is not developed fully, the bilirubin tends to build up in the blood, causing that yellowish tinge.

In most cases, newborn jaundice isn't serious and resolves itself within about two weeks, but your doctor will need to monitor your baby until the jaundice clears up.

If the jaundice is severe, your baby may have to stay in hospital for a while. He may receive phototherapy treatment, which involves placing him on a kind of sunbed with bright fluorescent lights for short periods of time until his jaundice starts to fade. If you go home rather than stay in hospital, your midwife or health visitor will keep a close eye on your baby's jaundice during home visits. As you care for your little yellow-tinged bundle of joy, keep the following points in mind:

  ✔ **Seek out the sun.** Exposure to sunlight is very beneficial, because it helps your baby to break down bilirubin. At home, expose him to as much daylight as possible, preferably while he's not wearing anything. Don't put him in direct sunlight, however, because he could overheat or get sunburnt very quickly.

✔ **Feed on demand.** This will make your baby wee more and thus excrete more waste products, helping to flush out his system. Breastmilk is a particularly powerful detoxifier.

In rare cases, bilirubin increases rapidly rather than reduces, suggesting that the jaundice is *non-physiological*. If your baby has sluggish reflexes and poor sucking, or the jaundice continues for more than two weeks, he may need treatment or further tests. Abnormally high levels of bilirubin need to be controlled in order to prevent a condition known as *kernicterus*, which can lead to brain damage if left untreated. Treatment of this kind of jaundice depends on the severity of the jaundice but may include phototherapy, drug therapy to cut down bilirubin production, and blood transfusion.

Combating colic: Every parent's nightmare

Bouts of inconsolable crying for hours at a time, with no apparent trigger, can have you climbing walls in desperation. But don't panic: Your baby's probably not seriously ill. The crying won't last forever, and it certainly won't cause your baby any long-term damage.

Although there's no true medical definition, colic is thought to be pain caused by the build-up of wind in the stomach or bowel. Another increasingly popular theory is that colic is caused by an intolerance to lactose, the natural sugar found in milk. Whatever the cause, if your baby has colic, you may see the following signs in addition to the non-stop crying:

✔ He'll cry out in pain for long stretches of time and be very difficult to settle.

✔ You may notice him drawing up his knees to his chest and going bright red in the face.

✔ His tummy may be swollen or bloated, as if he has swallowed a lot of air, and he may pass wind.

The good news – yes, there is some! – is that colic doesn't last forever. In the vast majority of cases, colic disappears at around three months of age.

Before diagnosing colic, rule out other causes of crying. Your baby may be hungry, overtired, or ill. If your baby has any other symptoms, such as a high temperature, diarrhoea, or a rash, then see your GP.

Calming the crying

Calming a colicky baby can be very difficult, but use trial and error to find out what comforts him most. Remember that what doesn't work today may be effective tomorrow. Here are a few ideas:

- **Work miracles with winding.** Halfway through and at the end of feeding, try winding your baby. Also, try not to let your baby cry for too long before you feed him, as crying can make him swallow lots of air.

- **Rock-a-bye baby.** Rock your baby gently, holding him close to you so he can feel your warmth and hear your heartbeat. Gentle repetitive movement can be very relaxing for your baby, even if it gives you arm ache! Alternatively, take him for a walk in the pram or a drive in the car.

- **Try old-fashioned remedies.** Colic drops are available over the counter at your pharmacy. Gripe water, which contains digestion-boosting dill seed oil, and bicarbonate of soda are other treatments that some mums swear by – but don't use them if your baby is less than four weeks old. Remember: Whatever remedy you decide to use, always read the label and never exceed the recommended dose.

- **Massage away baby's troubles.** Massage is a great way of helping to relieve trapped wind. Rub a little olive into your fingers. Then, using two fingertips, gently stroke your baby's stomach in a clockwise circular motion from the navel outwards. Make the circles gradually bigger, and then start again, repeating as many times as you like. Try this an hour before your baby usually starts to cry, but not just after a feed.

- **Calm down with camomile tea.** Some breastfeeding mums find the calming, slightly sedative effect of camomile tea is passed on to their babies if they drink it a couple of hours before they breastfeed. Even if a cuppa doesn't cure your baby of colic, it may make you feel calmer. If you're bottle-feeding, try putting a few drops of weak camomile tea in your baby's bottle or on a teaspoon.

- **Going over the counter.** Remedies such as Infacol and Colief are medicines specially designed to help with colic. You simply suck up the recommended dose into the dropper inside the cap, and pop it into your baby's mouth before feeds. These products don't work for all babies, but they can be invaluable. You can get them on prescription – ask your health visitor or GP.

- **Let him suck.** Babies find sucking very comforting, and you may find that a dummy helps him settle. Some research suggests that sucking can actually soothe pain in babies. If your baby uses a dummy, remember to keep it sterile – you'll need a good supply of dummies because they're guaranteed to end up on the floor on a regular basis. Try to wean your baby off the dummy before his teeth start to come through.

- **Take time out.** Try giving your baby some quiet time away from distractions such as siblings, toys, and bright lights. Take him to a quiet room, swaddle him, or carry him in a sling. Don't try to play with him or chat to him. Just create a calm, peaceful environment where you can be close.

✔ **Sit up straight.** Some experts believe that feeding your baby when he is in an upright position may help prevent the build-up of wind associated with colic. In countries where babies are carried upright and breastfed in slings, there is far less colic.

✔ **Watch what you eat.** If you're breastfeeding, you may be inadvertently giving your baby wind by eating certain foods. Try avoiding things that make you windy – onions and baked beans are common culprits – and see whether this helps.

✔ **Go small.** If you're bottle-feeding and your baby has only small feeds, try using 125-ml (4-oz) bottles instead of full-size bottles to stop your baby sucking in too much air when he's drinking. Look for a slow-flow teat, which will help stop your baby gulping in air. If you're worried that your baby's formula milk doesn't agree with him, talk to your GP or health visitor. They may suggest a soya formula as an alternative to dairy, but never switch your baby's milk without consulting your GP or health visitor first.

✔ **Go alternative.** Cranial osteopathy involves gentle manipulation of the spine, neck, and skull to make sure they're aligned properly. Some parents swear by it, especially if their baby had difficult births. Complementary remedies such as herbalism and homeopathy may also be beneficial in treating the symptoms of colic. Ask your GP for advice. (We talk about various complementary treatments Chapter 18.)

Surviving colic

Many parents believe, mistakenly, that somehow they're responsible for their baby's colic. But this maddening condition is to do with your baby's development, not yours. The best thing you can do to help your baby is to soothe him as calmly and rationally as possible. That can be a tall order and you will likely need a break at times. If you're left holding the baby 24/7, get your partner, a parent, or a friend to look after your baby while you relax in a warm bath or just sit in a quiet room for a while. If you're scared you may lose control and hurt your baby, put him safely in his cot, leave the room, and take ten minutes to sit and calm down. Contact a support group such as Crysis (020-7404-5011). Simply talking to someone who knows what you're going through can make all the difference.

Reflecting on reflux

Gastro-oesophageal reflux (GOR) is a common problem in the first year of life because the muscle at the entrance to your baby's stomach is still weak, allowing his milk to come back up again (and all over you). The condition usually appears in the first few weeks after birth, but in most babies it disappears again by the end of the first year.

The main symptoms of GOR are vomiting, regurgitation of feeds (your baby may constantly dribble milk from the mouth), crying, irritability, and, if the problem persists, failure to thrive. (We talk about failure to thrive in Chapter 7.)

If your baby is very troubled by reflux, see your doctor, who can perform tests for a definitive diagnosis and may also prescribe feed thickeners and anti-sickness drugs. If your baby is projectile vomiting large amounts, he may have pyloric stenosis, for which you need to see your GP (see Chapter 7).

Lots of babies use vomiting as a useful 'overflow mechanism', which is why you can often tell a new parent by the white stains down the back of their clothes! Many babies bring up a bit of milk with their wind, and most of them come to no harm whatsoever. This sort of vomiting is called 'possetting'. If your baby is feeding, pooing, passing water, and putting on weight normally, and doesn't seem troubled by his possetting, you don't need to be, either.

If your baby's vomit is bloodstained, see your doctor straight away.

Dealing with Delicate Areas

Every little part of your bundle of joy comes with its own care instructions. A few simple tips can make all the difference when it comes to your confidence in dealing with delicate areas. This section aims to reassure you that you don't need to worry – but also gives you an idea of when you should.

Caring for your baby's umbilical cord

Your baby's cord stump, where the umbilical cord was cut after delivery, will be clamped with a piece of plastic at birth. It can look a bit messy for a few days, as it's usually covered with dried blood, but it's not painful for your baby and it will come away within the first week or so. The area is best left alone. Never try to pull the stump off, but do keep it dry. Some doctors think cleaning the stump isn't necessary, unless there's a lot of gooey stuff around the base. If you do need to clean the stump, use a cotton swab dipped in cooled, boiled water to clean around the base.

The stump is usually quite sticky by the time it drops off, and it may leave a slight smear of blood on the cotton wool when you clean it – again, nothing to worry about. The navel underneath should be healed, but sometimes a little piece of inflamed tissue remains and weeps. This common symptom is harmless, but if it's big your GP will need to treat it by touching it with a silver nitrate stick to make it shrivel away – this is painless for your baby.

When you're putting a nappy on your baby, fold down the top of the nappy to keep the cord stump exposed to the air and clear of urine, which will help to minimise infection. Until the cord stump drops off, try to avoid getting the navel wet.

Speak to your doctor or midwife if you notice that the cord is particularly sticky, weepy, or smelly, the skin around the navel is red or spotty, or fresh drops of blood are coming from the navel.

Homing in on hernias

An *umbilical hernia* occurs when there's a gap or weakness in the muscles around the navel, causing part of the intestine to bulge though. Umbilical hernias are a common problem in newborns, especially boys. The condition isn't serious or painful, although you may notice that the bulge gets larger when your baby cries, laughs, strains, or coughs.

Most umbilical hernias disappear without treatment within the first three years of life, but if a hernia gets larger or has not disappeared by the age of five years, a minor operation can be carried out – usually as day surgery – to close the gap in the muscles.

Inguinal hernias occur when a gap in the abdomen wall allows part of the intestine to bulge through, causing a soft swelling just above the groin or scrotum. Around one in 20 babies is born with an inguinal hernia, and many more babies develop inguinal hernias in the first six months. This type of hernia doesn't disappear without treatment. Your doctor will likely recommend a simple operation to stop the risk of the hernia becoming strangulated, which can affect blood supply to the intestine.

Getting to the bottom of nappy rash

If you notice small spots or red patches on your baby's groin or bottom, which look sore and are sensitive to touch, then he has nappy rash. He's not alone: Nappy rash affects around 80 per cent of babies during the first year of life.

Nappy rash is caused by a chemical called ammonia in your baby's urine and stools, which can irritate and burn the skin. This inflamed area often gets infected with a yeast or thrush infection (yes, the same one that causes athlete's foot and sore, itchy ladies' nether regions).

Try the following to soothe or help prevent, your baby's mild nappy rash:

✔ Change your baby's nappies frequently and as soon as they are soiled. Even super-absorbent nappies should be changed as soon as you know they're wet.

✔ Wipe and dry your baby's bottom at each change. Warm water and cotton wool are the best thing for cleaning sore bottoms. Avoid wipes impregnated with chemicals and perfumes, as they can irritate sensitive or chapped skin.

✔ Whenever you can, leave your baby's nappy off for a while. Lay him on a thick towel to absorb any accidents. Always make sure your baby's completely dry before you put him in a new nappy.

✔ Use zinc and caster oil cream or Sudocrem to soothe the rash.

✔ Try different brands of nappies. You may find that his skin reacts better to certain types, because each type is made from slightly different materials.

If your baby's bottom gets very red and sore, or if it has raw patches with a scaly edge or lots of small red spots, see your GP or health visitor. Your baby may have a thrush infection in their nappy area. Your doctor can prescribe a cream.

Going gooey eyed

A slight yellowish or creamy discharge in your baby's eyes may be caused by bacteria picked up in the birth canal, or simply poor hygiene. If you clean your baby's eyes regularly, the discharge should clear up within a couple of days. If the discharge doesn't clear up, talk to your GP, because your baby may need antibiotic eyedrops to treat the infection.

Bathing your baby's eyes regularly with cooled, boiled water is the best way to deal with sticky eyes. Wash your hands before you begin. Then take a piece of clean cotton wool, dip it in the water, and squeeze it out. Wipe one eye from the inner to the outer corner. Do the same with the other eye, using a fresh piece of cotton wool.

Instead of using cooled, boiled water, you can use a drop of fresh breast milk to clean the eyes. Breast milk contains powerful antibodies that help to fight infection.

Thrashing out thrush

If you notice white patches like cottage cheese or milk curds inside your baby's mouth and on his tongue, he's probably got thrush, a yeast infection that affects a large number of new babies. If you suspect your baby has thrush, seek advice from your GP straight away. Thrush is very uncomfortable for your baby: He'll probably find sucking painful, which will disrupt his feeding.

Your GP may prescribe infant paracetamol for the pain and an oral antifungal cream to tackle the infection. The thrush will very likely clear up within a few days. Thrush can by trying for all of you – a hungry baby who finds it painful to feed is a very sad sight – but it's usually short-lived. Give your baby all the comfort he needs, and follow your doctor's instructions for pain relief and medicine, and the infection will pass.

It's very easy to mistake milk curds left in the mouth after feeding for thrush. Milk curds, unlike oral thrush, come off easily if you touch them with your finger, and they don't leave a red patch behind on the inside of the mouth. It's worth trying this simple test before you take your baby to the doctor.

Alert your doctor if the thrush doesn't seem to clear up after treatment or if your baby has a fever, as this may indicate a different infection.

If you're breastfeeding, apply the anti-fungal cream to your nipples too, so that you and your baby don't pass the infection to each other.

Diagnosing urinary tract infections

Urinary tract infections (UTIs) can be difficult to diagnose. Try to get to know the symptoms, however, as an untreated UTI can lead to kidney problems. If your baby has any of the following symptoms, see your GP:

- ✔ More irritable than normal
- ✔ A persistent or recurrent raised temperature (over 37.5°C/99.5°F) with no apparent cause
- ✔ Feeding problems
- ✔ Slow weight gain
- ✔ Persistent vomiting or diarrhoea

UTIs are caused by germs from your baby's bowel entering the *urethra*, the tube leading from the bladder that your baby wees out of. Your baby may be more prone to UTIs if he was born with an obstruction in his urinary system, such as urinary reflux, in which the urine flows back into the bladder or the kidney, increasing the likelihood of infection.

Always clean your baby from front to back when changing a nappy.

If your GP suspects your baby has a UTI, he will ask you to collect a sample of your baby's urine for testing. Your doctor will prescribe antibiotics if the test shows a UTI. If the infection persists, your baby may need further tests in case stronger medication is needed. Antibiotics usually work, however, and even if your baby has recurrent infections due to reflux, there's a good chance he'll grow out of them.

Part III
Raising Healthy Children

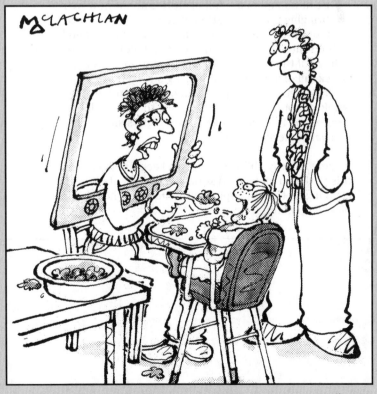

"It's the only way I can get her to eat."

In this part . . .

The newspapers are full of stories about how we're bringing up a generation of couch potatoes. There's no doubt that children today are getting bigger and bigger, as they eat more junk food and spend more and more time in front of the television or games station. This part is chock-full of advice about making sure your child has a healthy diet, and gets plenty of exercise. You'll also find a whole chapter devoted to ensuring that your child receives all the benefits of a good night's sleep. That way, you get some shuteye too.

Raising healthy children involves keeping them clean, so this part also includes tips on sterilising baby's bottle, cleaning teeth, and coping with nits and other nasties picked up at nursery.

Chapter 9

The Importance of Nutrition

A child's growing body depends on the nutrients in the food she eats for health and vitality, so it's not surprising that parents worry about food so much. Proteins, minerals, vitamins, fibre, fats, carbohydrates . . . there are so many things to remember to include – and in the right amounts – that working out what your child should and shouldn't be chomping on can be a minefield. It's easy to get lost in all the recommended guidelines, but the good news is that you don't need a degree in nutrition science to feed your child a healthy diet.

Healthy eating means a lot more than balancing a list of desirable nutrients. Eating's a social activity and a focal point of family life, and providing food is a way of expressing care and love, so mealtimes must be enjoyable for your child.

Meeting Your Child's Nutritional Needs

Believe it or not, making sure your child eats well can be relatively simple. After weaning, a healthy diet for your baby is basically the same as a healthy diet for you. Before the age of 2 years, fats should not be restricted – so use full-fat milk and yoghurts, for example – but from then on there's no reason to cook special meals for your child – as long as you don't live off takeaways and chips-with-everything.

Food contains calories, which supply the energy needed for growth and exercise and stop your child feeling hungry. Food also contains crucial vitamins and minerals. Among their many roles, vitamins help the body absorb other nutrients, aid growth and development, assist the body in fighting infection, and ensure organs and cells function normally.

Making sense of food groups

Your child cannot live off bread alone. Or carrots. Or chips. Or any other single food. She needs a varied diet in order to get all the essential nutrients her body needs to be healthy and function efficiently. There are five main food groups that are crucial for your child's health:

- **Carbohydrates,** found in bread, potatoes, cereals, rice, and pasta, are the body's most important and readily available source of energy.

- **Fruits and vegetables** contain essential nutrients, including vitamins, minerals, and fibre.

- **Proteins,** found in meat, fish, poultry, eggs, pulses, seeds, and nuts, are key to growth and help build and repair essential parts of the body.

- **Dairy foods** are an important source of protein, vitamins, and minerals, especially calcium, which is essential for healthy teeth and bones.

- **Fats,** such as butter and vegetable oils, are essential (in the correct form and quantity) for the development of healthy brain tissue and the maintenance of the central nervous system.

Playing a vital role: Vitamins

Vitamins are found naturally in foods from animal and plant sources and are also added to some cereals and juices. Different vitamins act on different parts and processes of the body – a healthy diet includes all of them. Table 9-1 gives a rundown of the vitamins and their sources and uses.

Table 9-1	Vitamins and Their Sources and Uses	
Vitamin	*Sources*	*Uses*
Vitamin A (including beta carotene and retinol)	Dairy products, eggs (carrots, red peppers, sweetcorn)	Essential for growth, fighting infection, healthy skin, vision and bones
Vitamin B complex	Yeast, egg yolk, wheatgerm, nuts, red meat, cereals, avocados, bananas, tofu, dark green veg	Essential for growth, healthy nervous system, aids digestion
Vitamin C (ascorbic acid)	Citrus fruits, strawberries, blackcurrants, potatoes, green leafy veg, peppers	Essential for tissue repair, healthy skin, absorption of iron, healthy immune system

Vitamin	Sources	Uses
Vitamin D	Tuna, salmon, sardines, milk, cheese, eggs; also formed in the skin when skin is exposed to sunlight	Plays a role in the absorption of calcium, which is essential for healthy bones
Vitamin E	Pure vegetable oils, wheatgerm, wholemeal bread and cereals, egg yolk, nuts, sunflower seeds	Protects tissues against damage, promotes normal growth and development, helps in formation of normal red blood cells
Vitamin K	Green veg	Helps blood to clot

In general, if your child eats a balanced diet and doesn't have special health concerns, she doesn't need vitamin or mineral supplements. If your child's a really fussy eater, however, you may consider giving her multivitamins – but ask your GP or health visitor first. The safest supplements are multivitamins that have been specially formulated for children. Always read the label and follow the instructions, as overdosing can be dangerous and even fatal.

Ruling out mineral deficiencies

Most vitamin and mineral deficiencies are uncommon in the UK because British people tend to eat a varied diet and many foods are also enriched with nutrients. Two common mineral deficiencies in the UK, however, are iron and calcium.

Pumping up the iron

Without iron, your child can't make enough red blood cells and her organs won't function well. Iron deficiency can also affect your child's growth and lead to learning and behavioural problems. Babies under the age of 1 year usually get enough iron, because breast milk is a natural iron source and formula milk is usually fortified with iron. Toddlers and young children are more prone to iron deficiency, because cows' milk is low in iron and can even decrease the absorption of iron. Good sources of iron include red meat, dark poultry, tuna, salmon, eggs, pulses, dried fruits, leafy green veg, and whole grains.

Iron-deficiency anaemia often has no symptoms to begin with because the body's supply is depleted slowly. But as the anaemia progresses, some of the following signs may appear:

✔ Fatigue and weakness

✔ Pale skin

✔ Rapid heartbeat

✔ Irritability

✔ Decreased appetite

✔ Dizziness or light-headedness.

If your child has any of the above symptoms, ask your doctor to do a simple blood test to find out whether your child has iron-deficiency anaemia. If she does have iron-deficiency anaemia, the doctor may prescribe iron supplements.

Excessive iron intake can cause health problems, so never give your child iron supplements without consulting your doctor first. Keep iron supplements well out of your child's reach, as accidental overdosing can be extremely dangerous.

Catching up on calcium

Without enough calcium, your child's bones and teeth won't grow strong and straight. Calcium also helps the body to absorb vitamin D, and so calcium deficiency is related to rickets and osteoporosis (brittle-bone disease) later in life. Good sources of calcium include dairy products, calcium-fortified orange juice, and white beans. If your child is on a dairy-free or vegan diet, you may find it a bit harder to provide the right amount of calcium. Vegetables contain calcium, but other important non-dairy sources include calcium-fortified soya milk, tofu processed with calcium sulphate, and nuts and seeds.

Giving your child milkshakes or yoghurt-based smoothies made from semi-skimmed milk is an excellent way to boost calcium intake.

Putting it all on a plate

To work out how much of each food your child should be eating, try to picture an empty plate. Put a generous helping of starchy food like pasta or potatoes on to the plate. Add an equally good helping of vegetables and fruit, with as much variety as you like. Next, add a smaller portion of food high in protein, such as meat or pulses, and finish the plate off with a helping of dairy food such as cheese. The plate now contains a healthy balanced meal. The only things that are missing are fatty foods such as butter and vegetable or animal fats, which can be added sparingly.

The number of calories each child needs varies according to size, growth rate, and activity level. A good rule of thumb for children up to the age of 5 years is around 1000 calories a day, with an extra 100 calories a day for each year after that until adulthood.

Many children don't eat large platefuls of food and prefer to snack or graze. Don't be concerned if your child does this, provided that her daily intake goes by the same principles as those listed above – plenty of carbs, fruit, and veg, and a good amount of protein and dairy. Snacking on nutritional food can actually be beneficial for young children because they need higher energy and nutrient levels than adults to fuel their rapid growth.

Establishing Healthy Eating Habits

The most effective way to teach your child healthy eating habits is to set a good example. Making nutritious food a priority in your life, limiting visits to fast-food restaurants, and teaching your child to prepare meals and snacks healthily will help steer your child in the right direction. The following sections offer some suggestions for fostering healthy eating habits.

Getting up for breakfast

Breakfast is the most important meal of the day for both you and your child. Compared with children who don't eat breakfast, children who do eat breakfast:

- Do better at maths and reading and have better concentration and behaviour.
- Are more likely to keep their weight under control and have lower blood cholesterol levels. Children who miss breakfast are much more likely to snack on junk food such as biscuits, crisps, and chocolate, before lunch.
- Are more likely to meet their nutritional needs, with adequate levels of minerals and vitamins.

Mornings are one of the worst times for busy families, but breakfast doesn't have to mean a home-made gourmet meal every day. Here are some suggestions for quick and easy breakfasts that are also nutritious:

- Cereal with fruit and milk.
- Toasted bagel with cheese.
- Fruit and yogurt.
- Toasted waffle topped with fruit and yogurt.
- Fruit smoothie (fruit and milk or yoghurt whizzed in a blender).
- Peanut butter on wholemeal toast.

Cereal can be one of the healthiest of breakfasts, providing slow-burning energy to last your child until lunchtime. It has the added advantage of getting milk into your child too! However, remember that some sweetened cereals are very high in sugar, so stick to the unsweetened (and preferably wholegrain) types. Make sure you set a good example by eating breakfast too – parents are their children's number one influence as far as diet, exercise, and lifestyle are concerned.

Stocking up on healthy foods

A good way to instil healthy eating habits is to control the supply lines – the foods that you serve for meals and have on hand for snacks. Here are some suggestions:

- ✔ **Keep the pantry full of fruit and veg.** The best option is fresh fruits and veg, but canned and frozen work just as well. With plenty on hand, you can easily work fruits and vegetables into the daily menu, aiming for the goal of at least five servings a day. Having ready-to-eat fruit and veggies, such as chunks of apples or carrot sticks, makes it easy for your child to choose healthy snacks.

- ✔ **Stock up on healthy snacks.** Good snacks include rice cakes, yogurt, celery smeared with peanut butter, and wholegrain crackers with cheese.

- ✔ **Choose wholegrain breads and cereals.** These contain more fibre than white bread.

- ✔ **Ditch the deep-fat fryer.** Limit your child's fat intake by using healthier cooking methods, such as grilling and steaming, rather than deep-fat frying.

- ✔ **Empty the fridge of sugary drinks.** Limit fizzy drinks and squash and try to get your child to drink water and milk instead.

- ✔ **Invest in a liquidiser or food processor to make smoothies.** Let your child help with preparing the ingredients for these healthy shakes. It's amazing what a wide selection of fruit (and sometimes vegetables) you can get your child to take that way!

Making food interesting

Having a plate of bland, colourless food shoved in front of you does little for your appetite (remember school dinners?). Food needs to be appealing to get your child to eat, so get creative. This doesn't mean concocting cordon bleu recipes in the kitchen. Here are some easy ways to inspire your child's interest in food:

- ✔ **Variety's the spice of life.** Children who eat a wide assortment of foods increase their chances of meeting their nutritional requirements, so serve foods from all the food groups, with plenty of carbs, dairy products, proteins, fruits, and veg.

- ✔ **Colours are cool.** A plate of food with lots of different colours not only looks appetising but also typically contains a good range of nutrients.

- ✔ **Food can be fun.** Whether your child is 7 months or 7 years old, food can be a shared source of enjoyment. Your child should see food as a pleasure rather than a chore, so get her interested by letting her help you prepare meals. Baked potato boats, vegetable hedgehogs, or yoghurt-filled halved peaches with raisin eyes and satsuma-segment smiles are great fun for children to help make, and they're more likely to eat them, too.

- ✔ **Junk the junk food – but be tactical.** As your child gets old enough to be tempted by the lure of junk food, you may find it difficult to avoid being nagged for chicken nuggets or fish fingers. In fact, skinless chicken breast or sliced, boned fillet of fish dipped in egg and breadcrumbs and shallow fried in just a teaspoon of olive oil feels deliciously naughty but is actually very healthy.

- ✔ **Bring out the artist in your hungry child.** Let your children loose with pizza bases and dishes of peppers, sweetcorn, cheese, tomatoes, olives, and home-made tomato sauce (just wash their hands well and be prepared to clean up afterwards!). In fact, make-your-own pizza is a wonderful activity for a birthday party, offering children the opportunity to compare notes and eat their own creations.

Eating together

The idea of family mealtimes often conjures up images of battlegrounds – but regular family dinners don't have to mean tin hats for all. Family meals are a great way to encourage healthy eating habits and offer the chance to introduce your child to new foods and to discover the foods that she likes and dislikes. Children also like the predictability of family meals. Studies show that compared with children who have few family meals, children who eat regularly with their family are:

- ✔ More likely to eat fruits, vegetables, and grains.

- ✔ Less likely to snack on unhealthy foods.

- ✔ Less likely to smoke, use marijuana, or drink alcohol when they are older.

Sitting in front of the television to eat, even if you're sitting at a table, means that your child won't be concentrating fully on her food, and is likely to eat more. So don't gawp – talk while you eat instead!

Whether it's a takeaway or a home-cooked meal with all the trimmings, strive for nutritious food and a time when the whole family can be there.

Ditching the junk food

If your child's a junk-food junkie, she's not alone. You only need to open a newspaper to see that the things our children eat are making them fatter and unhealthier than ever before. Obesity's on the rise, as are the related problems of diabetes and heart disease.

Junk or convenience food, which includes everything from burgers and chips to biscuits and cakes, is one of the most significant contributory factors towards child health problems. Ditching the junk is easier said than done if it forms your child's staple diet, but here are a few tips to help you on your way:

- ✔ Don't expect to be able to cut out the junk food overnight – it's easier to make small changes to your child's diet than to cut out all the food she's used to in one single stroke.

- ✔ If your child is old enough, explain to her why eating healthy food is so important. Get her to list all her favourite colours and match them up with fruit or vegetables to get her imagination going.

- ✔ If she has a favourite superhero or sporting celebrity, let her know that they only eat healthy food. Understanding the connection between eating well and being healthy and strong will inspire her.

- ✔ Convenience food doesn't have to be processed. A banana or an avocado needs no preparation – you can't get more convenient than that!

- ✔ Involve your child when choosing and preparing fresh food – would she prefer beans or peas, for example, with her meal? This involvement gives her a feeling of control over what she eats.

Of course, you can't stop your child from eating junk food altogether, but if junk foods dominate her diet she could lose out in the health stakes. Children are getting taller and heavier than ever before because they're consuming more than enough calories. But they're not getting healthier, as junk food provides plenty of calories but few nutrients. Junk food contributes to a number of modern-day health problems, including tiredness, lack of energy, irritability, mood swings, constipation, loose bowels, weight problems, skin problems, dark shadows under the eyes, frequent infections, and poor concentration.

Going hyper: Food additives and behaviour

The question of whether food additives cause behavioural problems in children is an area of concern for parents and nutritionists alike, especially as so much food aimed specifically at chidden contains additives. Food additives are subject to strict testing and regulation, but little is known about their long-term effects when they are used in combination.

Colours such as tartrazine (E102), sunset yellow (E110), carmoisine (E122), and ponceau 4R (E124) and the preservative sodium benzoate (E211) have been implicated in hyperactive behaviour in children. Hyperactivity is difficult to define and diagnose, but about 5 per cent of

children in the UK are believed to suffer from it. Much of the evidence on hyperactivity is anecdotal, but studies have linked additive intake with hyperactivity. The consensus still seems to be that more studies are needed.

Some UK manufacturers have bowed to consumer pressure and removed artificial colours, flavours, and preservatives from their processed foods. If you're worried about your child eating additives, the best thing to do is to steer as clear of processed foods as much as possible. Making home-made food is the obvious way of doing so. If you must use processed foods, read the labels carefully before you make your choice.

Nutritionists believe there's no such thing as bad food – just bad diet. So one packet of crisps will do no harm, but if crisps are a regular feature of your child's diet they may impact on her health.

Sussing out salt

Studies show that many children eat twice as much salt as they should – an alarming statistic, as high salt consumption is extremely dangerous for health. Salt has been linked with a whole range of problems, including high blood pressure and heart problems, so try to be salt-aware when it comes to your child's diet. Around three-quarters of the salt consumed by children comes from processed food such as crisps and ready-made meals.

Nutritionists make the following recommendations about the maximum amount of salt that is healthy for children to consume in a day:

- **Babies aged up to 6 months:** Don't give any salt at all.
- **Babies aged between 6 and 12 months:** No more than 1 g.
- **Children aged between 1 and 3 years:** No more than 2 g.
- **Children aged between 4 and 6 years:** No more than 3 g.
- **Children aged 7 years and over:** No more than 5 g.

Feeding fussy eaters

Having a child who refuses to eat or only wants to follow a very restricted diet can be really trying for a parent. The best thing you can do is to be patient. Don't give up on introducing new foods regularly, even if your child rejects them at first. Children are programmed to be suspicious of new foods: This is a self-protective mechanism to stop them eating anything poisonous. You may have to offer your child something many times before she agrees to try it, but don't give up.

A child who's fussy about her food or isn't eating in the way you expect her to is unlikely to have an 'eating problem'. Even the pickiest eaters rarely develop nutritional deficiencies, and food fads are usually temporary. Your child won't expire from vitamin deficiency just because she exists for a week or two on a diet of breadsticks dipped in fromage frais! Most of the nutrients she needs for healthy growth are stored by her body, so she can afford to do without them until the latest food fad passes, as long as you can get a reasonable variety of foods into her in the longer term. One of the best ways to tell whether your child has a serious problem is to look at her overall growth pattern: If she's following the expected course, you probably don't need to be concerned. If she's losing weight or you're at all worried, see your doctor.

Here are some suggestions for turning your picky tot into a happy muncher:

- **Stay calm:** Don't always insist on a clean plate.

- **Let her feed herself:** Some toddlers eat more if you let them do the honours.

- **Don't give food as rewards:** And don't say things like 'No pudding if you don't eat all your greens'. You could end up putting your child off eating veg altogether – plus you're reinforcing the idea that the pudding is more desirable than the vegetables.

- **Offer new food from someone else's plate:** This is less overwhelming than putting the food directly in front of your child on her own plate.

- **Limit her drinks in the hour before a meal:** Drinking too much liquid can lessen your child's appetite.

- **Present healthy food in a positive light:** Avoid categorising foods as 'good' or 'bad'.

- **Give small portions:** Your child won't be overwhelmed by the food in front of her.

- **Let her help you:** Give your child plenty of opportunities to be involved in preparing her food, and let her make choices about what to put on her plate.

Fat-finding: The Good, the Bad, and the Ugly

In recent years, fats have been accused of being bad things that must be avoided at all costs. But although some fats have nothing more to offer your child than a furred-up artery, certain fats are good for both you and your child and are an important part of a healthy diet. The trick is to sort out the good guys from the bad – and then make sure your child eats the right kinds. There are basically two groups of fats:

- ✔ **Saturated fats:** These are the fats responsible for giving fat a bad name. They're found in meat and other animal products, such as dairy products and lard, and in palm and coconut oils. Saturated fats are often used in commercial baked goods such as cakes and biscuits and in some margarines and snack foods and may be listed as *trans fats* or *hydrogenated fats*. If your child eats too many saturated fats, she will have an increased risk of becoming overweight or obese and of developing heart disease.

- ✔ **Unsaturated fats:** These fats are positively beneficial. They're found in plant foods and fish. The best unsaturated fats are monounsaturated (found in avocados and olive and peanut oil) and polyunsaturated (found in most vegetable oils). Omega-3 fatty acids (found in oily fish such as tuna, salmon, mackerel, and sardines) are another important group of fats, and are essential for the healthy development of nerves and organs: They have been found to boost children's brain power if their mothers eat them in pregnancy. There's no reason to believe that the benefits don't continue when your little darling can chew for herself.

Getting the best from fats

Fat has twice as many calories as protein and carbs, so keeping fat in check is the key. But fats are still a necessary part of your child's diet:

- ✔ Fats are essential for growth and development. Your child needs a certain amount of fat in her diet to help her brain and nervous system develop correctly.

- ✔ Fats provide fuel. They are the richest source of calories you can get, which is useful to your growing child.

- ✔ Fats aid the absorption of some vitamins. Vitamins A, D, E, and K are *fat-soluble*, which means they are absorbed only if there's also some fat in the diet.

- ✔ Fats are necessary for the production of hormones and for insulating the tissues of the nervous system.

Keeping the bad guys under control

Restrictive diets aren't recommended for your young child unless she's very overweight. Your child needs fat and cholesterol in her diet because they play an important role in brain development. If your child is under 2 years old, you shouldn't restrict her fat intake at all. However, try to ensure that your child eats the good fats rather than the bad ones. Here are some suggestions:

- Offer your child naturally low-fat foods, such as fruits and vegetables, whole grains, and lean meats. Foods such as avocados and nuts (don't give nuts to a child under 5) are rich in healthy fats.

- When cooking meat, grill or spit-roast it to allow the fat to drip away during cooking. Remove all skin from chicken and turkey before you put it onto your child's plate – it's full of fat, in contrast to the lean meat.

- Avoid low-fat biscuits and sweets, because they are generally packed with bulking agents and additives. One normal biscuit has fewer nasties.

- Pack school lunches and meals for family outings instead of relying on your child to make healthy choices at the school cafeteria or going to fast-food restaurants.

- Plan your child's meals ahead of time, because this can reduce your reliance on fatty foods.

Exposing the Bitter Truth about Sugar

In the UK, the average child's diet contains more than double the recommended amount of sugar. Sugar's not an essential nutrient – so despite what your child may claim, you can't die of not having enough sugar. Too much sugar, on the other hand, can cause serious health problems.

Foods that are high in added sugar, such as pastries, cakes, sweets, frozen desserts, and some fruit juices, also tend to be high in calories and low in other valuable nutrients. As a result, a high-sugar diet is often linked with bad health and obesity. Eating too many sugary foods can also lead to tooth decay. A high-sugar diet often means a deficiency in the recommended amounts of fruit and low-fat milk.

Sugar isn't addictive in the true sense, but it can condition your child's taste preferences and affect the chemicals in the brain. The more sugar your child consumes, the harder it is for your child to experience the sweet sensation that sugar provides – and so the more sugar she needs to satisfy her sweet tooth.

Seeing how sugar can affect your child's health

People often say that children get 'drunk' on sugar in the same way that adults do on alcohol. You only need to observe your child before and after chomping on a chocolate muffin to see what kind of effect sugar has – expect lots of noise and a child who's bouncing off the walls.

- ✔ **Mood swings:** You're probably well aware that letting your child binge affects her behaviour. When your child consumes sugary drinks or food, the sugar is converted into glucose, giving your child a rush of energy that can make her feel a little 'hyper'. The pancreas then produces insulin to stabilise the glucose, and your child's energy levels come crashing down, making her feel weak, tired, and unable to concentrate.

- ✔ **Tooth rot:** Frequent snacking on sugary foods and drinks damages your child's teeth. Every time she eats or drinks something sugary, the enamel on her teeth comes under attack for up to an hour. And if teeth are constantly bathed in sugary solutions, they will inevitably decay. Never give your child bottles containing sugary juice, even before their teeth emerge.

- ✔ **Weight gain:** If your child eats a lot of sugary food, she may be at increased risk of becoming overweight. Sugar is a source of calories; it also makes food more palatable, and so your child may overeat sugary foods. And if your child's calorie intake is higher than her energy needs, she'll gain weight.

- ✔ **Diabetes:** Obesity has serious affects on long-term health, increasing the risk of diabetes and premature death. Type 2 diabetes – a disease that in the past was seen only in older adults – is now being seen in children as young as 9 years old. Even a little puppy fat can make your child vulnerable to health problems in later life: Excess fat tissue makes the blood vessels inflexible and increases the risk of heart problems.

Hunting for hidden sugars

One reason for the over consumption of sugar is that many of our foods contain 'hidden' sugars. Vast numbers of processed foods contain sugar – from drinks, flavoured yoghurts, cereals, cakes, and confectionery to baked beans and tomato ketchup. Manufacturers realise that children like sweet things. Adding sugar to food has other benefits for manufacturers too – sugar masks the taste of poor-quality food, bulks out the product, and preserves it for longer.

Government guidelines recommend that no more than 10 per cent of our energy intake should come from foods (such as cakes and biscuits) that contain 'added' sugars. A couple of biscuits, a few cups of squash, and maybe a fruity yoghurt between meals are enough to put your child over the sugar limit.

A product whose label announces 'no added sugar' is not necessarily sugar-free. The word 'sugar' on food labels refers only to sucrose – but many other types of sugar are used to sweeten food, including honey, fructose, glucose, dextrose, concentrated fruit juice, and raw-cane hydrolysed starch. These all add sweetness and calories to food. Don't be tempted to give your toddler 'diet' and 'low-sugar' foods: They are highly likely to contain artificial sweeteners such as saccharine, which aren't necessarily any better than sugar for your child.

Ingredients must be listed in descending order of weight – so most comes first. The further up the list of ingredients one of these 'hidden' sugars appears, the more of it there is.

Cutting down on the sweet stuff

Yes, young children *can* be weaned off sugar. Studies show that if you give your child just a small amount of sugar between the ages of 2 and 4 years, she may not actually like sugar when she grows up and becomes exposed to more of it. Here are some suggestions for keeping down your child's sugar intake:

- ✔ Offer chopped fruit as a tasty alternative to sweet foods such as biscuits, which are low in nutrients and high in added sugar. Fruit is a naturally sweet carbohydrate-containing snack that also contains fibre and vitamins, which your child needs. Giving lots of fruit now can help set her up for a lifetime of healthy eating habits.

  Baby packs of raisins provide a great treat, and are an essential stand-by for the changing bag – you never know when your toddler is going to run out of patience.

- ✔ Restrict sweet foods at mealtimes. Offer only healthy snacks – for example, a cracker with cream cheese, chopped fresh raw fruit, a bread stick with hummus, or mashed banana on fingers of toast – between meals. This type of snack releases energy slowly and help avoid mood swings caused by yo-yoing blood sugar levels.

- ✔ Avoid using sugary foods as a bribe for your child eating up her meal or for good behaviour.

Of course, every child has sugar now and then, and adding sugar can enhance the taste of some foods that children may otherwise resist. The key to keeping your child's sugar consumption in check is moderation. A little sugar, particularly in a food that provides other important nutrients – cereals, for example – isn't going to tip the scale or send your child to the dentist.

A word about fizzy drinks

Sweetened drinks are the largest source of added sugar in children's diets. A 12-ounce (355-ml) serving of a carbonated sweetened soft drink contains the equivalent of ten teaspoons (49 ml) of sugar and 150 calories – and just one serving a day increases your child's risk of obesity by 60 per cent. One of the most effective ways to eliminate excess sugar in your child's diet is to cut out fizzy drinks and squashes altogether.

Instead of sweetened drinks – and that includes juice drinks, which often contain as much added sugar as fizzy drinks – offer your child low-fat milk, water, or 100 per cent fruit juice. Bear in mind that although there's no added sugar in 100 per cent juice, the calories from the natural sugars found in fruit juice can add up, so limit juice intake to 4–6 ounces (118–177 millilitres) for children under 7 years old and 8–12 ounces (237–355 millilitres) for older children and teens.

Raising a Healthy Vegetarian

A well-planned vegetarian diet can be very healthy for your child. The principles of a healthy veggie diet are the same as those for any healthy diet – offer variety and include things from all food groups. A balanced vegetarian diet can provide the right combinations to meet your child's nutritional needs, but be aware of potential nutrient deficiencies and figure out how you'll account for them.

A healthy vegetarian diet contains a variety of foods that provide enough calories and nutrients to enable your child to grow normally. Experts say a lacto-ovo vegetarian diet (eating dairy products and eggs, but no meat or fish) is a healthy choice for most children – although allergists recommend not introducing eggs until your child is older than 1 year. (For more on egg allergies, see Chapter 15.)

Pondering possible deficiencies

Certain nutrients can be particularly challenging to fit into your toddler's diet, especially if she's vegetarian. A vegan baby is particularly likely to miss out on vital nutrients unless you take special care to include them regularly in her diet. Table 9-2 shows the nutrients that vegetarians need to keep an eye on to make sure they get, and examples of the food sources in which they can be found:

Table 9-2	Nutrients That Must Be Included in a Vegetarian Diet
Nutrient	*Source*
Vitamin B12	Dairy products, eggs, vitamin-fortified products (e.g. cereals, breads, soy/rice drinks)
Vitamin D	Dairy products, calcium-fortified orange juice, vitamin-fortified products
Calcium	Dairy products, dark green leafy veg, broccoli, chickpeas, calcium-fortified products (e.g. orange juice, soy/rice drinks, cereals)
Protein	Dairy products, eggs, tofu, dried beans, nuts
Iron	Eggs, dried beans, dried fruits, whole grains, leafy green veg, iron-fortified cereals/bread
Zinc	Wheatgerm, nuts, fortified cereal, vegetables such as peas and beans

Doing dairy-free and vegan diets

As they come off breast milk or formula at the age of about 1 year (although vegans often breastfeed for longer), vegan children are at risk for nutritional deficiencies. This doesn't mean you can't bring up a child on a vegan diet, but you need to keep a close eye on the nutrients your child gets. A strict vegan diet may be lacking in essential vitamins and minerals, such as vitamin D, vitamin B12, iron, calcium, and zinc. Many of the 'non-meat' substitute sources of nutrients come from eggs and dairy products, cheese and fish. Some doctors recommend that parents do not give their children a strictly vegan diet, especially before school age.

If you feel strongly about raising your child as a vegan, serve her lots of fortified cereals and nutrient-dense foods. Your doctor may recommend vitamin supplements for your child if her vegan diet does not provide adequate nutrients. Toddlers are typically picky about which foods they'll eat. As a result, your toddler may not get enough calories from a vegan diet to thrive. And for vegan toddlers, the amount of vegetables needed for proper nutrition and calories may be too bulky for their tiny stomachs. During the picky toddler stage, make sure your child eats enough calories. You *can* get enough fat and calories in a vegan child's diet, but you have to plan carefully when excluding food groups. See the tables in this chapter for guidance on what nutrients are needed. For more information, contact the Vegan Society (www.vegansociety.com).

Chapter 10

Exercise, Activity, and Play

● ●

In This Chapter

▶ Getting the most out of exercise

▶ Finding activities to suit your child

▶ Enjoying relaxation time

▶ Looking at how TV affects your child's health

● ●

*E*very child needs exercise – it's essential for mental and physical health. For you, the word 'exercise' probably conjures up sweaty sessions lifting weights at the gym, but for your child exercise comes in many guises – from throwing a ball in the garden to riding a bike, from playing tag to going to a ballet class. Even if your child isn't naturally sporty, you can keep him active in lots of fun ways. Exercise can be a really pleasurable experience, and you may be able to find an activity you both enjoy. What a great way to bond and get healthy at the same time!

Looking at the Benefits of Exercise

Encouraging your child to be active from an early age teaches him good habits that help him stay healthy into adolescence and adulthood. Lack of exercise is linked with a whole host of diseases, not least obesity, which is reaching dangerous levels in the UK – one in four children is overweight or obese. Today's children are significantly heavier than ever before, not only because they eat the wrong food but also because they're far less active than their predecessors.

Getting off the couch and springing into action offers a whole range of benefits for your child's physical health. Physical exercise:

✔ keeps your child's heart and circulation healthy

✔ helps your child develop strong muscles and bones

✔ reduces body fat

✔ makes your child live longer

✔ reduces the chances of your child developing illnesses such as diabetes, heart disease, and osteoporosis later in life

Exercise also boosts your child's brainpower by improving circulation of oxygen to the brain and helping him stay alert and able to concentrate. Studies have shown that physically active children have better cognitive skills and IQs and do better at school than their inactive peers.

Exercising makes a positive impact on your child's wellbeing. During rigorous activity, the brain releases chemicals such as serotonin and endorphins – the body's feel-good hormones.

Doing well at a chosen physical activity helps build your child's self-esteem: Active children are less likely to feel lonely, shy, or depressed than inactive children. Joining in with sports and activities has social benefits too: Your child gets the chance to mix with other children, make friends, and learn about the give and take needed to keep play fun and fair.

Inspiring Your Child to Get off the Sofa

The key to getting your child involved in exercise is to make it part of his everyday life. Exercising's a great way to spend time together as a family, even if you're just walking in the park, playing in the garden, or splashing about in a swimming pool. And if being active becomes a natural part of your child's day, he's more likely to keep it up for the rest of his life – especially if you do it too. In addition to the everyday activities that you and your child can participate in together, your child can join in organised activities.

Family fun

The best way to get your child up and running is to do things together. If your little one sees you enjoying active pursuits, he's more likely to join in. Kids love playing with their parents. At least once a week, try to do an activity together as a family, such as swimming or cycling. Here are a few simple activities that make incorporating exercise into your lives easy:

✔ **Take walks:** We walk without even thinking about it – but most of us could do a bit more. Walking's an easy exercise to incorporate into your everyday routine. Simply walking instead of driving to the shops or to school every day really can make a difference – little and often is key.

Investigate your local 'walk to school' initiative. If you haven't got one in your area, why not set one up for yourself? Approach the school and ask about publicising a register of where children from your school live, and a rota of parents who can collect each other's kids en route, or meet at a designated house to walk to school together. Your kids then have the opportunity to make new friends and get exercise!

✔ **Get outside:** If you have a garden, make the most of it. Play equipment needn't take up too much space. If you can't afford new equipment, look for *safe* second-hand garden gear. Outdoor toys are a great way of encouraging creative play – an old tyre may look like just that to you, but for your child it provides hours of endless entertainment. A climbing frame, swing, or a rope hanging securely from a tree branch encourages your child to be active outdoors. Hula hoops, trampolines, bikes, roller skates, skipping ropes, balls . . . the list's endless.

✔ **Go to the playground:** Play equipment encourages younger children to develop their strength and coordination and makes for a great social activity too. For older children, a park or playground provides space to kick a ball about or play games such as chase and tennis.

✔ **Have a run:** A run in the park can do wonders for burning up excess energy – try it! Most children love to race each other. If your child's good at running, he may even be interested in taking it up as a competitive sport at school.

✔ **Learn to swim:** Knowing how to swim is an essential life skill, so the sooner your child masters it the better. Find out about classes at your local pool, or teach your child yourself. Swimming and splashing about in a pool is a great all-round exercise for your child.

✔ **Take up cycling:** This is another important life skill, and one that'll help your child's coordination, balancing skills, and muscle development. Cycling's also a useful way of getting around – and you don't have to worry about parking problems or traffic jams. Check your local paper for a cycling proficiency course near you.

Next time you book a holiday, consider going on an *active* holiday – believe it or not, it can be even more fun than lounging by the pool. Lots of adventurous activity holidays and outdoor breaks are suitable for families. A week spent learning to ski or sail may possibly spark off a lifelong interest for your child (even if your bank manager isn't too happy about the price).

If your child has previously done very little activity, he must build up slowly. This is also important if he's been unwell or out of action for whatever reason – even a slight cold can affect your child's strength and ability to breathe. Doing too much exercise too soon may exhaust him and run him down. Start by aiming for no more than half an hour's activity a day, which you can gradually increase until he's doing an hour or so every day.

Organised sports

Toddlers and preschoolers don't usually need encouragement when it comes to being active – it's part of their job description. As soon as your child's mobile, you may feel like he's permanently on the go. You can find loads of constructive ways to channel his natural energy. Music-and-movement and mini-gymnastic classes help your child develop a whole variety of skills, such as climbing and jumping, and encourage coordination, balance, and agility. Best of all, your child builds his muscles while having fun too.

If your child's at school, encourage him to join an after-school activity club. If his school doesn't offer what you're looking for, your local leisure club, community centre, or library have info on the clubs, games, and activities on offer in your area. The range of activities to choose from is enormous. What about some of these?

- ✔ **Team sports:** Football, netball, and other team sports can motivate your child. Being part of a team means he is supported by others around him and that people depend on him.

- ✔ **Gymnastics:** A mini-gym class is great for improving balance, coordination, and muscle tone.

- ✔ **Tennis:** Joining a children's tennis club can be a good way of making friends and getting fit at the same time.

- ✔ **Dancing:** Many children love to express themselves through dancing. Even if you don't go to a structured dancing class, just putting on some music and dancing around your living room together can be good fun and great exercise.

- ✔ **Martial arts:** This is an excellent form of exercise for your child. Martial arts can be particularly good for building confidence, body strength, flexibility, coordination, and self-discipline.

- ✔ **Yoga:** This is becoming more and more popular for children – it's a great way of toning muscles, improving flexibility, and de-stressing.

The more activities your child tries, the more likely he'll find something he enjoys doing. These trial periods can be frustrating (and expensive!), but to a certain extent you can avoid false starts by making sure that your child's really keen and knows what's involved.

Finding activities to suit your child

It may sound obvious, but ask your child what he wants to do first – and then go along to watch a session together before signing him up to a class. This also gives you a chance to check out how well the activity is run. You'll soon tell whether the children look as if they're having fun, whether the group leaders are friendly and encouraging, and whether the group takes individual needs and abilities into account. After your child's picked an activity, be prepared to ease him in slowly. Give him lots of praise and encouragement, particularly if he's learning a new skill. Keep the feedback positive and avoid pushing him too hard – the emphasis must always be on having fun.

Your child's personality is a factor in choosing a new activity. A naturally sporty child may flourish in a more competitive environment. But if your child finds it hard to be assertive, then games where he needs to be an active participant, such as football, may dispirit him. A swimming or riding club, where he can progress at his own speed, is probably a better choice. Similarly, take your child's likes and dislikes into account. You may love the idea of your little treasure learning how to tap dance, but there's no point in pressurising him if he was born with two left feet and a distinct lack of interest in anything musical.

Your child's far more likely to take part in a new activity if a friend goes with him, so ask the parents of his pals whether they'd be interested in joining too. An added bonus is that you may be able to share the responsibility for supervising the children and picking them up and dropping them off.

Maximising your chances for success

If your child's sedentary, prefers reading to roughhousing, and plays computer chess rather than cricket, try enticing him into being more physically active. The following suggestions can help:

- ✔ **Teach him basic skills, such as hopping, jumping, skipping, throwing, and catching, so he feels confident.** Some children don't participate in games because they feel self-conscious about their abilities. Helping your child overcome his diffidence means he's more likely to join in when the neighbouring children play outside.

- ✔ **Invite friends round to play.** Active games are far more fun with others, and between them they'll come up with double the number of games to play.

- ✔ **Limit the amount of time your child spends in front of the TV and computer.** An hour a day is plenty for most children. You may want to increase limits at weekends – who knows, one day you may even get a lie-in! Using television viewing as a treat to be earned by spending an equivalent time reading, or doing exercise, can give you a useful reward. Try not to use the removal of TV or computer privileges as a constant punishment, though – it just makes it more desirable!

- ✔ **Make exercise challenging but fun.** Invest in a pedometer, which measures the number of steps you take every day. Set challenges for your child or have a competition to see who walks the most steps in one day.

✔ **Be creative with items around the house.** Set up a circuit training course at home. Who needs a gym when you've got stairs, living-room furniture, and tins of beans at home? Using everyday items as exercise tools makes for creative fun. Jog up and down the stairs, do crunches with your legs on the couch, and try skipping in the porch. You may look a bit silly, but that makes it all the more fun for your kids.

✔ **Reward your child's effort.** Give your child lots of praise to keep him motivated. Try setting up a point system for exercise – keep a track of the whole family's exercise feats with a chart. Don't make it a competition, but reward the whole family's accomplishments, for example with a trip to the cinema (don't reward your child with food though).

School-age children find almost any activity more attractive if their parents involve themselves as well. Putting the emphasis on fun and family participation can inspire even the most sedentary child. If your child sees the value you attach to being out and about and on the move, he's more likely to see it as worthwhile.

Exercising an overweight child

One of the most important things you can do to help your overweight child is let him know that he's fantastic whatever his weight. Children's feelings about themselves often centre on their parents' feelings about them. If you accept your child at any weight, he'll be more likely to accept and feel good about himself. Talk to your child about his weight and allow him to share his concerns with you. He probably realises better than anyone else that he has a weight problem. Your overweight child needs support, acceptance, and encouragement from you.

Don't set your overweight child apart as 'the one with the problem' – don't expect him to eat less or exercise more than other family members. He's already going to feel different – overweight children may be made to feel self-conscious at an early age by other children at school. Making him feel he's being treated differently at home only does more damage to his self-esteem. Family involvement helps your child develop healthy habits and builds his confidence by not singling him out.

Regular physical activity combined with healthy eating habits is the most efficient and healthy way to control weight and is an important part of a healthy lifestyle. To help your overweight child, focus on gradually changing your whole family's physical activity and eating habits. Consider the following suggestions:

> ✔ **Switch off the TV.** Reduce the amount of time you and your family spend in sedentary activities, such as watching TV and playing on the computer.
>
> ✔ **Be active together.** Make the most of the opportunities you and your family have to be active. For example, instead of taking the lift in the shopping centre, walk up the stairs together.

Be sensitive to your child's needs. Your overweight child may feel uncomfortable about participating in certain activities, especially competitive team sports, so help him find physical activities that he enjoys and that aren't embarrassing or difficult for him such as cycling, walking, or Frisbee. Encourage your child to be confident that he can come to you with any worries about negative behaviour he may receive at school.

Working out how much is enough

To maintain a necessary level of fitness, experts recommend that children of all ages need to have at least one hour of moderate activity every day. Examples of moderate activity include brisk walking, swimming, dancing, active play, cycling, and most sports.

An hour a day may sound challenging, but children prefer, and are more suited to, short bursts rather than sustained periods of activity. For example, a child who walks briskly to and from school, plays outside most days, does a regular activity such as football or dancing, and joins in with family activities at weekends is probably averaging the recommended level of exercise over the week.

Taking Sensible Precautions

You can do plenty of things to ensure that your child isn't at risk of injuring himself while he's exercising. Take steps to see that his surroundings and equipment are safe, and that he gets a healthy diet to keep muscles and bones well-nourished, and supplied with plenty of energy. These simple things really can help to keep your little athlete in tiptop condition.

Minimising the risk of injury

Your child's safety is your first concern when he's exercising. Exercise-related accidents are common, but most are not serious. You can still take steps to reduce the risk of accidents happening:

✔ Ensure that organised sports are conducted with appropriate attention to safety and injury prevention – children shouldn't be pushed to the point where injuries may occur.

✔ Don't let your child do vigorous exercise if he's ill, in pain, or taking medication, unless your child's doctor gives the okay.

✔ Make sure that your child wears the appropriate protective equipment: Footwear that provides appropriate support and traction, and a helmet if he's cycling are musts.

✔ Minimise the chances of your child pulling a muscle by seeing he does stretching and warming up exercise. Children's bones often grow at a faster rate than the adjacent muscles and tendons, predisposing them to muscle tightness, especially at the hamstrings and quadriceps, so stretching and warming up is particularly important.

✔ Ensure that play areas are away from traffic and free from debris.

✔ Keep your child well hydrated: Children are more vulnerable than adults to dehydration. Teach your child to drink fluids before, during, and after exercise, without waiting to become thirsty.

Eating and resting

Your child will flag without regular rest and food. He'll enjoy activities far more if he feels energetic, so fuel him up about an hour before a big exercise session and make sure that he eats a good breakfast before leaving for school in the morning so he doesn't run out of energy before playtime. Kids burn up calories incredibly quickly, so offering your child a nutritious snack such as a banana is a good way to keep him going.

Growing children get tired easily, so plenty of rest is important for recharging run-down batteries. Between the ages of 5 and 11 years, children need at least nine hours of sleep a night. But don't expect your child to go to sleep immediately after running around for hours: End the fun and games well before bedtime, so he gets a chance to wind down.

Balance periods when your toddler's expending physical energy with quieter times when he can recharge his batteries. Children aren't aware of their own limits and can find it difficult to wind down. Overactive children can become sleep-deprived, which may in turn lead to behavioural problems. Incorporating calm, relaxing activities into your child's day to balance the more physically demanding activities helps him maintain his energy levels and good humour.

Massaging: The facts

Massage is a great aid to relaxation and eases aches and pains. Sports massage is a rapidly expanding field and is popular among both professional athletes and fitness enthusiasts – and your child can benefit too. Muscle and joint massage can assist training, prevent injury, and aid healing of injuries. Massage can be used both before and after exercise as a way of reducing muscular tension. If your child has been rigorously active, massage his muscles afterwards to reduce the likelihood of soreness or aching the next day. Suggested techniques include:

✔ Slow, rhythmic strokes on the affected area are particularly good for the calf and shoulder muscles. Massage in the direction of blood flow, towards the heart – for example, from wrist to shoulder, or from ankle to knee – gradually applying an increasing amount of pressure.

✔ For tension or knotted muscles, try kneading or pressing the muscles, alternately tightening and loosening your grasp.

Before physical exercise, massage gets the blood moving to assist in the warm-up. Massage after exercise is shown to reduce waste products such as lactic and carbonic acids, which build up in the muscles after exercise and cause cramping and discomfort – it can also really help your child with growing pains. Some evidence suggests that massage enhances the immune system and aids recovery from injuries by increasing blood circulation to injured areas.

Understanding the Impact of Television on Your Child

TV affects your child in many different ways. Lots of parents worry that their children watch too much telly or spend vast amounts of time on the computer – and they're right to be concerned. Statistics show that children in the UK watch an average of four hours of TV a day, and more than half have televisions in their bedrooms. And with the advent of digital TV, with all those extra channels, your tot can in theory spend every waking hour watching children's programmes.

Snuggling up with your child on the sofa to watch a favourite programme is unlikely to affect him adversely, but there's growing evidence that spending hours at a time in front of a screen on a regular basis can damage your child's health.

TV or not TV: The adverse affects of too much telly

Several studies have shown that spending too long in front of the TV is contributing to children becoming fatter and unhealthier. Children who watch a lot of telly – three hours or more a day is considered 'a lot' – or have tellies in their bedrooms have a greater risk of obesity in later life because they're less active and more likely to snack rather than have regular meals. As TV viewing increases, time spent in active work and play decreases. Studies have found a number of other worrying effects of TV, including the following:

- ✔ According to many speech and language therapists, watching too much television can affect your child's communication skills. Small children learn to speak by hearing familiar adults speak to them, and constant background noise from the telly doesn't help.

- ✔ Children's social skills may not develop properly if they have less chance to play and interact. Many children now have TVs in their bedrooms and often watch it alone rather than indulge in it as a family activity.

- ✔ Watching telly can have a detrimental effect on sleep. Research points to late-night TV viewing as a prime cause of disturbed sleep. Winding down with a familiar story is best at bedtime.

- ✔ Many experts believe a link exists between aggressive behaviour and TV watching. Although the jury's still out on the matter, many reports have linked aggressive behaviour in children to seeing it on TV. There's also concern that inappropriate programmes can make tiny couch potatoes aggressive and prone to nightmares, and delay their speech development.

Problems with concentrating can ensue from watching too much TV, because it can affects your child's attention span. Some research suggests that watching TV at a very young age may be linked to an increase in the risk of developing attention deficit/hyperactivity disorder (ADHD). You can read more about ADHD in Chapter 16.

Love it or loathe it, television's a part of our everyday lives. Of course, it's not all bad news. Children need chill-out time, and there's nothing wrong with your child watching several short amounts of telly or playing a game on the computer. Television's also a valuable source of information – watched selectively, it can broaden your child's outlook on the world. Computers, too, play an important part of everyday life, and information technology is a large part of the National Curriculum. But if you leave your child to his own devices, he may spend hours mesmerised in front of the screen.

Television-watching for children under 2 years

Many experts don't recommend television at all for children under the age of 2 years. Replacing shared time between baby and parent with television viewing can impact on the baby's physical and mental development. TV can also be damaging for young children because they're likely to miss out on a range of social, emotional, and learning skills. When you're caring for a toddler at home, with many hours to fill, you may be tempted to turn to passive activities such as watching TV. But limiting your child's TV intake is a good way to keep him physically active. A toddler can get much more out of fiddling with a shape sorter, playing on a swing, or listening to a book read by a caring adult. If you do put the telly on, watch it together so that you can discuss what you're seeing.

Even educational programmes aren't as enriching as real-life activities, such as working out how a toy functions or playing games and singing songs together. If you choose to allow a little TV time for your tot, try to limit it to a maximum of one hour of quality children's programmes per day. If possible, choose non-commercial channels, which don't have lots of adverts pushing low-nutrient snacks and drinks.

Age-appropriate DVDs and videos that invite your child to play along are much better than endless children's cartoons. So if you do want your child to watch TV, it's worth investing in a few.

Keeping control of the small screen

The obvious worry is that your child may be viewing unsuitable material. Many computer games have aggressive themes, and violence appears regularly on our TV screens. Of equal concern is that a child who is sitting indoors in front of a screen all day is inactive and solitary. To control how much and what kind of TV your child watches, try the following:

- ✔ **Have TV-free days.** One of the problems with television and computer games is that they become a habitual part of the day-to-day routine, so make sure that it doesn't become the norm.

- ✔ **Set viewing limits.** Don't let your child watch TV for hours at a time. TV's a great occasional babysitter when you need a break or have to get something done, but don't leaving your child glued to the screen for hours on end – viewing for long periods can leave him feeling irritable and lethargic. Allow your child a reasonable period of time each day, or a certain number of hours a week, for watching programmes or playing on the computer. Use an egg timer to prevent arguments when time's up.

✔ **Go communal.** Keep TVs and computers in a family room rather than your child's bedroom, so that you can monitor what he's watching or playing.

✔ **Keep to the age limit.** Allow your child to watch only programmes devised specifically for his age group. Check that the programmes your child is watching are suitable for him, and don't let him play computer games that are unsuitable for his age.

✔ **Watch from start to finish.** Viewing an entire film or programme with characters, a storyline, and an ending can be far better than watching snippets or several short programmes in a row.

✔ **Watch TV together.** That way, you can explain to your child anything puzzling as it crops up. Television then becomes a social activity and provides an opportunity for you to spend close time with your child.

✔ **Switch it off!** Turn the TV off when the programme finishes – don't leave it on as background noise.

✔ **Play with it.** Use ideas from programmes to develop imaginative play, such as making things or acting out the plot of something you've seen.

Chapter 11

Dozing Off: The Importance of Sleep

*I*s sleep your obsession? If so, join the club – parents crave it, particularly in the early years. Sleep's a precious commodity for parents – and most of us want more than we get. In fact, parents ask health visitors about children's sleep – or lack of it – more than any other subject. And for good reason, because without sleep no one can function. You're probably only too well aware of what sleep deprivation can do to both you and your child. Sleep affects every aspect of our lives: Good sleep's vital for physical health and has a major impact on mood, learning, and behaviour.

Uncovering the Mysteries of Sleep

The exact role of sleep has baffled scientists for centuries, but it clearly has many health benefits. Loads of stuff happens while your child sleeps:

- ✔ Cells in her body multiply rapidly and her growth hormones jump into action.

- ✔ The calories from her milk or food are converted into energy for growth and warmth, helping to build muscle as well as strength.

- ✔ Her body produces white blood cells, which are essential for fighting infections. Studies show that lack of sleep increases vulnerability to illnesses such as colds and flu, because the immune system does all its repair work during sleep.

✔ Her brain expands and makes new connections, plugging in to her long-term memory things that she learned during the day. Sleep is also essential for the development of cognitive skills such as speech, memory, and thinking.

Looking at sleep stages

When we sleep, we go through two distinct stages, which have various effects on the brain and body:

✔ **Dream sleep:** As you watch your child sleeping, you may notice her eyes flickering beneath the lids and her body twitching. They are signs that she's dreaming, a sleep stage known as rapid eye movement (REM) or dream sleep. Research suggests that this kind of sleep is the most crucial for the development and maintenance of the brain – in this stage, the brain does its filing ready for the next day. Newborn babies spend around half their time in REM sleep, but this reduces after the first few months of life, so that in later childhood and adulthood only around 20 per cent of sleep time is spent in REM.

✔ **Dreamless sleep:** Non-REM or quiet sleep is more peaceful than REM sleep, and the brain is less active in this stage. Dreamless sleep consists of four phases of gradually deepening sleep: drowsiness, light sleep, deep sleep, and very deep sleep. Everyone goes through these phases, or *sleep cycles*, with alternating periods of REM and non-REM sleep, throughout the night.

Each sleep cycle lasts around 90 minutes (60 minutes for a baby). Every time you comes out of a sleep cycle you wake up briefly, although you're unlikely to remember this awakening unless you feel insecure in your surroundings or something's disturbing you.

One of the main causes of sleep problems in babies and young children is that they can't lull themselves back to sleep when they come out of a sleep cycle. They're used to being rocked, cuddled, or fed to sleep by you, so when they wake up briefly they wonder where Mum or Dad has gone and start to cry. The section 'Establishing Healthy Sleeping Habits' later in the chapter offers some suggestions for helping your child to go back to sleep on her own.

Working out how much sleep your child needs

Every baby is different – even from their brothers and sisters! Just because your first baby slept through the night by four months old and the second is still waking every three hours doesn't mean anything's wrong with either of them. How much sleep does your child need? The following is a very rough guide – but bear in mind that your child's unlikely to be average!

- **Newborn:** At this stage a baby has no regular pattern, but an average new baby sleeps for about 16 or 17 hours out of 24. It may not feel like that to you though! A new baby's unlikely to sleep for more than two or three hours at a stretch, and she'll wake up throughout the day and night to be fed.

- **Three months:** At three months, night-time sleep averages about nine hours, with around five hours' worth of naps throughout the day.

- **Six months:** Your baby may now sleep for 10 or 11 hours at night, with around four hours of daytime naps. She'll sleep for longer stretches at night – say, six hours – because she no longer needs night-time feeds.

  If your baby doesn't naturally drop her night feeds, try gradually decreasing the amount of milk you give during the night: Reduce breast-feeds by a minute each time, or give 1 fluid ounce less of bottle-feed every night. If your baby wakes up before feeding time, comfort her but don't hold her or feed her, as this habit can become harder and harder to break.

- **Twelve months:** Total night-time sleep is now about 11½ hours, with two or three hours' worth of naps.

- **Toddlers:** The need for daytime naps starts to taper off around the age of 3 years, although many children continue to nap until the age of 5 years.

- **Three years and over:** Your child probably needs around 11 hours sleep per night.

- **School age:** Your child will sleep for about ten hours a day.

The best way to judge how much sleep your child needs is to go by her signals. If your child's a year old and sleeps for just ten hours a day, don't worry as long as she's happy and healthy and not displaying signs of overtiredness such as irritability and mood swings.

Giving your baby a really good feed at the end of the evening can often help her to sleep for longer, but you may find that you don't have much milk. Try expressing in the morning, when you have more milk (read Chapter 6 for more tips on expressing milk). You can then let your partner feed the baby last thing at night – helping your baby to sleep better, giving dad a little bonding time, and you some well-earned rest!

Establishing Healthy Sleeping Habits

When you've got a new baby, it's all you can do to master the art of feeding and nappy changing, so it's not surprising that many parents get into a bit of a pickle over the whole sleep issue. You want to attend your baby's every need, and if that includes letting her fall asleep in your arms, or having to go to her 10 times a night, so be it. But at some point most of us decide we can no longer carry on like this, and you may want to introduce a bit of discipline into the night-time proceedings. Gentle but effective ways exist of encouraging good sleep habits in your baby or child, so don't despair.

Fixing broken nights

Broken nights are the most common thing parents complain about, especially those with babies and toddlers. To prevent disrupted nights for the whole family, the key is to help your baby or child learn how to sleep by herself – which means putting her to bed while she's still awake. Climbing in with her and nodding off won't do her – or you – any favours, no matter how tempting it seems after a long day. Even young babies can benefit from being able to lull themselves to sleep.

In the very early days, sleep is intricately bound up with feeding, so your baby wakes frequently for sustenance – she needs to do this until she's around 6 months old. However, from around 3 months, when her body clock adjusts to a night-day pattern, you can start to lay the foundations for good sleep patterns. For example:

1. Instead of rocking your baby to sleep or letting her doze off while she's feeding or in your arms, make sure that she's still awake.

2. When she's drowsy, put her into her cot or bed, say goodnight, and leave the room. If she cries, go back and comfort her for a few minutes but don't pick her up or let her get out of bed. When she settles, leave the room. If she cries again, leave her for a few minutes before going in and soothing her again.

3. When she's calm, leave the room again. If she continues to cry, leave it a little longer than last time before you go in to calm her and leaving again. You may have to do this many times, gradually increasing the amount of time you leave your baby by a minute or so.

4. If she wakes in the night, feed her if she is under six months (after which, most babies don't need a night-time feed).

You may need to persevere with your sleep plan for several nights before your child starts to sleep through. It can be exhausting at first, because you may have to get up several times in the night. If you're consistent, ultimately the plan will benefit the whole family. It may be worth warning the neighbours in case they worry unnecessarily, otherwise you may be unpopular! Remind them that you're doing the sleep plan to reduce the number of times your baby disturbs all of you in the long run.

By following a sleep programme, you're not being cruel to your child or making her suffer. In the long run, you're helping her because she'll benefit from unbroken sleep as much as you will. The programme teaches your child that you haven't abandoned her. She learns that you're there for her and her needs are important to you, but she's safe to go to sleep without you.

Getting into a routine

I cannot overemphasise the benefits of having a well-established bedtime routine for your child. A routine helps make your child feel secure at bedtime, which is crucial to a good night's sleep. Babies and young children soon learn to predict and anticipate what is going to happen next, reading the signals that the day's over and it's time to go to sleep. A routine can also be an enjoyable and fulfilling part of your relationship for many years to come.

Babies under the age of 8 months or so still have feeding incorporated into their bedtime routine, but after 8 months it's a good idea to feed your child before starting your routine – say, half an hour before bedtime – to help her disassociate sleeping with feeding. Try some or all of the following in your child's bedtime routine:

1. Give her a wash or bath. Warm water's relaxing and a great way of helping your child wind down. Remember to clean her teeth too.

2. Take her to her bedroom, dim the lights, draw the curtains, and dress her in her pyjamas. Keep noise and distractions to a minimum.

3. Tell your child a story or look at a book together.

4. Give her a cuddle and a kiss before you lift her into her cot or tuck her into bed.

5. Say goodnight and leave the room.

Solving Common Sleep Problems

Occasional disruptions to your child's sleep patterns are inevitable. A lot of sleep problems are temporary or developmental, so rest assured that in time your child'll grow out of them.

Never be tempted to give your child over-the-counter medications that cause drowsiness in an attempt to cure her sleep problems. If sleeplessness is severe, arrange to see your doctor or health visitor.

Helping your unwell child sleep

If your child's ill, her nights (and yours) will probably be punctuated by frequent awakenings. Discomfort from vaccinations, fever, pain, coughing, and a stuffy nose are all contenders for keeping your child awake at night, and so she's going to need soothing, cuddling, drinks, medicine (if appropriate), and lots of comfort. You may find it easier to sleep in your child's room with her while she's ill: She may need extra reassurance and she'll probably settle better with you close by.

Temporary changes to bedtime routines and night-time sleeping arrangements during illness are unavoidable. Try to re-establish your routine as soon as possible after the disruptive period in order to avoid long-term problems. If your child remains unsettled after everything else has returned to normal, you may need to retrain her.

Colds and snuffles

Colds can be very disruptive to your child's sleep patterns. A blocked nose forces her to breathe through her mouth, which can interfere with self-soothing techniques such as thumb-sucking. Feeding can be difficult if your child has a blocked nose, and she may give up before she's satisfied – which means she is going to be hungry again quickly.

If your baby has a cough, it may get worse when she lies down to sleep because the excess mucus drips into and irritates the back of her throat. Try raising her head on an extra pillow. For safety reasons, never use pillows under the head of a baby under a year old. Instead, put a folded towel or thin pillow under the head of her mattress.

Try a cool-mist humidifier in your child's room to keep her nasal passages clear, or put a few drops of an over-the-counter menthol inhalant (check age suitability) on a hanky near her bed or cot. You can buy a nasal sucker from your pharmacy to suck her blocked nose gently clear before you put her down or feed her.

Ear infections

Ear infections can have a profound impact on your child's sleeping habits. Ear infections often go undiagnosed, but they're a major cause of disturbed nights in babies and young children. An ear infection is painful and may wake your baby or child frequently. Pain is caused by the build-up in the middle ear of fluid that cannot drain away adequately when your child's lying down, so she may benefit from sleeping on some extra pillows to help raise her head (put under the mattress for babies under a year).

The correct dose of children's paracetamol or, if indicated for her age, ibuprofen liquid, can help to soothe earache. If your child has earache for more than a day or so see your doctor, because she may need other medication as well.

After the ear infection has cleared up, your child should sleep normally again.

Working through wee problems: Bedwetting

By about the age of 3 years, most children are toilet-trained and dryness usually follows soon afterwards. But as many as one in six children frequently wet the bed until the age of 5 years or older. If your child still wets the bed after you've toilet-trained her, she may simply be a bit later than average in developing the ability to wake up when her bladder's full. The problem is likely clear up as she matures.

Bedwetting is thought to be related to an immature bladder or a deep sleeping pattern: Some children sleep so deeply that they're not aware of the messages the bladder sends to the brain saying it's full. Bedwetting can also run in families. Children with learning disabilities and allergies seem more likely to be bedwetters.

Help your child by offering positive support, understanding, and encouragement. Reinforcing your child's negative feelings about her bedwetting may only serve to make the problem worse.

Medical treatment for bedwetting usually consists of drugs to improve sleeping patterns and to help the smooth functioning of the muscles around the bladder. Sometimes, antidiuretics can be given in the form of a nasal spray to help your child's body make less urine. All medication has side effects, however, and should be used only as a last resort.

Behavioural treatment is often more effective than medical treatment. Although behavioural treatment may take longer to show results, the improvement is usually permanent. Several methods have been proved helpful, including the following:

- **Star chart:** Use a star chart to offer rewards for a certain number of dry nights.

- **Fluid timing:** Give your child plenty of fluids over the course of the day, but if she tends to drink a lot just before she goes to bed, cut out or limit pre-bedtime drinking to improve her chances of staying dry.

- **Night-lifting:** You wake your child periodically throughout the night, walking her to the bathroom to wee, and then returning her to bed. By teaching your child to wake up to empty her bladder many times during the night, eventually she may stay dry.

- **Moisture alarms:** A useful and successful way to treat bedwetting is by using moisture alarms, but they may take many weeks to be effective. You attach a clip-on sensor probe to the outside of your child's bedclothes. An alarm then goes off if she starts to wet the bed. The alarm wakes your child, who then gets up to go to the loo. This slowly conditions the brain to respond appropriately during sleep.

- **Hypnosis:** By listening repeatedly to a hypnosis tape, your child's brain is reprogrammed so that she responds to a full bladder when she's asleep in the same way she does when she's awake. Hypnosis can be an extremely effective treatment for bedwetting.

- **Retention and control training:** The doctor may ask your child to control her urinating during the day by postponing it, at first by a few minutes and then gradually increasing the length of time. This can strengthen the muscle that holds back urine.

Never try to get your child to control her urine without first seeking advice from a doctor a GP or paediatrician.

Almost all children outgrow the habit of wetting the bed. As they mature, their muscles become stronger and their bladder capacity increases. They also tend to sleep less deeply, so they're more sensitive to the messages the bladder sends to the brain.

If your child starts to wet the bed after having been dry for some time, she may have a urinary tract infection (UTI). Signs of UTI include pain when urinating, being unusually thirsty, and smelly urine. She may also have fever or vomiting. See your doctor if you suspect your child is suffering, as it may need to be treated with antibiotics (if it's left untreated, it can cause kidney problems). Give her lots of fluids to help flush out the bacteria. To help prevent UTIs, always wash her genitals from front to back, to avoid spreading bacteria from her bottom.

Getting help for your child's sleep problems

If you're having problems getting your baby or child to sleep, your health visitor may be able to refer you to a sleep clinic, which can give you support and advice. NHS and private sleep clinics are located throughout the UK.

Sleep clinics are not normally recommended for babies under 6 months old: Night-time feeds are still a biological necessity at this age, and expecting such a young child to sleep through the night is unrealistic. If you have an older baby or child with sleep problems, a sleep clinic can be great for getting some moral support through what can be a trying time. You may meet other parents facing the same problems – just realising that you're not alone can really help. Sleep clinics are run by qualified specialists who help you work out the problems and break poor sleep cycles by retraining the parents and the child. After an initial consultation, the clinic normally gets you to write a detailed diary of your child's sleeping habits so that new routines can be suggested in order to help train your baby or child to sleep.

A sudden onset of bedwetting may also be due to some kind of stress – perhaps your child's just about to start school, for example. If your child starts to wet the bed, reassure her and be sympathetic. Try to work out whether she's under stress – and if she is, take steps to reduce it.

If bedwetting continues for more than two weeks or you can't identify the source of the problem, see your doctor or paediatrician. And if she continues to wet the bed after the age of 6 years, talk to your doctor about referring your child to a specialist.

Try not to make a fuss, tell your child off, or punish her for wetting the bed – it isn't her fault. In the meantime, use a waterproof sheet and get your child to help you change the sheets – although make sure that she realises she is helping you, and it isn't a punishment. She may feel more secure if she wears disposable pull-ups in bed for a while.

Sleepwalking and Monster-spotting: Nightmare Scenarios

All children have nightmares. These scary dreams may relate to something that happened during the day or to fears that come to the surface in the way of images or dreams. If your child has a nightmare, she may wake up afraid and crying. Comfort her as quickly as possible – she needs lots of reassurance from you. Ask her to talk about the dream, and then try making up a happier ending. Stay with her until she's calm.

Although distressing for you and your child, nightmares are rarely serious. By the time she's 5 years old or so, your child will be better able to understand that these images are only dreams.

Dealing with night terrors

Night terrors are far less common than nightmares. Although experts remain unsure why they occur, they may be triggered by a number of factors, including over-tiredness, irregular sleep patterns, or anxiety. They appear to happen if a child is woken at a particular sleep stage; the brain is only partially aroused. They tend to happen most frequently during preschool years. If your child's having a night terror, she'll appear to be wide awake, even though she's not. She'll be upset, perhaps crying, screaming, or thrashing, but she won't respond to you. She'll have no recollection of the night terror the next day.

Try holding your child and reassuring her during a night terror, but don't attempt to wake her because you may aggravate her fear even more. After a while, she'll settle and go back to sleep.

Night terrors are not damaging and they soon pass. They're often more scary for the parents to witness than for your child to experience. Your child will almost certainly stop having them as she gets older, although even adults get night terrors occasionally.

Looking after your sleepwalking child

Like night terrors, sleepwalking occurs when a child partially comes out of a deep sleep. You don't need to rouse your sleepwalking child – in fact, it may alarm her if you do. Instead, gently guide her back to bed. Most children grow out of sleepwalking by the age of 6 years, although very occasionally it can last into adulthood.

If your child sleepwalks, ensure that your home is safe, with window locks and safety gates. Don't leave hazards such as toys lying around, which your child can trip over. You could also hang a bell on your child's bedroom door so you can hear if she leaves her room.

Getting rid of monsters under the bed

A child's imagination can run riot at bedtime. Silly as it may seem to you, you must take your child's fears seriously and let her know she's safe if she's frightened there may be monsters under the bed – they're very real to her. Turn on the light and show her that her room at night is just as cosy as it is during the day. Do a thorough monster check of the cupboards and under the bed so she can see there's nothing to be afraid of. Your child may prefer to keep her light on at night, or you can leave a light on outside her door or use a nightlight.

Be patient with your child if she's feeling insecure in her room. Make sure that she's happy by spending lots of fun time in her room together. And don't send her to her room as punishment because she'll associate it with bad feelings.

To sleep, perchance to snore . . .

You may have thought it was only great big heavy blokes who snored, but some of the loudest nocturnal noises can come from the smallest sources. About 1 in 10 children snore, and that number's even higher if the parents smoke.

Snoring's most common between the ages of 3 and 6 years, but it can show up a lot earlier. Young babies often snore or make throaty noises in their sleep because they still have soft flexible airways. The noise tends to disappear as your child matures.

Snoring in an older child can be a sign that her adenoids or tonsils are enlarged, which often happens when she's fighting an infection such as a cold or tonsillitis. Persistent allergies may also cause problems. Sometimes the adenoids and tonsils become enlarged for no apparent reason. Snoring alone is not a cause for concern, as it tends to diminish as the tonsils and adenoids stop growing and begin to shrink at about the age of 8 years. Occasionally, a child needs to have her tonsils or adenoids removed to resolve the problem.

If your child suddenly starts making strange breathing sounds, seems to struggle for breath in her sleep, or momentarily stops breathing, see your doctor immediately. Always ask your doctor to check any significant breathing irregularities, snores, gurgles, or pauses in your child's breathing. Although such symptoms are unlikely to be serious, your doctor does need to rule out other causes, such as obstructive sleep apnoea (episodes where he stops breathing).

Making Sure That Your Baby Sleeps Safely

Working out where your child sleeps takes a lot of thought. Experts agree that new babies are better off sleeping near their parents during the early weeks, in a cot or Moses basket by the bed.

Sleeping in a cot

Your baby's cot must be safety-approved, which means it should conform to British Standard EN716. Modern cot designs are required by law to meet certain standards. Cot bars should be no more than 6 centimetres apart so your baby can't get her head or limbs stuck. There should be no horizontal bars, as your baby may be able to climb them and fall out. If the cot has a drop side, the catch mechanism must be really sturdy.

Keep your child's cot or bed well away from windows, blinds, cords, curtains, radiators, and electrical appliances.

If your baby sleeps in a cot, check that the cot is locked every time you put her in it. Never leave her in the cot with the side down.

Bed sharing

The Federation for the Study of Infant Deaths (FSID) advises against sharing a bed with a baby under 3 months of age because of the risks of overheating and suffocating. If you want to sleep near your baby, consider buying a bedside cot – a cot with one detachable side so that your baby's bed becomes an extension of yours.

Reducing the risk of cot death

Most parents with a young baby worry about the possibility of cot death, or sudden infant death syndrome (SIDS). It's important to remember that the risk of cot death striking is very small, particularly if you adhere to the recommended guidelines below; but around 300 babies still die every year.

The causes of this tragic syndrome are not fully understood, but it is more common in babies under the age of six months. The following guidelines can significantly reduce the risk of SIDS happening to your baby, but for more details and advice, visit www.sids.org.uk or call 027 233 2090.

- ✔ Always put your baby to sleep on her back. Since the FSID started giving parents this advice, the number of cot deaths has fallen significantly. If your baby turns on to her stomach during the night, don't worry – she's at much less risk of cot death once she can roll over by herself – but turn her on to her back again when you go in to check her.

- ✔ Never smoke around your baby, and keep her away from smoky atmospheres. Babies exposed to cigarette smoke are at a higher risk of dying from SIDS. Smoking anywhere in the house – not just your baby's room – increases her risk of chest infections and cot death.

✔ Keep your baby's bedroom at the right temperature (around 18°C). Overheating is life-threatening, because your baby cannot regulate her own body temperature during the early months of life. Feel her tummy or the nape of her neck to see whether she feels hot or clammy, and remove layers accordingly if necessary. Buy a nursery thermometer to help you make sure that the bedroom is at the right temperature.

✔ Prevent your baby from slipping under the covers and suffocating by placing her with her feet at the foot of her cot, Moses basket, or cradle. Always keep her head uncovered. Never use a pillow for a baby under one year old.

✔ Never use duvets, quilts, or thick blankets. Soft bedding can cause your baby to become overheated, so best to use a sheet or one or two layers of thin blankets, securely tucked into the sides and foot of the mattress no higher than your baby's chest. In warm weather, take off a layer or remove the bedcovers altogether. Don't use cot bumpers because they can contribute to overheating. Never use hot water bottles or electric blankets.

✔ Don't put soft toys in your baby's cot or put her to sleep on top of a cushion, beanbag, or waterbed.

✔ Never go to sleep with your baby on a sofa.

✔ Use a firm mattress and clean and air it regularly. Make sure that there are no gaps between the edges of the mattress and the sides of the cot.

✔ Seek medical advice immediately if your baby is unwell.

A recent study suggests that the risk of cot death is reduced if babies use dummies. However, more research needs to be done before experts actively recommend dummies for all babies, especially because it seems that a baby who usually has a dummy but is not given one for a night (perhaps because a parent forgets to give it, or it falls out and is lost) is known to be more at risk of cot death.

Monitoring your baby's breathing

A breathing monitor is an electronic pad that fits under your baby's mattress and registers your baby's breathing. An alarm goes off if it detects a pause in her breathing. Monitors aren't routinely recommended because they can serve to increase anxiety because of the many inevitable false alarms. They also increase your chance, and that of your baby, of having regularly disturbed sleep. However, if your baby is at high risk of SIDS – if she's diagnosed with apnoea attacks (episodes where he stops breathing), perhaps – you may be advised by your doctor to use one.

Breathing monitors do not prevent SIDS. Far better to practise the preventive sleeping methods talked about in this chapter than to rely solely on electronic monitors.

Chapter 12

Basic Hygiene and the War on Germs

*L*et's face it: Germs have a lot to answer for. Germs cause many of the most common diseases in children (and adults), from food poisoning to meningitis. Germs come in many guises, including bacteria and viruses. Most germs enter the body by being inhaled or from hand-to-mouth contact. After entering the body, germs make themselves at home, multiplying at an alarming rate and damaging or destroying healthy cells. As germs use up the body's nutrients and energy, they produce waste products, or toxins, which cause symptoms such as sniffles, sneezing, coughing, diarrhoea, high fever, increased heart rate, and even life-threatening illness.

Hygiene How-Tos

Your child can pick up germs in several ways, including touching dirty hands, eating contaminated food, breathing in somebody else's cough or sneeze droplets, and touching contaminated surfaces such as a toilet seat or table-top. Your child then needs only to touch his eyes, nose, or mouth to transfer the germs to those places. After your child's infected, the whole family is likely come down with the same illness. But by abiding by the basic rules of hygiene, you reduce the risk of your child being infected.

Dishing the dirt on hand-washing

Although we need to come into contact with some germs in order to build up our immune systems and help fight infection, exposure to some germs can lead to nasty illnesses. The best way of preventing exposure to germs is to practise good hygiene and cleanliness – most notably, by keeping your hands clean.

Hand-washing is by far the best way to prevent germs spreading and reduce the chances of your child becoming sick. Hand-washing is the first line of defence against the spread of many illnesses – not only the common cold but also more serious illnesses such as hepatitis A and diarrhoea. In fact, good hand-washing can stop a vast array of illnesses in their tracks.

 Your child needs to understand how to wash his hands properly, so show him how to do it. Try washing your hands together several times a day so that your child realises how important the habit is. Always use warm water and soap, and make sure that you get in between the fingers and under the nails, where uninvited germs like to hide. Don't forget to wash the tops of your hands and your wrists. Ideally, wash for at least 10 seconds. Always rinse and dry well with a clean towel. Not drying hands properly significantly increases the number of germs on your hands, because germs thrive in warm, moist conditions.

To reduce the risk of germs passing around your family, make frequent hand-washing a rule for everyone, especially:

- ✔ Before eating and cooking.
- ✔ After using the toilet – the number of germs on your child's fingertips doubles if he doesn't wash your hands after going to the loo.
- ✔ After touching animals, including pets.
- ✔ After nose-blowing, coughing and sneezing.
- ✔ After being outside or using public transport.
- ✔ After taking care of an unwell person.

Understanding sterilising

When your baby is under 12 months, you should sterilise all his feeding equipment to prevent bacterial contamination. Babies are particularly vulnerable to infections because of their sensitive digestive systems and undeveloped immune systems. The germs that breed in milk curds are particularly nasty. Warm, milky bottles and teats are favourite breeding grounds for bacteria, which can multiply rapidly within half an hour of being in a bottle, causing nasty stomach upsets that can be life-threatening, so never give your baby a half-drunk bottle. Health experts recommend sterilising all your baby's feeding utensils for at least the first 6 months of life – and preferably for up to a year.

Sterilising helps kill potentially harmful bacteria and germs. Before sterilising became the norm, gastroenteritis caused thousands of infant deaths every year. Even today, the majority of baby tummy bugs are the result of inadequate sterilising procedures.

Getting it right

Sterilising's really very simple. Follow these steps:

1. **Before sterilising, wash everything (bottles, neck rings, teats, and tops) separately in hot soapy water.**

   Use a bottle brush and teat cleaner so that every trace of milk is removed. Rinse well and leave to dry or use a clean tea towel or kitchen towel to dry. Remember that germs thrive on used, wet tea towels, so avoid these when drying your baby's feeding equipment.

   Always check bottle teats thoroughly to make sure that they're not clogged with milk. If you use latex teats, pour a little salt in the teat, grind it between your fingers, and rinse thoroughly before sterilising to unclog any milk lurking there. (This is not suitable for silicone teats – just wash them in soap and water.)

2. **Sterilise the bottles using one of the methods listed in the following section.**

3. **Allow the bottles to cool down.**

4. **Fill them with formula and store.**

Selecting a sterilisation method

You can sterilise your baby's feeding equipment in a number of ways:

- ✔ **Get boiling.** This is the simplest and cheapest way to sterilise. Select a large pan and use it solely for sterilising. Don't use the same pan for cooking – your baby won't appreciate the remains of yesterday's baked beans in his bottle. Fill the pan with water and bring it to the boil. Then immerse all the bottle parts fully, ensuring that bottles and teats contain no air pockets.. Cover the pan and leave to boil for at least 10 minutes. You can leave the bottle parts in the covered pan until you're ready to use them again, or you can dry everything with a clean tea towel. The main drawback to boiling is that it can make the teats feel sticky. Also, the bottles tend to go cloudy after a few boils. When this happens, replace the teats and bottles, which you should do every couple of months anyway.

✔ **Use your dishwasher.** Dishwashing's convenient, and is a popular method of sterilising. But it's only effective if you select the right temperature – the water must be at least as hot as 80°C. The main drawback is that bottles won't remain sterile for long after using the dishwasher, so you need to fill them straightaway with formula milk or pumped breast milk.

✔ **Try steaming or microwaving.** Steaming's another simple and efficient way to sterilise. And quick too – most steam steriliser cycles take less than 15 minutes. Microwave steamers are even quicker. Another advantage of this form of sterilising is that no chemicals are involved and so there's no smell or aftertaste. If you keep the lid on the steriliser, the sterilised items will remain sterile for up to 3 hours. Make sure that you place bottles and teats upside-down in the steriliser so they're sterilised fully.

✔ **Use sterilising liquid or tablets.** This is a good way of sterilising when you're on holiday. You can buy sterilising tablets from supermarkets and pharmacies. Fill a large container with water, add the recommended number of tablets or liquid, and totally immerse the equipment, making sure that no air bubbles remain. Leave for about 30 minutes. Rinse with cooled, boiled water before use.

✔ **Keep cooked and raw meat well separated, even in the fridge.** Never let the juices from raw meat drip onto and other food (especially not cooked meat).

Preventing food poisoning

Basic food hygiene's essential for everyone, but especially babies and young children. A lot of the rules involve basic common sense, but be aware of how easily food can be contaminated accidentally.

Following a few simple rules on food safety and hygiene each time you prepare a meal ensures that your child stays in the best of health:

✔ Wash your hands thoroughly before preparing food.

✔ Wash fruit and vegetables before preparation and cooking. (Here's a nice thought for you: All these foods have been handled by someone else before they reach the supermarket shelves . . . and there's no telling where they've been.) Pat dry with clean kitchen towel before serving. For babies, always peel and wash fruit and veg.

✔ Use separate chopping boards for meat and vegetables to help prevent cross-contamination of bacteria. Plastic chopping boards are more hygienic, easier to clean, and less likely to harbour bacteria than wooden boards.

✔ Cook food thoroughly. Always cook meat, fish, and poultry well in order to kill off bacteria and parasites. Meat that has not been cooked thoroughly can be a source of salmonella or listeria food poisoning. To check that meat is cooked properly, stick a skewer or knife into the centre. If it's ready, the juices run clear.

✔ Use clean dry cloths or paper towels for drying up. And remember: Germs multiply on damp cloths and tea towels.

✔ Keep kitchen surfaces clean, including highchairs, fridge door handles, and bin lids, to minimise bacteria growth. After use, thoroughly rinse kitchen cloths and sponges and hang out to dry.

✔ Keep pets away from areas where you prepare food. Never let cats walk on work surfaces or tabletops, as they can pass on lethal germs and infections such as toxoplasmosis.

✔ Place unused food in sealed containers or cover with cling film and place in the fridge. Store raw meat at the bottom of the fridge to stop meat juices dripping on to other foods.

✔ Don't keep half-used jars of baby food from which you've fed your baby, as saliva can quickly contaminate the food. Far better to transfer some food into a bowl and put the rest back in the fridge.

✔ Don't give your baby opened food that's been left in the fridge for more than 24 hours.

✔ Never refreeze cooked food that's already been frozen before: Refreezing can cause bacterial contamination.

The risk of food poisoning increases in warm weather. Always put things back in the fridge when you've finished using them.

Treating food poisoning and tummy upsets

The most important part of treating a baby or child with food poisoning is replacing fluids lost through vomiting and diarrhoea. Make sure that your child drinks lots of fluids – avoid sugary drinks and fruit juice, because they can irritate the stomach. Water is best. Drinking little and often is a good rule of thumb. Even if your child vomits the fluid, some of what he drinks is likely to remain his body, so continue to offer fluids even if he's vomiting. Look out for symptoms of dehydration. If your baby is under 6 months old, continue to breastfeed or bottle-feed him and offer extra drinks of cooled, boiled water between feeds. (See Chapter 13 for more on dealing with dehydration.)

If your child is over 6 months old and has mild to moderate dehydration, your doctor may prescribe oral rehydration powders. But *never* give your child any other medicines to stop diarrhoea or vomiting. Most anti-diarrhoea medicines are not suitable for children and may cause side effects such as drowsiness and skin reactions. Antibiotics are not normally necessary either, unless your child gets a specific bacterial infection.

If your baby is less than 6 months old and shows signs of a stomach upset, such as watery, green poo or vomiting, call a doctor. If your child becomes severely dehydrated, he will need urgent hospital treatment and possibly intravenous fluid replacement, which helps your child's body to absorb fluids and salts. Signs of severe dehydration include pale skin, a sunken fontanelle, and a dry nappy for several hours.

Talking about your pet subject

Having a pet has many benefits. For example, studies show that children with furry friends seem less likely to suffer from allergies and appear less stressed than children without pets. But hygiene must be your number-one priority: All animals can carry infections, and some of these infections are dangerous to humans. Two of the most common and potentially harmful infections that animals can pass on to humans are toxoplasmosis and toxocariasis:

- ✔ **Toxoplasmosis:** This infection is caused by bacteria present in cat and dog faeces. The same bacteria can also be transmitted via raw meat. The symptoms of the disease are similar to those of glandular fever. In rare cases, toxoplasmosis causes blindness if the bacteria passes to the eye. Toxoplasmosis is also dangerous to pregnant women, as it can cause deformities, including brain and eye damage, in the unborn baby. Always wash your child's hands after he's handled an animal and discourage him from eating and handling pets at the same time.

- ✔ **Toxocariasis:** Dogs and, less commonly, cats carry the worms that cause toxocariasis and can pass on the infection to humans. Almost all puppies are born with toxocariasis. The infected animal excretes the worm eggs in its faeces. Worm your dog or cat regularly and scoop up and dispose of faeces carefully. Many children don't present any symptoms of the disease, and may not need treatment, but in severe cases it can cause fever, wheezing, and swollen glands. It can also affect your child's eyes, causing damage to the retina. Your doctor can take blood tests to determine whether your child has the condition, which can be treated with medication.

Keep pets well away from areas where you prepare and cook food. Don't let your pet poo where children play. Clear up any dog mess immediately.

Nursery Nasties

After your child starts mixing regularly with other children, he is going to be exposed to a lot more germs and bacteria than before. Coughs and colds spread easily in nursery environments, but a few other things pass around too.

Nitpicking

Having a load of tiny insects living in your child's hair is probably not what you had in mind when you hoped he'd make friends at nursery. But before you freak out, let's set the record straight: Head lice are *not* a sign of bad hygiene. Lice are notoriously unfussy about the hair they live in – they happily survive on any head (apart from completely bald ones). Unfortunately, head lice are incredibly common among young children. Head lice spread by head-to-head contact. Youngsters often play with their heads close together, and so they're pretty likely to pick up lice. If your child has head lice, try to keep him away from other children until you've treated the problem.

Head lice are tiny grey or brown insects. The adults reach around 2 mm in length – about the size of a sesame seed. The lice live on your child's scalp, feeding by sucking blood. The females lay eggs (nits), which look like tiny white or brown dots sticking to your child's hair. Nits take 7–10 days to hatch, and the insects take another 7–14 days to become fully mature. They then can mate and lay eggs.

Itching isn't necessarily a symptom unless the lice have been living in your child's hair for a while. The only way you can be sure is by looking for lice and eggs in the hair.

The best way to get rid of head lice is to wash your child's hair, put on loads of conditioner, and then comb through with a special nit comb. You can buy a nit comb at your pharmacy. A plastic comb with closely spaced teeth is best so they catch the head lice. After each stroke, wipe the comb on a tissue or run it under a tap until all the lice have gone – they normally just slide off. You can get battery-operated combs, although many people don't find them very effective.

If your child has lice, you must check and treat the whole family, in order to avoid spreading the lice to and from each other.

You can also use a specially formulated insecticide lotion to kill the lice. Ask your pharmacist to recommend a lotion suitable for your child. Many of these lotions contain powerful chemicals, so repeated use is not recommended. Health shops and pharmacies supply several natural remedies for lice. Whatever treatment you use, read the label and follow the directions carefully. If the eggs continue to hatch, use wet combing with conditioner instead.

Wet combing is effective in removing the lice, but ordinary combing doesn't remove the eggs. Therefore, you must wet comb every 3–4 days to catch any new lice that have hatched – the trick is to catch the lice before they mature and lay eggs. If you wet comb consistently, the lice should be cleared within 2 weeks.

Worrying about worms

As if head lice aren't enough to contend with, your child is likely to get some unwelcome visitors down the other end, too. In fact, nearly half of all children under the age of 10 years have worms at some point. The good news is they're not harmful – but they can be extremely itchy and uncomfortable, and they need treatment.

By far the most common form of worm children catch is the threadworm. Threadworms look like fine white threads of cotton up to 10 mm in length. They cause itching at night, when the female worm comes out to lay eggs around your child's anus. You may see worms in your child's stools, or be alerted by complaints of an itchy bottom. The itching may be worse at night, when your child is warmest; and he may itch in his sleep and the eggs caught under his fingernails. Then, if your child put his fingers in his mouth, the eggs can be transferred back into his body, re-infecting your child all over again. They can also be spread to other children your child comes into contact with.

If your child has threadworms, go to your GP and get a single tablet (or liquid) for the whole family. On the day of treatment, vacuum all carpets and damp-dust all smooth surfaces in the house. Wash around your child's anus every morning to get rid of eggs, and let the school or nursery know, so that they can check their hygiene. You don't need to keep your child at home.

Threadworms, unlike head lice, can survive for up to two weeks away from a human host. That's why, unlike with a head lice infestation, you need to wash all clothes and bedding if your child is infected. Help prevent future worm infections by keeping your child's nails short and well scrubbed and encouraging everyone in the family to wash their hands after going to the toilet, and before preparing and eating food. Be vigilant about hand-washing! You can also help get rid of worm eggs at home by washing clothes, bed linen, and pyjamas on a hot wash and getting your child to wear underpants in bed and change them in the morning.

Dealing with sticky eyes

Sticky eyes – known more correctly as conjunctivitis – is a condition caused by a bacterial or viral infection in which the protective transparent membranes of the eye become red and inflamed. Conjunctivitis passes easily from one eye to the other, and from one person to another. Keeping the eye clean is essential. You also need to keep your child away from nursery or school until the infection has cleared up.

Red itchy eyes are the most obvious symptom. The lower part of the eye becomes sticky with a discharge that may cause the eyelids to become crusted and stuck together, especially after your child has been asleep.

Before treatment, always wash your own hands. Bathe your child's eyes with clean cotton wool dipped in cooled, boiled salt water. Wipe from the inner to the outer part of the eye. Use a fresh piece of cotton wool for each stroke and each eye. And – of course – always wash your hands after treatment as well. If the condition doesn't clear up within a day or two, see your GP, who can prescribe some antibiotic eyedrops.

Tackling Teeth

Looking after your child's teeth during the early years has lifelong health benefits. Healthy baby teeth help make strong adult teeth, and oral hygiene is essential to prevent problems such as gingivitis (gum disease). As well as brushing your child's teeth regularly, you can do plenty of other things to help keep his teeth strong and healthy. Chapter 7 includes information about teething.

Getting protective

You don't need to be a trained dentist to be aware that the main cause of tooth decay is sugar. Present in so many foods and drinks, sugar is the number-one enemy of teeth, so you need to keep a close eye on your child's intake of the sweet stuff. But don't panic! You don't need to ban all sweet treats altogether, so your child still loves you.

Letting your child have sugar little and often may sound sensible, but is actually far more harmful than giving lots of sweets in one sitting. Frequent contact with sugar, even in small quantities, is extremely damaging to tooth enamel. The less time sugar is in contact with your child's teeth, the less chance there is of decay.

Of course, all children love sweet things. It can be difficult to keep your child's cravings under control. The following tips can keep your toddler – and his teeth – happy.

- ✔ **Stick to mealtimes.** Save cakes and puddings for mealtimes and encourage your child to finish off with a small mouthful of cheese afterwards to help neutralise harmful acid. It normally takes 20 minutes for saliva to neutralise acid formed by eating sugar, but eating something savoury like cheese can reduce the neutralising time to 10 minutes.

- ✔ **Have a sweet time.** Introduce a once-a-week sweet day so your child has his sweet ration in one hit. Encourage him to eat his sweets quickly: A handful of sweets finished off in 10 minutes is better than one sweet every couple of hours. Choose your child's sweets carefully: Sugary fragments from chewy sweets can get stuck on his teeth for ages, and lollipops are just as bad because they last such a long time. Chocolate's the best choice.

- ✔ **Choose snacks carefully.** Dried fruit may be healthier than sweets, but it contains lots of sugar and, like chewy sweets, can stick to your child's teeth for ages. Keep dried fruit for mealtimes only. Fresh fruit – especially apples – also has a high sugar content, so clean your child's teeth afterwards whenever possible.

- ✔ **Think about drinks.** Drinking juice or milk from a bottle or baby beaker is harmful for your child's teeth and is a primary cause of tooth decay. The liquid washes around the teeth for longer than when your child simply swallows liquid straight from a cup. Wean your child on to a cup as soon as possible and keep juice and milk for mealtimes only. Plain water between meals will quench his thirst.

Keeping teeth clean

Tooth decay occurs when the natural bacteria in the mouth mix with sugars in bits of food left on the teeth. The bacteria produce an acid that then attacks the tooth's protective layer of enamel. Brushing your child's teeth regularly is crucial to keeping them healthy and decay-free.

You need a toothbrush – for babies and young children, a small, soft-bristled brush is best – and a specially formulated child's toothpaste.

Consider investing in a rechargeable electric toothbrush to make cleaning easier and more fun.

Have your child brush his teeth twice a day – after breakfast and before bed. To brush your toddler's teeth, put a pea-sized amount of toothpaste on his brush and follow these steps:

1. **Sit your child on your lap facing away from you, or stand behind him. Gently hold his forehead to keep him still.**

2. **Gently massage his teeth and gums with the brush.**

   Pay special attention to the molars (the 'chewing' teeth at the sides) as food can easily stick to their irregular surfaces. But don't put too much pressure on any of the teeth.

   Brush for 2–3 minutes – use an egg timer if it helps!

3. **Encourage your child to spit when you've finished so he doesn't swallow too much fluoride.**

Too much fluoride is not good for your child (or you). Never let a child under the age of 7 years use adult toothpaste, because it contains too much fluoride. Encourage your child to spit out rather than swallow the toothpaste. In a few parts of the UK, fluoride is added to drinking water. As there have been some concerns about the health risks of too much fluoride, you may wish to ask your dentist or doctor for advice.

If your child refuses to open his mouth and let you brush, have a few tricks up your sleeve. Try asking him to brush your teeth for you first – then he can let you do his. Promise your child a song or a story while you brush. And let him choose his own toothbrush – crazy, colourful brushes work just as well as boring ones and can make brushing much more fun for a child.

You need to brush your child's teeth until he's at least 7 years old. He won't have the manual dexterity to brush his teeth properly until he's mastered reasonable handwriting.

Visiting the dentist

After your child's first teeth come through, you should take him to the dentist for regular checks, so that any problems with decay can be detected early and also helps your child get used to the whole dental experience. Talk to your child about the trip so he knows what to expect: Tell him that the dentist will look in his mouth, count his teeth, and use his fingers and maybe a tiny mirror to check that all's well. On the day, if your child's nervous, let him sit on your lap in the dentist's chair. The session won't last more than a few minutes.

Going over the top: Our germ-free world

Antibacterial soaps, detergents, toys, and even clothes – the list keeps growing. With so many antibacterial products out there, you'd imagine that the war on germs had been won. But unfortunately, the reality is that all these germ-killing products may end up leaving us even more vulnerable to infection. Overuse and misuse of antibacterial products may kill off good bacteria, such as those that aid digestion, and weak bacteria, leaving behind the strongest, most resistant bacteria.

Exposure to germs – and getting infected by some of them – strengthens the body's natural immune system against allergies. Many experts regard our use of disinfectants and antibacterials as interfering with our early exposure to germs and disturbing the body's system for recognition and response to bacteria and viruses. The unused immune system, which is keen to do its job, therefore sees dust and pollen as dangerous invaders and responds in a way that causes asthma and allergies (they're discussed in more detail in Chapter 15).

Antibacterial products appear to offer little protection against the most common germs that cause illness anyway, which is good news for parents, who don't really want to spend all their time cleaning and disinfecting. Soap and water wash away most harmful germs perfectly adequately.

Part IV
Symptoms, Illnesses, and Treatments

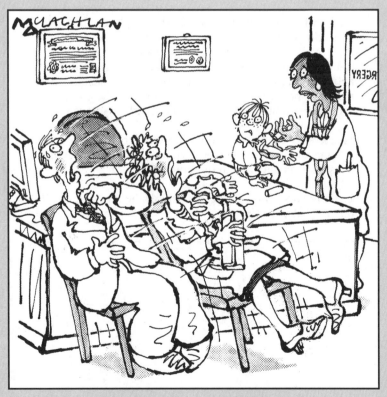

"Now, Simon, I hope you're all right with needles......"

In this part . . .

When your baby or child is ill it is distressing for both of you, especially if you're not sure what's wrong with your little precious.

This part helps you to diagnose what might be the problem, and offers solutions to make your child feel better. Chapter 13 covers all the aches – headaches, earaches, tummy aches, and sore throats. Chapter 14 gives tips about coping with common infections from measles to mumps, and you can use this chapter with the colour section to identify any rashes your child may develop.

This is also the part for you if want to know more about asthma and eczema, and behavioural and emotional problems such as autism and hyperactivity.

If you're concerned about your child's health, don't hesitate to visit your GP.

Chapter 13

Symptoms and What They May Mean

*A*ll children suffer from minor illnesses at some stage – which doesn't come as much comfort when your little treasure's poorly. Having an ill child is one of the most worrying aspects of being a parent: Is your child seriously ill or simply fighting off a bug? Should you dial 999 or just administer a little infant paracetamol and lots of TLC? The rule of thumb is that you should always call a doctor if you're at all concerned about your child's health – you understand your child better than anyone else and your instinct's likely to be right.

In this chapter, you can read about how to spot the signs of some of the most common complaints that affect children, such as tummy pain and headaches, and what you can do to help soothe them.

Tackling Headaches Head-on

Although headaches are rare in young children, they become more frequent as they get older. By school age, most children have complained of at least one headache. Because a headache is often difficult to work out exactly where it's hurting, your child may find it hard to describe what she's feeling.

Headaches don't occur in the brain – there aren't any sensory nerves there. Rather, headache pain is located in the membranes surrounding the brain or in the muscles and blood vessels beneath the scalp.

Causes of headaches include all sorts of things, from colds and fevers to stress, hunger, and overactivity. By far the most common type of headache in children is psychogenic or stress headache, which can be caused by anything from reading for too long to worrying about something. This sort of headache tends to come on gradually during the day and is felt all over the head rather than in one particular area.

Your child (and you) can get headaches because of eye strain, which becomes more likely when she's reading, or looking at a blackboard at school. Headaches caused by eye strain are usually felt around the eyes and/or the temples, and you may also spot that your child tends to screw his eyes up or sit very close to the television. If you have any doubts about your child's eyesight, you must get it checked. If she's under five years old, your health visitor can arrange for an eye check with an optician at the hospital. All children under the age of 16 are eligible for free eye checks at high street ophthalmic opticians.

In extremely rare cases, a headache is a sign of a serious brain infection such as meningitis. Chapter 14 introduces you to the symptoms of these rarer diseases.

A headache without other symptoms, such as fever, usually passes in a few hours and is rarely serious, especially if it improves after giving infant paracetamol and some TLC.

Finding and solving the problem

Simple and common triggers of headaches include missing a meal, which can affect blood-sugar levels and cause irritability as well as headaches, being in a smoky room, spending too long in hot sunshine, dehydration, and reading or sitting in front of a television or computer screen for a long time.

If your child has a headache:

- ✔ Suggest she lies down in a quiet room and draw the curtains. Put a cool, damp towel on her forehead and give her plenty to drink and a snack if she's missed a meal. You can give infant paracetamol to take the edge off the pain.

- ✔ Check her temperature with a fever strip or thermometer. If her temperature's high (38°C or more), cool her down by removing layers of clothing and reducing the room temperature by switching central heating off (a common cause of headaches). Also, you can give her the correct dose of infant paracetamol. For more on fevers and how to treat them, go to Chapter 17.

✔ Look for other symptoms, such as a stuffy or runny nose, which indicate that your child has a cold or bug. If your child's getting over a cold and the pain's around the top of her nose and eyes, and is worse when she wakes up, she may have sinusitis (for more on the subject look at the later section 'Sussing out sinusitis').

Managing migraine

If your child gets frequent headaches on one side of the head, feels nauseous, vomits, isn't feverish, and wants to be in a dark room, she may suffer from migraine. *Migraine* is a throbbing ache that tends to affect the front of the head and the temples, often on only one side of the head. Visual disturbances, problems with hearing or smelling, nausea, and vomiting are quite common during migraine. The best thing you can do is give your child infant paracetamol and let her lie in a darkened room and sleep it off.

Sussing out sinusitis

Sinusitis is an inflammation or infection of the membrane lining the sinuses. Sinusitis is common in older children. The *sinuses* are situated around the bones of the face and filter and pre-warm air before the air is transferred to the lungs. The sinuses that most commonly become infected are those in the forehead between the eyes and in the cheekbones on either side of the nose.

Sinusitis usually follows a bacterial infection or a viral illness such as a cold. The condition develops when the drainage holes that lead from the sinuses into the back of the nose become blocked. Sinuses may also become infected as a complication of the swelling of the mucous membranes associated with allergic rhinitis. Some children get an attack of sinusitis with every cold, but others are never affected. Sinusitis is more common in children older than 10 years.

Symptoms of sinusitis include thick yellowish or white nasal mucus, pain or tenderness around the forehead, nose, and eyes, and sometimes a fever. To ease the pain of sinusitis, follow the same steps for a headache (more details are in 'Finding and solving the problem' earlier in the chapter). Your child's doctor may prescribe antibiotics or a nasal decongestant to reduce the inflammation and allow the sinuses to drain.

 Put a vaporiser in your child's bedroom, or prepare a wide-bottomed bowl of warm water and let your child breathe in the steam. You can add herbal decongestant drops if you wish. Sit your child at a table and drape a towel over her head to direct the steam towards her face. But don't leave her alone while she's inhaling. If your child is prone to sinusitis, use a vaporiser or give regular steam inhalations whenever she gets a cold. Show her how to pinch her nose when she jumps into water to prevent water being forced into the sinuses.

When a headache's an emergency

Occasionally, a headache's a sign that your child needs immediate medical help. Consult your doctor in the following situations:

✔ Your child's headaches are severe and/or recur frequently.

✔ Your child's headaches wake her up or are worse when she wakes up.

✔ Your child seems listless.

In the following situations, call an ambulance or go to the hospital immediately:

✔ Your child has a fever, is vomiting, is intolerant of bright lights, has pain when bending her chin to chest, and is drowsy or distant. If your child shows the above symptoms, the cause may be meningitis or encephalitis (inflammation of the brain).

✔ Your child has had a recent bang on the head and complains of a headache – she may have a head injury. Other signs of head injury include confused or odd behaviour, drowsiness, vomiting, and difficulty breathing.

Mum, I've Got Earache!

If you're the parent of a screaming baby or a noisy toddler, you may think it's only *you* that suffers from earache. But if your child complains from earache, she may have an ear infection. Earaches often start during or shortly after a cold or other bug. The infection spreads to one or both ears, making them swollen, blocked, and painful. Children under the age of 6 years are particularly vulnerable to earache – in fact, earache is one of the most common reasons for children to visit their GP. If your child has an allergy, she may be more susceptible to earache. And if she goes to day nursery or has just started school, she may be even more prone, because she'll be exposed to many more infections.

Two main types of earache in children are:

✔ **Outer-ear infections.** Also called *otitis externa* and swimmers' ear, outer-ear infections are usually caused by water getting into the ear through swimming or bathing, causing infection and inflammation. Your child will have earache and possibly discharge from the ear. If your child suffers from otitis externa, always rinse her hair with a shower attachment, to avoid tipping her whole head back into the bath.

✔ **Middle-ear infections.** (Also known as *otitis media*.) These occur when the eardrum fills with pus. They are very common in young children because their Eustachian tubes, which connect the ears with the back of the throat, are still very narrow and short, making it easier for bacteria and viruses to travel from the nose and throat to the middle ear. Risk factors for getting a lot of middle-ear infections include having a parent or other family member that smokes, having another family member who had a lot of ear infections, and drinking from a bottle while lying down. Ear infections are less common in babies who breastfeed, possibly because of the semi-upright position involved, but also because of the infection-fighting antibodies present in breast milk.

Sometimes, during a severe middle-ear infection your child's eardrum may 'burst' or perforate because of the build-up of pressure. After the eardrum bursts, your child's pain reduces dramatically. The hole in the eardrum normally heals in about a week, but your child should avoid swimming and should cover the ear when washing for at least a month afterwards.

Spotting the symptoms

If your baby has an ear infection, she may tug at her ear or rub the side of her face. She's miserable, off her feeds, and may be feverish. She may have vomiting and diarrhoea. Her sleep is also disrupted.

Your older child will probably complain of a throbbing ache or a sharp, stabbing pain in her ear, which can be excruciating. She may say her ear feels 'full' or blocked. The pain may follow a cold or cough, and your child may be feverish. If the pain stops suddenly, the eardrum may have ruptured. You may see pus, sometimes streaked with blood, oozing out of your child's ear.

In both babies and older children, you may also find a red scaly area around the opening of the ear and yellow discharge from the ear. Earwax is a yellowy-brown secretion produced by glands in the ear canal to clean and moisten the canal. Most children produce only small amounts, but some children make so much that it blocks the canal. The sudden appearance of runny wax in the canal may be a sign of a middle-ear infection.

In rare cases, ear infections can lead to a severe complication called *mastoiditis*, which affects the mastoid bone around the ear. If your child gets mastoiditis, she's very unwell, often with a high fever (over 39 degrees). She may also have redness of the ear or behind the ear, and the area behind the ear may be extremely tender to touch. If you suspect your child may have mastoiditis, seek medical help immediately.

Treating the infection

If your child is suffering from an ear infection, try the following to ease her discomfort:

✔ Gently wash off any sticky or crusted discharge on her ear lobe with warm water and cotton wool. Never wash inside your child's ear, as doing so can re-infect the ear.

Always leave your child's ear canal well alone – never put anything in the ear that's smaller than your elbow! If necessary, gently wipe wax off the earlobe with cotton wool and warm water, but never try to remove wax from the canal with a cotton bud – you may impact the wax and make the condition worse.

✔ Check your child's temperature. If she is running a high temperature, give the correct dose of infant paracetamol and consult your doctor.

✔ Try to stop your child from touching or scratching her ear. Wipe away any discharge from the outside – but leave the ear canal well alone.

✔ To relieve your child's pain, warm a soft cloth on a radiator and place it on your baby's sheet or your older child's pillow to lay her head on, with the affected ear against the cloth. Alternatively, suggest your child rests her cheek against a thickly covered hot-water bottle.

✔ If your child gets regular ear infections, consider visiting a homeopath. Homeopathy is becoming increasing recognised for its effectiveness in treating ear problems.

✔ Most ear infections are caused by viruses and clear up without treatment. However, your doctor may prescribe antibiotics if she considers the infection is caused by bacteria, especially if the infection takes more than a week to clear up.

✔ Wait until your child's ear infection has cleared before letting her go swimming. If possible, don't wash her hair if her ear is infected – if you really have to wash it, use a shower cap or earplugs to protect her ear and stop water or shampoo getting in.

A young child with earache may not want a doctor to look at her ear with an *otoscope*, an instrument for examining the ear. Ask the doctor to examine your child's less painful ear first or even to look in teddy's ear first (wait until you're out of the surgery before you laugh though!).

Flying or travelling through a deep tunnel can give your child intense earache, especially if she has a cold, because of the change in air pressure. On takeoff and landing and when travelling through tunnels, give your child a sweet to suck or a straw to drink through or breastfeed your baby.

Getting All Gummed Up about Glue Ear

Glue ear (also known as *otitis media* with effusion) is extremely common in children and can cause distressing partial deafness. You may find that the condition comes and goes as the ear clears itself and then becomes blocked again. Most children recover from glue ear within six months, and the deafness always clears on its own eventually. Some children, however, get glue ear on and off until they're 10 years old or so.

Bouts of glue ear can start in early infancy and can be very disruptive for your child. The two peak ages are around 1–2 years and again at 5 years, when your child starts school and is exposed to a large number of bacteria and viruses. You must get treatment for your child's glue ear: The condition tends to affect children at important developmental stages, and if she can't hear properly her speech, behaviour, and reading may be affected.

The lining of the middle ear produces mucus to fight infection. If it produces too much mucus, the mucus can cause a blockage in the ear tubes. Normally, mucus drains away down the Eustachian tube to the back of the throat, but problems with this drainage system are common in children because the tubes are so short and do not slope downwards as steeply as in adults, making it easy for bacteria and viruses to collect and travel from the throat and nose into the middle-ear cavity. If your child gets repeated infections, the Eustachian tubes can become blocked. The problem may be made worse if your child's adenoids are also swollen, because they can block the entrance to the tubes. If the tubes are blocked, mucus collects in the middle ear, thickens, and becomes gluey, making it difficult for your child to hear properly.

The effects of glue ear vary from day to day, so many parents wonder whether their children hear when they 'want to'. In fact, a child with glue ear hears when she can.

Spotting signs of glue ear

If your baby has glue ear, she may have the following symptoms:

✔ She may not respond to your voice or turn to a noise.

✔ By 9 months of age, she may become really distressed when you're out of sight, or she may jump when you appear suddenly because she can't hear you approaching.

✔ She may be unusually clingy and difficult, and her sleep may be disrupted.

✔ She may be more prone to catching colds.

If your older child has glue ear, you may notice the following:

- ✔ She may watch intently as she lip-reads or observes gestures.

- ✔ She may behave badly: In a few children, the most obvious sign of glue ear is disruptive behaviour, often borne out of sheer frustration and poor concentration.

- ✔ She may sit very close to the television and have the volume too loud.

- ✔ She may find it hard to sit still and concentrate, especially in a group.

- ✔ She may complain of pain. Glue ear isn't usually painful, but some older children complain of a blocked ear. The condition is usually worse for a few weeks after your child's recovered from a cold. Glue ear is usually more continuous in winter.

Working out what to do

If you suspect your child is deaf, even intermittently, see your doctor (or your health visitor if your child's under 5 years old). Your doctor or health visitor may also refer your child to an audiologist to test her hearing. If your child is in pain, see your GP rather than your health visitor, in case your child has an infection.

Antibiotics usually clear the 'glue'. Eventually, however the glue returns. Your doctor may prescribe your child mild steroids to reduce any inflammation and to stimulate the Eustachian tubes to open, so that air pressure on either side of the eardrum is equalised.

Allergy-prone children seem to suffer more from glue ear than other children. If your doctor feels that the cause of your child's glue ear is allergic, she may suggest ways to reduce your child's exposure to certain *allergens* (the substances that cause allergy). Your doctor may also recommend antihistamines to dampen the allergic reaction.

If your child's hearing is significantly affected over several months, she may be referred to an Ear, Nose and Throat (ENT) surgeon at the hospital. The surgeon may recommend a straightforward operation under general anaesthetic to cut a slit in the eardrum, drain the glue, and maintain an open airflow into the middle ear. Your child may have her adenoids removed in the same operation to help prevent glue ear returning (this operation is much less common than it used to be, because it rarely helps).

During the operation, the surgeon may insert grommets into a tiny slit in one or both eardrums. *Grommets* are tiny plastic tubes, shaped like mini cotton reels, which allow air to flow in and out of the middle ear and normalise air pressure behind the middle ear. Grommets often produce a dramatic improvement in hearing. Grommets can stay in place for up to a year before they fall out. If your child is expected to need grommet treatment repeatedly or over a long period of time, she may have a special type of grommet fitted that remains in place much longer. The hole in the eardrum heals up quickly, but if the glue returns the grommet may need to be replaced.

Prevent water from getting through the grommet into your child's middle ear, where it can cause an increase in pressure and possibly an infection. Watertight earplugs for hair-washing are essential, to avoid gettting soapy water in the ear. Swimming on or just below the surface of a pool is fine (preferably with earplugs), as the pressure isn't enough to force water through the grommet, but avoid diving and underwater swimming because they put much more pressure on the eardrum.

Grommets are not magic cures for ear infections. Although they do help many children, some children continue to get ear infections.

Coping with glue ear

To communicate with your child with glue ear, talk to her face to face. Give simple clear instructions and be ready to repeat them. Turn off the radio or television while talking so your child hears only one source of sound. Choose a playgroup or nursery with small groups and structured activities.

Read to your child, sing songs with her, and help her repeat rhymes to build up her speech. If her speech is affected, ask your health visitor to refer your child for a speech therapy assessment.

If your child is 3 years old or more, show her how to blow her nose, one nostril at a time, to keep the middle ear aerated.

Getting to the Bottom of Tummy Ache

For your child, 'tummy ache' can be a catch-all term for many problems. Tummy ache results from all sorts of causes – most aren't anything to worry about, but you should always investigate, just in case your child's tummy ache is a sign of something serious. Common causes of tummy ache range from viruses, constipation, and wind, through urinary tract infections, to anxiety and food sensitivity. Tummy ache can also be a sign of an underlying childhood infection, as most illnesses can cause abdominal pain – even minor respiratory infections such as colds and sore throats can cause the lymph glands around the body to enlarge, and the glands in the abdomen can become uncomfortable as part of this generalised reaction, leading to abdominal pain. Although the pain normally settles without specific treatment, infant paracetamol or ibuprofen and drinking plenty of fluids can help.

The causes of abdominal pain may not just be physical – abdominal pain can be triggered by emotions such as stress or anxiety. For example, if your child is worried about something – perhaps going to school or the dentist – she may complain of tummy ache. This is a real pain – the gut and bowel are affected by anxiety and tend to tense up when your child's stressed, causing the painful symptoms.

Symptoms of a possible urine infection include strong or offensive smelling urine; dark coloured or cloudy urine; or tummy pain associated with vomiting or a fever. Remember that young children may not get, or may not be able to describe, the symptoms grown-ups associate with urine infections (such as burning pain on passing urine, or the need to pass urine much more often). If your child gets any of these symptoms, see your GP.

Helping to soothe away the pain

As a symptom on its own, tummy ache usually disappears without any treatment. Sometimes you can guess at the cause – for example, your child may have eaten too much or too quickly and simply have indigestion. Often, however, you never find of the cause of your child's tummy ache.

But tummy ache can be a sign of a serious illness, so keep an eye on your child for any other signs of illness or worsening of the pain.

If your child does complain of a tummy ache, the following can help her:

- ✔ Let your child lie down if she wants to. Give her water to drink, but avoid food and other drinks, as they can aggravate the problem.
- ✔ A covered hot-water bottle can help ease your child's tummy pain, but never leave your child alone with a hot-water bottle because of the risk of burning.

Your child may complain of tummy ache to express stress, worry, or even deep unhappiness. If you see a pattern to her symptoms, probe her gently for any worries or concerns she may have, such as school problems.

Consult your doctor if your child's tummy pain is so bad that she's bent double or crying persistently, if she vomits for more than an hour or so, if the pain keeps recurring, if the pain continues for more than six hours without any improvement, if you detect any tenderness of swelling in the groin or testicles, or if she vomits but the pain continues.

Diagnosing constipation

Often, tummy ache is simply a sign that your child needs to do a poo. Signs of constipation include the following:

- ✔ Fewer bowel movements than normal (your child may not have a movement for several days).

- ✔ Pain and strain when doing a poo. If your child hasn't been to the toilet for a long time, her poo will be hard, dry, and difficult to pass. Your child may say it hurts.

- ✔ When your child does go to the toilet, she may pass her poo in small, dry pellets.

- ✔ She may seem anxious or upset when trying to go to the toilet.

- ✔ She may have a sore bottom. If your child has to strain, the skin around her anus can tear and become sore and cracked and you may see streaks of blood in her stools.

See your doctor if you're worried about your child's constipation, as it can get worse if you wait. Your doctor may prescribe laxatives to get your child's bowels moving, but they are a last resort.

Never give laxatives to your child without seeking advice from your doctor.

If your child's constipated, the most important thing you can do is increase her fluid intake. One of the major causes of constipation is dehydration, so give her lots of water or diluted fruit juice, and keep offering her drinks. Here are some other suggestions:

- ✔ Increase the amount of fibre your child eats. Foods high in fibre help her pass stools more easily. Good sources of fibre include fresh fruit and vegetables and wholegrain cereal. Prunes, raisins, oats, and bran are particularly good.

- ✔ Encourage your child to be as physically active as possible. Activity helps boost her circulation and increases the oxygen supply to her vital organs, keeping them functioning well and more able to pass food through the digestive tract.

✔ Massage her tummy in a clockwise direction. Massage can also be nice and soothing, and may ease discomfort by getting rid of trapped wind.

✔ Try to stay relaxed about your child's toilet habits – don't put her under pressure to perform.

Sometimes, constipation can be psychological rather than physical. Children who have recently been potty- or toilet-trained often go through a phase of 'holding on' to their poo. This fear of letting go is quite normal, and you'll need to be patient but encouraging at the same time.

Contact your doctor if you see blood in your child's stools. Your doctor may recommend an anaesthetic gel to relieve any tears in your child's anus.

Beating tummy bugs

Simple hygiene measures will reduce the risk of your child getting tummy bugs, but they can't eliminate it. You *will* end up clearing up vomit and runny poo at some point in your child's early years!

A tummy bug, or gastroenteritis, is inflammation of the stomach and intestines. One of the most common causes of gastroenteritis is a virus called rotavirus, which is highly infectious. Virtually every child in the UK will suffer from a rotavirus infection by the age of five, and catching it once won't necessarily give her immunity. Fortunately, most cases of gastroenteritis, including the kind caused by rotavirus, settle down on their own within a few days, without causing any lasting harm.

Gastroenteritis can be passed easily from one child to another, by droplets in the air or via unwashed hands touching food that is then eaten by another child. A significant number of cases of gastroenteritis are caused by food poisoning, particularly in the summer. Signs of food poisoning include fever, vomiting that lasts up to three days, and diarrhoea – your child may need to go to the loo several times a day.

Symptoms of gastroenteritis often settle after a few days or so as the immune system usually clears the infection. Try to do the following until your child's symptoms ease:

✔ **Give lots to drink.** This is the most important thing you can do – it's essential to avoid your child dehydrating. Water is by far the best fluid to give, although oral rehydration solution can be useful for older children. Even if your child is vomiting or feels sick, still give her frequent sips, as she will absorb some of the fluid. Ice lollies are a useful extra source of fluid, preferably home-made from juice or very dilute squash.

Doctors (and old wives!) used to advise that flat fizzy drinks or sweetened drinks were helpful for gastroenteritis, but experts now consider that this advice is wrong. In a few cases, very sweet drinks can actually suck fluid out of your child's blood and into their gut, increasing the risk of dehydration and making them more ill. If your child really doesn't like water or oral rehydration solution, use a watered-down squash or juice, but it should be as weak as possible.

If you're breastfeeding or your baby is under one year old and bottle-fed, continue to feed her normally. If possible, give extra fluids to prevent dehydration. Frequently offer water from a bottle, or even from a sterilised spoon.

✔ **Give rehydration drinks.** Only give them on a doctor's advice. Your doctor may recommend oral rehydration salts if she's concerned about the risk of dehydration in your child. You can give rehydration drinks instead of or in addition to normal drinks. Rehydration drinks are made up from sachets of powder that you buy from your pharmacy: Add the contents of the sachet to the correct amount of water to provide your child with a perfect balance of water, salt, and sugar. Rehydration drinks are better than water alone because the small amount of sugar and salt helps the body absorb the water. They don't stop or reduce diarrhoea, but they're the best drinks to prevent or treat dehydration.

Don't use home-made rehydration drinks, as the quantity of salt must be exact.

✔ **Let your child eat as normally as possible.** You don't need to 'starve' your child when she has gastroenteritis. Withholding your child's food used to be advised but is now thought to be wrong. However, if your child doesn't want to eat, don't force her to. Drinks are the most important thing – food can wait until her appetite returns. Offer some food every now and then. Soups and food high in carbohydrate such as bread, pasta, rice, and potatoes are best to start with.

See a doctor if you suspect your child is getting dehydrated. Your child is unlikely to get dehydrated if she's over 1 year old. Babies under 6 months are much more at risk. Symptoms include being floppy and listless, with sunken eyes, and having dry nappies and/or no bowel movements for 12 hours or more. If you suspect your child is dehydrated, or if they have blood in their poo, seek medical help.

Never give over-the-counter anti-diarrhoea medicines to your young child. They aren't suitable for children and can cause damage.

Regular hand-washing using warm water and soap after going to the lavatory and before eating is one of the most effective ways to prevent your child getting gastroenteritis. Hand-washing is particularly important if your child's recovering from a gastric bug.

Checking for appendicitis

Recognising the symptoms of appendicitis and how they differ from those seen in run-of-the-mill tummy aches is important. Appendicitis isn't a very common cause of abdominal pain, but if your child does have appendicitis she must have immediate medical attention.

Appendicitis is an acute inflammation of the *appendix*, a small tube-like organ that's attached to the large intestine in the right-hand side of the abdomen. The inside of the appendix forms a kind of cul-de-sac that usually opens into the large intestine. If this opening is blocked, the appendix swells and can become inflamed or infected with bacteria. Although the cause of appendicitis isn't always known, it often results from a build-up of faeces in the appendix, which causes a blockage. In very young children, appendicitis can worsen very rapidly. If the infected appendix isn't removed, it can burst and spread bacteria and infection throughout the abdomen, which can lead to serious health problems.

Recognising appendicitis

The signs of appendicitis are:

- ✔ Sharp pain in the tummy, near the navel, moving down to the right-hand side of the groin. Your young child may not be able to say exactly where the pain is.

- ✔ Nausea, and sometimes vomiting and diarrhoea. Your child may not want to eat anything.

- ✔ Your child may find moving around, sneezing, and coughing make the pain worse. She may not want anyone to touch the lower right part of the abdomen because it feels so tender.

- ✔ Slight fever is often present, so appendicitis is sometimes mistaken for gastroenteritis to begin with.

If your child has appendicitis, she needs urgent medical attention. Don't give her any food, drink, or paracetamol, as she may need surgery. Just let your child lie still and call a doctor.

Treating appendicitis

If the doctor suspects appendicitis, she'll send your child to hospital immediately for observation and tests, including urine tests, ultrasound scans, and possibly a chest X-ray. If your child has appendicitis, a surgeon removes the inflamed appendix. The surgical procedure is known as an *appendectomy* and is performed under a general anaesthetic. The procedure is very quick – it takes little more than ten minutes. Speed is essential to stop the appendix bursting and causing a blood infection. If your child's appendix bursts, the surgeon washes the affected area, inserts a tube to drain off any pus, and gives your child a course of antibiotics. The operation leaves a small scar on the right-hand side of your child's groin.

Your child can eat and drink the day after the operation. Any drainage tubes are removed after two days, and then she can go home. After about two weeks she will be well enough to go back to school, but until the stitches have completely healed, she must avoid playing games that may knock the operation site.

Soothing a Sore Throat

On average, young children get around four sore throats a year. Most sore throats are caused by viruses, but some are a result of infection with the streptococcus bacterium, which tends to cause particularly severe symptoms. A sore throat is a sign that your child's fighting an infection of some kind. Infection that spreads from the pharynx into the Eustachian tubes can cause a middle-ear infection. If the infection also causes inflammation of the tonsils, it's called *tonsillitis*.

Symptoms of a sore throat include feeling generally unwell, lack of interest in food, fever, and swollen glands on either side of the jaw. Swallowing may hurt. You may notice that your child has bad breath.

Most sore throats get better in a couple of days. Your doctor finds it difficult to distinguish between a viral and a bacterial sore throat. If your child suffers from persistent sore throats, your doctor may take a swab to decipher the cause. If the cause is bacterial, your doctor may prescribe antibiotics – but they are effective only for bacterial infections.

Give your child regular doses of infant paracetamol and offer warm soothing drinks. Choose her favourite drinks to encourage her – it's important that she drinks, even if she only sips. Warm lemon and honey (for children over the age of a year) or milky drinks can ease the discomfort, especially if alternated with cold drinks. If your child doesn't want to drink, give her ice cream, yoghurts, or ice lollies instead.

To examine your child's throat, sit her under a good light and get her to say 'aaah' or 'baaa' while you gently hold town her tongue with the handle of a clean fork or spoon. If her throat issore, the back of her mouth may be bright red. Her tonsils, which are at either side of the back of the throat, may look swollen.

Don't expect your child with a sore throat to eat for a day or two, but consult your doctor if she stops drinking. If your baby misses more than one feed, call the doctor. Also phone the doctor if your child has difficulty breathing or her sore throat isn't better after three or four days.

Chapter 14

Common Childhood Illnesses

Although you may feel panicky at the first signs that something's wrong with your child, the likelihood is that he's picked up a common childhood infection that'll run its course.

This chapter describes the most common childhood infections, the symptoms to look out for, and the treatments you can rely on. Also mentioned here are a few of the less common, but more dangerous childhood diseases.

Your child is exposed to a number of infectious diseases throughout childhood. Most of them are caused by viruses and can't be treated with antibiotics. If an infection is caused by bacteria, your doctor may prescribe antibiotics. The appropriate dose of infant paracetamol or ibuprofen helps relieve pain and fever in most cases.

Chickenpox

Chickenpox is a common and highly contagious childhood illness. The infection is caused by a member of the herpes virus family. Chickenpox usually runs its course without problems within a week or so and rarely causes complications in children.

Refer to Image 3 in the colour section, and look out for the following signs of chickenpox in your child:

✔ Itchy spots or blisters on your child's body and head that spread to the arms and legs and turn into scabs after a couple of days

✔ A high temperature fever (38°C or over)

If your child has chickenpox, he should stay at home until the crusts have fallen off the spots and the blisters are no longer weeping, as he will be contagious until this has happened.

Contracting chickenpox in the early stages of pregnancy can cause serious harm to your unborn baby. If you come into contact with a case of chickenpox when you're pregnant and you're not sure if you had the disease as a child, see your GP. The doctor may do a blood test to check if you're immune – if you're not, he may prescribe a medicine called immunoglobulin to reduce your chances of catching the disease, or at least reduce the severity of the disease.

The worst part of chickenpox is the itching. It'll drive your child crazy – and watching your child scratch relentlessly will drive *you* crazy. Continually reopening the scabs can lead to infection or scarring. Here are a few tips to stop the itching:

- ✔ **Soothe your child's skin with calamine lotion or calamine aqueous cream.** Dab the lotion or cream directly on the spots to soothe the irritation.

- ✔ **Keep your child cool.** Being warm makes itching worse, so try tepid baths and just use sheets to cover him at night (as long as the weather isn't freezing outside!).

- ✔ **Consider using an antihistamine.** Consider asking your GP or practice nurse to prescribe an antihistamine to relieve the itching. Some antihistamines also cause drowsiness, which can help your child sleep.

If your child just won't stop scratching, try to minimise the damage. Some parents have success with the following tricks:

- ✔ Keep your child's nails trimmed short.

- ✔ Cover your child's hands with socks or mittens at night, when it'll be harder for him to stop himself scratching.

- ✔ Tell your child to slap rather than scratch the itch. Sometimes the sting of a quick slap does the trick – making it less likely to pull off the scab.

- ✔ Distract your child: Doing something fun (such as playing a game or watching a DVD together) can help him forget the itching.

Some diseases – including chickenpox – give lifelong immunity. At least nine out of ten people in the UK have had chickenpox, even if they don't know it – sometimes the symptoms are so mild that nobody notices. If you nurse your child with chickenpox, you're unlikely to catch the infection yourself.

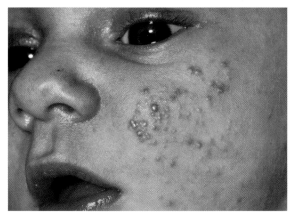

1. Milia (Ch 8): These pin-prick spots are caused by an excess of oil and are usually harmless.

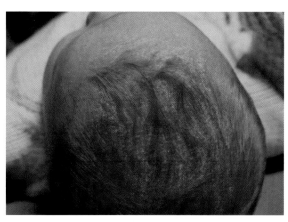

2. Cradle Cap (Ch 8): These thick scales do not harm your baby and usually clear up without treatment.

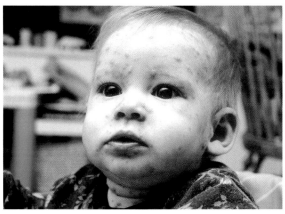

3. Chicken Pox (Ch 14): The spots are very itchy but usually disappear in a week.

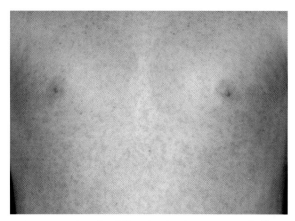

4. German Measles (Ch 14): Also known as rubella, this virus is infectious but not dangerous.

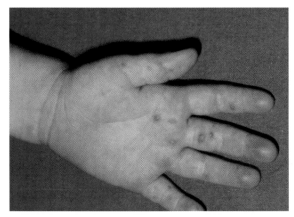

5. Hand, foot, and mouth disease (Ch 14): Spots and blisters indicate that the disease is still contagious.

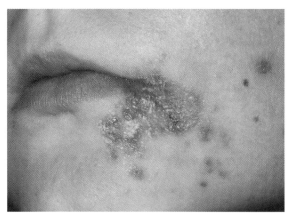

6. Impetigo (Ch 14): This common bacterial infection is easily treatable with antibiotics.

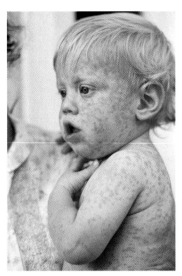

7. Measles (Ch 14): The rash begins around the ears. Measles is contagious and can be dangerous.

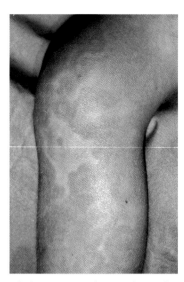

8. Nettle rash (urticaria) (Ch 14): The rash can be itchy but usually disappears within a day.

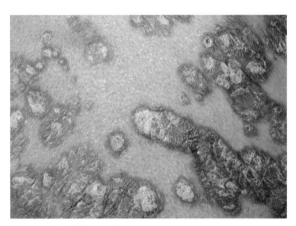

9. Psoriasis (Ch 14): This disease can be mild or severe but is not contagious.

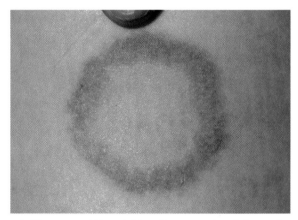

10. Ringworm (Ch 14): Usually transmitted through contact with animals, ringworm is itchy but not harmful.

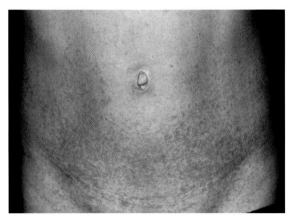

11. Scarlet fever (Ch 14): This rash appears in the groin or armpit and is treatable with antibiotics.

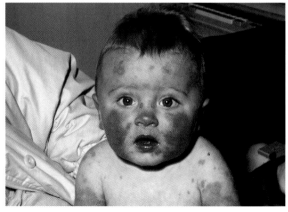

12. Slapped cheek syndrome (Ch 14): This mild viral infection clears up untreated, within two weeks.

Colds

A cold is the most common viral infection – and you may feel your baby has the snuffles constantly. Many children have up to ten colds a year because their immune systems aren't as well developed as adults' immune systems.

Your child's symptoms of a cold are just the same as yours. Look out for the following:

- ✔ Blocked or runny nose
- ✔ Sneezing and coughing
- ✔ Sore throat
- ✔ All-over muscle aches and pains
- ✔ High temperature

Doctors haven't found a cure for the common cold, so don't take your child to the doctor for a cold: Your doctor can offer sympathy but no medicine to cure the illness. Most colds are mild and your child should be better within a week.

Serious infections such as pneumonia occasionally cause the same symptoms as a cold in the early stages. If your child develops any symptoms suggestive of pneumonia (more details are in 'Pneumonia' later in the chapter), call the doctor.

Try doing the following to make your child more comfortable:

- ✔ Give him plenty of fluids such as fruit juice. Fluids help to prevent dehydration, which can be a problem if your child sweats off lots of fluid because of a fever.
- ✔ Stick to soft puréed foods to make eating easier. Your child may not feel like working his sore jaw muscles too hard.
- ✔ Paracetamol isn't strictly necessary if your child doesn't have a high fever. But you may consider giving a dose of infant paracetamol if your child's miserable and can't tell you why, as the drug reduces the all-over aches that often accompany a cold.

Cold Sores

Cold sores are a very common illness caused by the herpes simplex virus (HSV). The virus invades the skin cells, causing fluid-filled blisters to appear.

The blisters usually appear around the lips and are often tender or painful. The blisters heal without scarring but have a tendency to recur in the same place. There are two types of the virus:

- HSV1 – the most common type – causes cold sores.

- HSV2 causes genital herpes. It is unlikely to be an issue for your child, as the virus is caught only through sexual contact.

HSV is transmitted by close personal contact such as kissing. Most children come into contact with HSV between the ages of 3 and 5 years but don't show any symptoms until after puberty. A bad cold can reactivate the virus and cause the blisters to return.

Look out for the following symptoms in your child:

- **Your child complains of an unpleasant tingling in the skin.** The tingling sensation often precedes the arrival of the blisters.

- **Fluid-filled blisters appear.** The blisters become covered by scabs that usually fall off after eight to ten days.

- **Your child develops general symptoms of illness.** The virus affects the mouth and throat and may be accompanied by a fever and general aches and pains.

Make sure that your child washes his hands regularly after touching his lips and try to stop him picking his cold sores, as this can spread the virus to other parts of the body. See that he eats a varied diet, exercises, and gets plenty of sleep to help boost his immune system. Cold sores can be treated by an cream containing the drug aciclovir, which your doctor can prescribe (never give cream containing aciclovir without medical advice). This drug shortens an attack of cold sores, but it works only if you start treatment within a couple of days of the cold sore appearing – and preferably as soon as the symptoms appear.

Cold sores are highly infectious from the moment the tingling starts. Make sure that your child doesn't share towels or too many cuddles with other people in the household.

Very rarely, infection with HSV spreads to the brain and causes encephalitis (see 'Encephalitis' later in this chapter). If your child has any symptoms of encephalitis, get medical help immediately. Encephalitis is an extremely serious condition, but doctors can treat it if they diagnose it early enough, although there is a risk of permanent brain damage.

Croup

Croup is a nasty chest infection that is usually caused by a virus localised in the throat and surrounding tissues. The condition develops quickly in children. Croup usually occurs in children under the age of 5 years. Most cases clear up within a few days.

If your baby has had croup before, the condition may recur when he has a cold. After the age of 4–5 years, the symptoms of croup aren't so severe.

Look out for the following symptoms in your child:

- ✔ **Harsh, barking cough:** Many parents describe the cough as the sound of a barking seal.

- ✔ **Hoarseness and noisy breathing:** This often occurs at night when your child's been lying down for a couple of hours.

- ✔ **Fever:** Your child's temperature may be quite high (over 38.5°C), but if it settles, follow the simple measures described in Chapter 17.

If your child has croup, try the following:

- ✔ Keep him calm. The best way to do so is simply by being a good mum: Give him lots of soothing and cuddling, and remember to stay calm yourself.

  A croupy cough is one of the most unusual things you're likely to hear – imagine a sound that's a cross between a love-struck seal and Grandpa trying to clear a chicken bone from his throat – but panicking only upsets your child even more.

- ✔ Sit your child up so he can breathe more easily.

- ✔ Take your child to the bathroom, close the door, and run the hot tap into the bath. Inhaling steam may ease his symptoms because it reduces inflammation in his airways. Keep him well away from the hot water, and never leave him alone in the bathroom.

- ✔ Keep meals light and encourage your child to drink lots. He probably doesn't feel like eating much, but he's lost lots of fluid through sweating and fever.

- ✔ If your child has a fever, dress him in as little as possible and don't put him under warm bedclothes.

Croup usually clears up without any problems within three to four days, although the coughing may last a while longer.

Croup tends to settle on its own but occasionally it obstructs your child's breathing, especially if he's under 2 years old. If your child is having significant problems breathing, call the doctor.

Ear Infections

Ear infections are extremely common in childhood, for two reasons: First, children pick up all sorts of infections in the first few years of life. Second, the structures in children's ears are small, and so they are blocked easily. Chapter 17 describes the ins and outs of ear infections.

Encephalitis

Encephalitis, or inflammation of the brain, is a rare but extremely serious condition. Occasionally encephalitis is the complication of a more common childhood disease, such as mumps, German measles, or cold sores.

Look out for the following symptoms of encephalitis in your child:

- Drowsiness or a reduced level of consciousness
- Seizures or convulsions
- Fever
- Symptoms of meningitis (read more about 'Meningitis' later in the chapter)

Encephalitis is always a medical emergency. Take your child straight to hospital if you suspect he has encephalitis.

Flu (Influenza)

Flu is a highly contagious viral infection that affects the respiratory system. Symptoms of flu include the following:

- High temperature (up to 39°C)
- Loss of appetite
- Muscular aches and pains
- Pain over the sinuses and eyeballs
- General weakness and exhaustion

Many people say they have 'a touch of flu' when in fact they have a cold. There's no such thing as 'a touch of flu'. Real flu always makes you feel extremely unwell. Fortunately, most children recover completely from flu within a week or so, with no lasting effects.

If your child has flu, let him rest in a warm, well-ventilated room. Give him plenty of fluids to prevent dehydration.

Flu can be complicated by pneumonia. If your child develops any symptoms of pneumonia (see 'Pneumonia' later in this chapter), call a doctor.

Flu viruses are spread by coughing, sneezing, and skin contact. The flu virus survives for a short period on skin, so wash your hands regularly and show your child how to do the same. Hand-washing's especially important if you have a cold and you're handling your baby.

German Measles (Rubella)

German measles is caused by a virus. Every three to four years an epidemic of German measles breaks out in the UK, but the disease is less contagious than chickenpox or measles. German measles is pretty rare these days, as the MMR (measles, mumps, rubella) vaccine protects children against catching it.

Refer to Image 4 in the colour section and look out for the following symptoms of German measles in your child:

- ✔ A rash of tiny pink spots, first around the ears but then spreading all over the body. The rash changes hourly – it may spread rapidly or look more severe – and disappears after two to three days.

- ✔ Your child may develop a light cold and/or swelling in his neck and at the base of his skull.

Your child with German measles doesn't need any special treatment – apart from a few days' rest in bed. Remember that the disease is infectious and can be passed on to the rest of the family.

If you're pregnant, keep away from anybody with German measles, as the disease can damage your unborn baby. If you do come into contact with German measles, contact your doctor immediately. Most teenage girls in the UK are vaccinated against German measles to prevent rubella-related problems during pregnancy.

Most children recover from German measles without any complications. Encephalitis is a very rare complication. Get medical help immediately if your child has any symptoms suggestive of encephalitis.

Glandular Fever

Glandular fever is a viral infection caused by the Epstein–Barr virus. The disease is transferred from one person to another by saliva, which is why it's commonly called 'the kissing disease'. Glandular fever can also be spread by airborne droplets. The symptoms are similar to those of flu, so look out for the following:

- ✔ Sore throat
- ✔ Swollen lymph nodes and swollen tonsils with a white coating
- ✔ Fever
- ✔ Muscle pains
- ✔ Extreme tiredness

Children aged 10 years and older are most vulnerable to glandular fever. The illness usually passes without any serious problems. Your GP can diagnose the disease based on your child's symptoms and by taking a blood sample or throat swab.

If your child contracts glandular fever, keep the following tips in mind:

- ✔ Encourage him to drink plenty of liquids. Hot drinks can ease a sore throat.
- ✔ Get him to rest and avoid doing anything too physical. He should wait four weeks after feeling better before resuming physical activity.

Glandular fever usually takes two to four weeks to disappear. There's no cure, but you can ease the symptoms with the correct dose of paracetamol, lots of fluid, and plenty of rest. Just occasionally, your doctor may prescribe steroids for your child to bring down swelling in the throat. About 3 per cent of cases of glandular fever last for longer, and in rare cases it causes complications such as pneumonia. Having glandular fever once gives your child lifelong immunity against the disease.

Hand, Foot, and Mouth Disease

Hand, foot, and mouth disease is a common childhood infection caused by the Coxsackie type A virus. Symptoms include a large number of small spots and blisters, especially around your child's mouth, feet, and hands (see Image 5 in the colour section). Your child may also have a slight fever for a few days.

Your child doesn't need any treatment, but you may consider giving him infant paracetamol if his blisters are sore. See that he drinks plenty of fluids and washes his hands well after going to the toilet. If his mouth ulcers are really bad, try mashing up his food so he can eat more easily.

Hand, foot, and mouth disease is contagious if your child still has blisters and spots. Keep him at home, away from other children, until the blisters have gone – usually within a few days.

Impetigo

Impetigo is a common skin infection in children. It's extremely infectious and spreads quickly among young children, whose sticky fingers get everywhere. Fortunately impetigo doesn't cause serious complications, but it's unsightly and uncomfortable (take a look at Image 6 in the colour section). Impetigo's caused by a germ called *Staphylococcus aureus* – aureus means 'golden' and refers to the golden crusts that form on the skin in impetigo.

Look out for the following symptoms in your child:

- ✔ A rapidly spreading scabbed area, usually on the face. The scabby area tends to become covered with a yellow-golden crust.
- ✔ Your child feels well, but he may be tired and grumpy.

Impetigo is caused by a bacterial infection, and so your doctor can treat it quickly and easily with antibiotics. Your doctor may prescribe an antibiotic cream to apply to your child's skin if the infection is confined to a small area, or liquid or tablet antibiotics if the infection is more widespread. Keep your child out of school or nursery until the scabs have cleared – usually within a few days.

Measles

Measles, caused by the paramyxovirus, is one of the most contagious, unpleasant, and dangerous of the common childhood diseases. Measles is less common before the age of 1 year, because most mothers are immune to the disease and some of their antibodies stay in the child's system, from being in the womb and from breastfeeding, for a year or so.

Since the introduction of the MMR (measles, mumps, and rubella) vaccination, measles has become uncommon in the UK (for more on MMR, go to Chapter 3). It's important to remember that measles is a serious illness: as many as 1 in 15 cases result in complications which can include bronchitis and pneumonia, convulsions, and, rarely, encephalitis (inflammation of the brain).

Refer to Image 7 in the colour section and look out for the following symptoms in your child:

- ✔ Fever above 39°C
- ✔ A cold
- ✔ Barking cough
- ✔ Sore throat and sometimes swollen lymph nodes
- ✔ Red eyes
- ✔ Sensitivity to light
- ✔ Greyish spots inside the cheeks in the mouth
- ✔ A rash that starts around the ears and spreads to the rest of the body within a couple of days
- ✔ Spots of a brownish-red colour, which may join together to form large blotches

If your child is suffering from measles, keep him in a cool room away from bright light. Give the correct dose of infant paracetamol and sponge your child with tepid water to reduce his fever and general discomfort (for more guidance read 'Fighting a Fever' in Chapter 17). Measles is caused by a virus, and so it has no effective cure – you and your child simply need to sit it out.

Complications of measles include meningitis (covered in the next section), pneumonia, and febrile convulsions (covered in Chapter 17). All three are medical emergencies – so seek medical help immediately.

Meningitis

Most parents find meningitis a scary illness – understandable given that meningitis is an inflammation of the lining of the brain and the spinal cord and can be very serious. A number of different viruses and bacteria cause meningitis. One of the biggest worries with the disease is that it develops so quickly: Your child can be fine one minute and extremely ill a few hours later. Both you and your doctor may find it difficult to distinguish the symptoms of meningitis from those of other, less serious illnesses. Encephalitis, or inflammation of the brain, can cause similar symptoms to meningitis.

Look out for the following symptoms in your baby or young child:

- ✔ Fever
- ✔ Vomiting
- ✔ Refusal to feed
- ✔ Moaning, crying, and irritability
- ✔ Drowsiness

Your baby may also have a tense or bulging fontanelle (the soft spot on the top of his head), blotchy pale skin, rapid breathing, and a floppy body.

The early warning signs of meningitis in children often include cold hands and feet, abnormal skin colour, and leg pains. These are early signs of septicaemia, or blood poisoning. These may occur hours before the child develops a rash and sensitivity to bright light. Septicaemia is a medical emergency that needs urgent treatment, so consult your doctor immediately if you suspect your child has meningitis.

Look out for the following symptoms of meningitis in your older child:

- ✔ Severe headache
- ✔ Stiff neck
- ✔ Aversion to bright lights
- ✔ Fever and sickness
- ✔ Dark red rash that doesn't blanch when you press a glass on to the skin

If you suspect your child has meningitis, see your doctor immediately. If the doctor diagnoses your child with meningitis, he'll probably give your child an injection of antibiotics and then admit your child to hospital straight away. The hospital doctors may do various tests on your child, including a *lumbar puncture*, in which the doctor inserts a needle into your child's spinal cord and drains a small amount of fluid for examination. The lumbar test is distressing for both child and parents, but it is absolutely essential for the doctors to confirm the cause of your child's meningitis in order that they use the right antibiotics.

Since 1992, most babies and older children between the ages of 15 and 17 years receive routine vaccination against type C meningitis. This vaccination has reduced the number of cases of meningitis C by over 90 per cent, but it's important to remember that there are many strains of meningitis; this jab only protects against one particular strain. If your child is immunised, his risk of getting meningitis is very low. Check out Chapter 3 for the low-down on vaccinations.

Mumps

Until the introduction of the MMR jab, mumps was a common childhood illness caused by the paramyxovirus. The virus enters your child's body through his airways and moves through his bloodstream, ending up almost everywhere in your child's body. Of all the childhood diseases, mumps has the longest incubation period: It may take three weeks from infection to outbreak. Mumps is the least contagious of the childhood diseases. Close physical contact is necessary before it can be passed on. Mumps is most common from the age of 2 years onwards, although younger children can get it. Nowadays, most children are vaccinated against mumps between the ages of 12 and 18 months (read Chapter 3 for more on vaccinations).

If your child contracts mumps, he may have the following symptoms:

- ✔ High temperature (up to 40°C)
- ✔ Discomfort in his jawbone and swollen cheeks
- ✔ Sticking-out earlobes, making his face look very swollen
- ✔ Pain on opening his mouth

The swelling usually lasts three to four days but can go on for a week or more. The best remedy is to get your child to stay in bed and rest while his swelling and temperature are high.

Mumps can cause serious complications, including encephalitis and meningitis. If your child has mumps and develops any symptoms suggestive of encephalitis or meningitis, seek urgent medical help. In older boys, mumps can cause painful swelling of the testicles – see your doctor immediately if you detect this in your child.

Nettle Rash (Urticaria)

Nettle rash is reddish itchy wheals or swellings on the skin (see Image 8 in the colour section), much like your child would get from contact with a stinging nettle. The rash varies in shape and size and can be itchy, although it usually disappears within a day. Nettle rash may occur repeatedly or as a one-off. In most cases, there's no apparent cause although it can be due to an allergic reaction.

If your child has nettle rash, try to work out whether any of the following is the culprit:

✔ Foods that cause allergies – for example, eggs, nuts, seafood, or strawberries

✔ Contact with pollen

✔ Insect bites

✔ Contact with stinging nettles or stinging animals, such as jellyfish

✔ Common household products, perfumes, preservatives, colourings, nickel, or tar

In acute nettle rash, the attack begins within an hour of your child being exposed to the precipitant, so you can usually work out what's caused it. You don't need to call your doctor unless your child has severe nettle rash. If the symptoms are severe or persistent, your doctor may recommend antihistamine medicine for your child.

Pneumonia

Pneumonia is an inflammation of the lungs, normally caused by infection. Pneumonia is fairly rare in children, but you must take it seriously if you suspect your child has the disease. Pneumonia may come on rapidly and with no warning – your child may change from being completely healthy to having typical symptoms of pneumonia. Pneumonia may occur as a complication of a cough or cold, so even if the doctor gives your child the all-clear take him back if he develops new symptoms suggestive of pneumonia. Nobody can predict which cough or cold is going to develop into pneumonia, so your GP initially may have no indication that complications would set in.

Symptoms of pneumonia include the following:

- Fever (usually high, above 38.5°C)

- Constant tiredness, floppiness, and lethargy (not, as with many coughs and colds, being lethargic one minute and bouncing back with lots of energy within a couple of hours)

- Shortness of breath, rapid breathing, and seeing your child's ribs very clearly as he breathes in

- Going blue around the lips

If you suspect your child may have pneumonia, call your doctor. In some cases, pneumonia can be treated at home with antibiotics. In more serious cases, your child may need to be admitted to hospital, where he'll probably have a chest X-ray and blood tests. He may stay in hospital for a couple of days so he can have antibiotics through a drip.

Psoriasis

Psoriasis is a recurrent chronic skin disease that runs in families. Doctors aren't sure what causes psoriasis, but it isn't caused by an infection and it isn't contagious. Your child's more like to have psoriasis if you also have it.

Your child may experience mild psoriasis and not even be aware he has it, or he may have a severe outbreak that's socially disabling. Children of all ages can get psoriasis, but it tends to be most common between the ages of 16 and 22 years.

Look out for the following symptoms of psoriasis and refer to Image 9 in the colour section:

- Your child develops red spots or patches that grow bigger and become covered with silvery scales.

- The upper scales fall off but the lower scales remain.

- The edges of the spots are quite clearly marked out. Your child may have a few large irregular patches – *plaque psoriasis* – or may small round patches – *guttate psoriasis*.

- Plaque psoriasis classically affects the front of the knees and the back of the elbows. It can also affect the scalp and, in young children, the nappy area.

- If your child scrapes the skin, you may see small bleeding points.

✔ Your child may have small ridges in his fingernails. If his psoriasis is severe, his nails may thicken and crumble away.

✔ Red itchy patches under his armpits or on his stomach, groin, or buttocks.

If your doctor suspects your child has psoriasis, he'll examine your child's skin. The doctor may take a *biopsy* – a small portion of your child's skin – and test it for psoriasis. Treatment for psoriasis varies depending on the age of your child and the severity of his condition, but often your doctor prescribes a cream that you apply regularly to your child's skin.

Natural sunlight can improve psoriasis. However, remember that excessive exposure to the sun increases the risk of skin cancer later in life.

Ringworm

Ringworm is a fungal skin infection affecting the scalp, skin, fingers, toenails, and feet (see Image 10 in the colour section). Your child may come into contact with the ringworm fungus from three main sources – soil, animals, and humans – but animals are the usual culprits, including dogs, cats, hamsters, and guinea pigs.

Children are particularly susceptible to ringworm although adults can also become infected.

Look out for the following symptoms of ringworm in your child:

✔ Red, scaly patches of skin that are ring-shaped or oval with red, scaly edges.

✔ Inside the ring, the skin may be scaly but looks normal otherwise. The ring is usually quite itchy.

Your doctor can probably diagnose ringworm based on your child's rash. He may also take a sample of your child's skin for analysis. Depending on the severity of the infection, your doctor may prescribe your child antifungal cream or tablets.

Ringworm may be unsightly, but your doctor can treat it easily, it rarely causes any symptoms apart from the rash, and is not particularly easy to catch from contact with other children. Children naturally love animals, and keeping your child away from all things furry may do more harm in the long term than a short-lived case of ringworm.

Roseola

Roseola is a common viral illness most common between the age of 6 months and 2 years. If your child has roseola, he may develop a sudden high temperature (over 39°C) which may continue for a few days. Following a temperature , a pink rash on his body develops that lasts for up to a week. He may be fussy or irritable and have no appetite. You may see swollen glands in your child's neck. When the fever breaks, your child develops a pink-red rash on his tummy, spreading over the rest of his body. The rash spots turn white when you touch them, and they may be surrounded by halos. The spots last from a few hours to several days.

If your child has roseola, try the following measures to make him more comfortable:

- ✔ Undress your child so he isn't too hot.
- ✔ Give your child the correct dose of infant paracetamol to control his temperature.
- ✔ Make sure that your child drinks plenty of clear fluids so that he doesn't dehydrate.

Roseola is highly contagious during the whole period of the disease, so don't let your infected child mix with other children under the age of 3 years until the disease is over. You don't need to consult your doctor unless your child develops a high fever.

A rapid-onset fever triggers *febrile seizures* – convulsions caused by a high fevers – in about 10 per cent of young children. Consult your doctor immediately if your child starts jerking or twitching in his arms, face, and legs or loses bladder control.

Scarlet Fever

Scarlet fever is a rash accompanied by a sore throat caused by the streptococcus bacterium. Symptoms include a slight to moderate fever, a sore throat, and a rash in your child's armpit or groin (take a look at Image 11 in the colour section). Your child's skin may peel where the rash was, and he may have a coarse pink tongue known as *strawberry tongue*.

If your child has scarlet fever, your doctor can treat him with antibiotics. Complications of scarlet fever are rare. If your child has scarlet fever, keep him at home and don't let him mix with other children. Scarlet fever's contagious for the first few days of infection, but after taking antibiotics for three days your child is no longer infectious.

Scarlet fever is a *notifiable disease* in the UK. You or your GP must tell your local health authority if your child contracts scarlet fever so they can monitor the spread of the disease.

Slapped-Cheek Syndrome (Fifth Disease)

Slapped-cheek syndrome is a mild viral infection that usually occurs in children aged between 4 and 12 years. Symptoms include red specks on your child's cheeks, nose, arms, thighs, and buttocks (see Image 12 in the colour section). Your child may describe the specks as feeling numb, as if he's been slapped – hence the name of the illness. Slapped-cheek syndrome doesn't usually cause a fever. The disease can last for up to two weeks.

There's no treatment for slapped-cheek syndrome, which disappears by itself. If your child is uncomfortable, keep him in a cool room and apply a cold cloth to his skin.

If you're pregnant, avoid contact with children with slapped-cheek syndrome as infection with the virus in pregnancy can cause miscarriage. If you come into contact with a child suffering from the illness, consult your doctor, who may prescribe medicine to reduce the risks to your baby.

Sore Throat

Sore throats are incredibly common among children. Most sore throats are the sign of a viral infection and tend to settle on their own. If your child has a sore throat and a cough or cold, try giving him the correct dose of infant paracetamol or ibuprofen to relieve his symptoms while his body fights off the virus.

If your child has a cold, he's likely to be a bit off his food. If he also has a sore throat, food's likely to be the last thing on his mind. Try giving him soft, easy-to-swallow foods such as soup, yoghurt, and puréed fruit and vegetables. Don't worry if he doesn't want to eat – he'll make up for it when he's better. Do encourage him to drink lots of water though, to prevent dehydration.

Tonsillitis (covered in the next section) and streptococcus infection ('strep throat'), also cause sore throat, but the symptoms are usually more severe than a normal sore throat. Strep throat may cause a tummy pains and red rash, especially under the arms and in skin creases. If your child has symptoms of tonsillitis or strep throat, contact your GP because your child may need antibiotics, but by no means all throat infections can be cured with antibiotics.

Tonsillitis

Tonsillitis is an inflammation of the tonsils at the back of the throat. The cause is a viral infection in at least half of cases. The remainder of cases of tonsillitis are caused by a bacterial infection, such as with the streptococcus bacterium.

If your child has tonsillitis, his throat is sore and he almost certainly has a fever. Look out for the following clues, which suggest your child has a bacterial infection that your doctor can treat with antibiotics:

- Sore throat without an accompanying cold or cough
- High fever (above 38.5°C)
- Difficulty swallowing – saliva drooling out of the mouth is a sure sign of this
- Swollen glands in the neck
- White pus at the back of the throat.

If your child has three or more of these symptoms, take him to the doctor.

Surgeons used to be all too ready to take out a child's tonsils. These days, doctors appreciate that, especially in young children, removing the tonsils carries risks because it involves a general anaesthetic. Your doctor's unlikely to recommend removing your child's tonsils unless:

- Your child is having frequent attacks of tonsillitis that affect his schooling.
- Your child's tonsils are so big that he has problems breathing at night.
- Your child develops a serious complication of tonsillitis called *quinsy* – an abscess on the tonsils. Symptoms of quinsy are similar to those of a severe attack of tonsillitis – and your child will be very unwell and floppy.

Tuberculosis (TB)

TB is an infectious disease of the lungs that spreads from the lungs via the blood to the rest of your child's organs. TB may occur in the covering of the lungs, the bones, the urinary tract, the sexual organs, the intestines, and the skin. TB caused up to a quarter of all deaths in Europe in the 19th century. As living conditions have improved, medicines have advanced, and most children are now vaccinated against TB, the disease is far less common today,

Tuberculosis meningitis is a rare life-threatening form of meningitis, most common in children under 4 years old. The infection begins in the lungs and travels through the body. Symptoms are vague and last for 2–8 weeks – they include non-specific aches and pains, low fever, headache, and feeling generally unwell. Always consult your doctor if your child has a persistent cold.

Whooping Cough

Whooping cough is an extremely contagious bacterial infection. If your child hasn't been vaccinated against whooping cough, he can catch the disease simply by being in the same room as an infected person. Whooping cough lasts up to ten weeks – much longer than most other childhood illnesses. Due to a vaccine, whooping cough is now rare in the UK.

Whooping cough begins with a cold and mild cough, and then the characteristic coughing bouts set in. These coughing fits leave no air in the lungs and may occur up to 40 times a day. The name of the disease comes from the deep intake of breath your child makes as air passes through his windpipe. Your child may cough up phlegm or vomit, but his temperature is usually normal.

Whooping cough is a very serious infection in babies under a year old. Before the whooping cough vaccine was introduced, children often died of whooping cough. Whooping cough is highly infectious, so keep your infected child away from children who haven't had the disease or been fully vaccinated against it.

If you breastfeed your baby, he's protected against most common childhood infections – but not whooping cough.

In most cases, whooping cough needs no specific treatment. But you should do the following:

- ✔ Monitor your child: If he's having problems breathing (more on this in 'Pneumonia' earlier in the chapter) or if he suffers from asthma, take him to hospital.
- ✔ Make sure that your child gets lots of fresh air.
- ✔ To reduce the risk of your child vomiting, feed him little and often.

We recommend that you have your child vaccinated against whooping cough. Your child is vaccinated at 2, 3, and 4 months. After the first two inoculations, protection is almost 100 per cent. For more about vaccinations, go to Chapter 3.

Chapter 15

Allergies, Asthma, and Eczema

*W*hat do dust, cockroaches, cat saliva, and mould all have in common? Yes, they're all rather unpleasant. But they're also among the most common triggers of allergic reactions – a major cause of illness in children. In fact, allergies seem to be more prevalent than ever before – one child in four is thought to suffer from an allergy, although the jury's still out as to why. The good news is that the vast majority of children grow out of their allergies by the time they reach their teens.

Understanding Allergies

In a nutshell, an allergy is an overreaction of the immune system to a substance that's harmless to most other people. The body's immune system treats the substance (an allergen) as a threat and reacts to it in the same way as it would react to a poison or germ, causing symptoms that can be anything from irritating to seriously harmful.

In an attempt to protect the body from something it finds threatening, the immune system produces antibodies called *immunoglobulin E* (IgE). These antibodies trigger the release of chemicals called histamines into the bloodstream. Histamines cause the symptoms of the allergic reaction, affecting the eyes, nose, throat, lungs, skin, and gastrointestinal tract, as the body attempts to rid itself of the invading allergen. Future exposure to the same allergen triggers the allergic response again.

Children in families with a history of eczema, asthma, food allergies, and hayfever are at particular risk of developing allergies. And if your child's allergic to one substance, she's more likely to be allergic to other substances as well. Some children develop allergies even if they don't have a family history, so don't ignore symptoms of allergies without talking to your GP.

Exploring why allergies are on the increase

Theories abound for the increasing diagnosis of allergies. The one thing experts seem to agree on is that a combination of factors is likely to be involved. Increased air pollution is often quoted as a trigger, for example, but our modern-day obsession with cleanliness may also be a culprit. Overuse of antibacterial cleaning products, such as household cleaners and handwashing solutions, means people have much less exposure to bugs, so our immune systems aren't getting enough practice at fighting germs. Our immune systems then weaken and become more likely to react to the environment. Other contributory factors include smoking, overuse of antibiotic drugs, and dietary habits.

Most allergens are in the air, and in our food, although insect stings and chemicals used in things from soap powder to industrial cleaning fluids are also common culprits. The following sections expose the common allergy triggers.

Floating around: Common airborne allergens

Airborne allergens cause hayfever (also known as *allergic rhinitis*) and asthma. Sneezing, itchy nose and/or throat, nasal congestion, coughing, and wheezing indicate a reaction to an airborne allergen. Here are some of the common culprits:

- ✔ **Dust mites.** These microscopic insects are one of the most common causes of allergies. Dust mites live all around us and feed on the millions of dead skin cells that fall off our bodies every day (yum!). Their faeces are airborne, and are a major cause of respiratory problems.

- ✔ **Pollen.** Trees, weeds, and grasses release tiny particles into the air to fertilise other plants, triggering reactions such as sneezing and sore eyes. Pollen allergies occur seasonally: If your child's allergic to tree pollen, which is profuse in early spring, she'll get her symptoms in the spring. Grass pollen, on the other hand, is usually in the air during the early summer months.

- ✔ **Mould.** This fungus thrives inside and out in warm, moist environments. Outdoor moulds grow in poor drainage areas, such as piles of rotting leaves and compost heaps. Indoor moulds thrive in dark, poorly ventilated places, such as bathrooms and damp leaky basements. Many moulds, especially those indoors, grow year-round.

✔ **Pet fur.** Allergens from warm-blooded animals cause problems for many children. When your household pet licks itself, it gets saliva on its fur or feathers. As the saliva dries, protein particles become airborne and work their way into fabrics in the home. Cats are the worst offenders because they tend to lick themselves more than other animals.

✔ **Cockroaches.** These lovely creatures aren't a major household allergen yet, but cockroaches are on the increase, especially in inner cities. Experts agree that, like dust mites, cockroach faeces and saliva contain potential allergens.

Digesting the facts about food allergies and intolerance

Real food allergies are much less common than people presume – in some studies, 10 times more people believed they had food allergies than actually turned out to have them. Nonetheless, there does seem to be an increasing problem with food allergies, especially to nuts and eggs. Nut allergies are rare but can be life-threatening.

Diagnosis of food allergies and intolerances is increasingly popular among a small number of nutritionists who use dubious tests and often recommend expensive supplements – not to mention repeat private visits. Some nutritionists are highly qualified and work to ethical standards, but there is no specific qualification to becoming a nutritionist – unlike a state-registered dietician, who must sit stringent exams and follow an ongoing educational programme. It's only advisable to visit a private nutritionist if a doctor personally recommends one.

Food allergies

With a true allergy, your child suffers severe symptoms after coming into contact with even the smallest amount of the offending food. Common symptoms of a food allergy include an itchy mouth and throat (some children have *only* this symptom, called 'oral allergy syndrome'), hives (raised, red, itchy bumps), runny and itchy nose, and abdominal cramps accompanied by nausea and vomiting or diarrhoea.

Food intolerances

Food intolerances are much more common than food allergies. A food intolerance is a reaction to a food that causes unpleasant but generally not harmful and not life-threatening symptoms. Symptoms include bloating, pain in the tummy, and diarrhoea. Food intolerances tend to be temporary – a bout of diarrhoea, for instance, may often be followed by a few weeks of lactose intolerance as your child's gut wall recovers from the infection. Food intolerance is usually caused by a lack or shortage of an enzyme. Lactose intolerance, for example, develops when there isn't enough of the enzyme lactase to break down and digest the lactose sugar in milk.

Allergies and intolerances may have similar symptoms, but symptoms of an intolerance tend to be mild. If your child has an intolerance, she can probably eat a small amount of the offending food without a problem. Larger quantities of the problem food may lead to rashes, flushing, tummy pains, flatulence, vomiting, diarrhoea, and palpitations.

Common culprits of food intolerances and allergies

Here are some of the more common causes of food intolerances and allergies:

- **Peanuts and tree nuts.** Peanuts are one of the most severe food allergens, often causing life-threatening reactions. Half of children allergic to peanuts are also allergic to tree nuts, such as almonds, walnuts, pecans, and cashews, and sometimes sunflower and sesame seeds.

- **Eggs.** An egg allergy can pose big challenges for parents, as eggs are used in many of the foods children eat. Eggs are 'hidden' ingredients in many processed foods, making egg allergy hard to diagnose. An egg allergy usually begins soon after a child is weaned, but most children outgrow the allergy by the time they're 5 years old. Most youngsters with an egg allergy are allergic to the proteins in egg whites, but some can't tolerate the proteins in the yolk either.

- **Fish and shellfish.** The proteins in fish can cause various allergic reactions, including gastrointestinal problems leading to diarrhoea and vomiting. Children can also have skin reactions to fish, including itching and dryness.

- **Cows' milk and other dairy products (including yoghurt and cheese).** The proteins in cows' milk can cause food allergies and intolerance in young children. Symptoms range from stomach problems, including spasms and diarrhoea, to coughing and wheezing. Lactose intolerance, unlike true cows' milk allergy, tends to cause only diarrhoea and sometimes stomach cramps.

- **Soy and soy products (including tofu).** Soy allergies are more prevalent among babies than older children. Some 30–40 per cent of infants who are allergic to cows' milk are also allergic to the protein in soy formulas. Soy is present in an increasing number of foods: ingredients such as hydrolysed vegetable protein and lecithin are derived from soy, so read food labels carefully.

✔ **Wheat.** Wheat proteins are found in many different foods – but some are more obvious than others. A true allergy to wheat is pretty rare, but temporary intolerance is quite common. Coeliac disease, a permanent form of wheat allergy, is caused by a sensitivity to gluten, which is found in wheat, oats, rye, and barley. It is a condition that can cause damage to the small intestine, and typically develops between the ages of 6 months and 2 years, although it may not be diagnosed until much later, especially if the symptoms are relatively mild.

If your child's diagnosed with a food allergy, you need to take stringent measures to ensure that she doesn't come into contact with that food. After your baby's system has become sensitised to a food allergen by being exposed to it, her body's reaction to future exposure usually becomes more severe.

If you suspect your child has a food allergy, make absolutely sure that she isn't exposed to the food again, even in tiny amounts, until you've had a diagnosis. See your GP for advice as soon as possible. Your doctor may refer your child to a paediatrician with an interest in food allergies, who can carry out tests, refer you to a dietician for advice, and discuss how to manage accidental exposure in the future. See the section 'A word about anaphylaxis' for more details.

If you find that your child has a food intolerance, make a routine appointment with your GP. Be aware, though, that many food intolerances, such as lactose intolerance after a tummy bug, settle down of their own accord within a few weeks.

Looking at other common allergens

Other common allergens include insect stings and medicines. You probably won't have any trouble diagnosing these allergies because your child will have an immediate reaction and may need urgent medical attention (see the section 'A word about anaphylaxis' later in the chapter, for more information). Other triggers include cleaning products such as soaps and laundry detergents, which contain chemicals that can trigger an itchy rash or breathing problems. Dyes and garden pesticides can also cause allergic reactions. Allergies to these are often harder to diagnose as it may not be obvious what has triggered the allergy. You may need to use a process of elimination to decipher what's causing your child's reaction.

If you accepted every article about allergies and chemicals in the newspapers today, you'd probably want to leave the planet, let alone the country. Try to get scare stories into perspective. All chemicals can cause problems if you or your child is exposed to them in excess, but most are fine if you use them sensibly. Soap powder, for instance, is often blamed for childhood eczema – but is rarely a problem if you rinse clothes thoroughly. Aerosols used in the home have also received a lot of bad publicity, but the studies that have attributed them to increases in childhood illness have often been flawed. One study showed that aerosols increased breathing problems in babies but failed to take into account that parents who smoke use more aerosols to cover up the smell and that it was almost certainly the smoking that was the real culprit. The message, then, is to use products in moderation.

Some children have allergic *cross-reactions*. For example, if your child is allergic to birch pollen, she may have a reaction when she eats an apple because the apple contains a protein similar to a protein in birch pollen. Children who are allergic to the latex in surgical gloves and some hospital equipment are more likely to be allergic to kiwis and bananas.

A word about anaphylaxis

Also called *anaphylactic shock*, anaphylaxis is a rare but potentially fatal condition. Anaphylaxis is a severe allergic reaction that spreads rapidly throughout the body, causing shock with a sudden drop in blood pressure and narrowing of the airways. Anaphylaxis can be fatal unless it is treated immediately. If your child develops an extreme sensitivity to a specific allergen, she may be more at risk for anaphylaxis.

Anaphylaxis is most commonly triggered by insect stings and certain drugs, such as penicillin. Some foods, such as strawberries, may also trigger anaphylaxis. Up to 80 per cent of anaphylactic reactions, however, are caused by peanuts and tree nuts.

Symptoms of anaphylactic shock include the following:

- Difficulty with breathing.
- Swelling, particularly of the face, throat, lips, and tongue in food allergies.
- Light-headedness and dizziness due to a rapid drop in blood pressure.
- Unconsciousness.
- Hives – a blotchy rash that comes up very quickly, usually over much of the body.
- Tightness of the throat and sometimes a hoarse voice.
- Nausea and/or vomiting and diarrhoea.
- Abdominal pain.

Anaphylaxis can happen seconds after your child is exposed to the triggering substance, or it may be delayed for up to 2 hours if the reaction is to a food. If your child shows symptoms of anaphylaxis, dial 999. Emergency treatment involves an immediate injection of adrenalin. Your child may also be given injections of antihistamines or corticosteroids, together with intravenous fluids.

If your child is thought to be at risk from anaphylaxis, or if she has had a previous anaphylactic attack, your GP may give your child injectable adrenalin, often in the form of an EpiPen, which she should carry with her at all times. The adrenalin must be injected into the thigh as soon as possible after exposure to the triggering substance. You then need to take your child to a hospital emergency department, where she can receive any necessary additional treatment. Up to a third of anaphylactic reactions have a second wave of symptoms several hours after the initial attack, so your child may need to stay in hospital for a few hours, even if she seems well.

The good news is that only a small group of children experience severe or life-threatening allergies. Each year, about 30 anaphylactic reactions per 100,000 people occur. Children with eczema, asthma, or hayfever are at greater risk of experiencing severe or life-threatening allergies. With proper diagnosis, preventive measures, and treatment, most children keep their allergies in check and live happy, healthy lives.

Diagnosing and Treating Allergies

Some allergies are easy to identify because the pattern of symptoms makes it hard to miss. Other allergies are less obvious because they can masquerade as other conditions.

If your child has cold-like symptoms for more than a week or two or develops a 'cold' at the same time every year, consult your doctor, who is likely to ask questions about your child's symptoms and when they appear. Based on the answers to your doctor's questions and a physical examination, your doctor may be able to make a diagnosis or may refer your child for allergy tests.

Uncovering the culprits

To determine the cause of an allergy, an allergist may perform skin tests for the most common environmental and food allergens. Although these tests can be carried out on babies, they're more reliable in children over the age of 2 years. There are several methods of diagnosing allergies:

✓ Skin-prick testing is the most common method. These tests are usually carried out at a hospital but sometimes a GP will do them. The doctor places a drop of solution of the suspected allergen on to your child's skin, usually inside the lower forearm, and then pricks the skin. A positive reaction normally occurs within minutes in the form of an itchy swollen lump with a white weal in the centre, like nettle rash. The final diameter of the lump indicates the severity of the allergic reaction.

✓ Patch testing is usually used to diagnose eczema. The allergens are applied in a soft paraffin jelly to small discs, which are attached to your child's back with hypoallergenic tape for 48 hours. The doctor then examines your child's skin for signs of redness and swelling.

✓ Less commonly, the doctor tests your child's blood for levels of IgE produced in response to the suspected allergen. This test is usually carried out only if skin-prick and patch testing are inappropriate or impractical, for example if your child suffers from severe dermatitis or eczema.

✓ A diagnostic test for food allergy is to use exclusion and elimination diets. You restrict your child's diet to foods least likely to cause allergic reactions, such as chicken, pears, carrots, and rice, and then slowly add other foods back into your child's diet. By methodically introducing new foods, you can recognise the source of the problem when a reaction occurs. You must make sure that your child continues to eat a healthy balanced diet (check out Chapter 9 for the ins and outs of good nutrition), so use an elimination diet only after consulting a dietician or your GP.

Controlling your child's allergy

Unfortunately, there's no real cure for allergies. You can relieve your child's symptoms though. The first thing to do is to reduce or eliminate your child's exposure to the allergens. As soon as your child can understand, talk to her about the allergy and the reaction she'll have if she comes into contact with the offending allergen. Inform all of your child's caregivers, including childcare personnel, teachers, extended family members, and parents of your child's friends, about her allergy. If necessary, make sure that your child carries injectable adrenalin with her at all times, and make clear to all her caregivers the symptoms of anaphylaxis and how to inject the adrenalin (see the section 'A word about anaphylaxis' earlier in the chapter).

If reducing exposure isn't possible or is ineffective, your child's doctor may prescribe medications, such as antihistamines and inhaled or nasal spray steroids.

Reducing your child's symptoms

Some of the measures discussed below – such as breastfeeding your baby and not exposing your child to smoke – benefit every child, regardless of whether she has allergies. Some of the measures won't make a big difference on their own, but they may be useful if they address a particular problem, such as allergy to mould, dust mites, or pollen.

- ✔ **Breastfeed your baby:** Breastfeeding's one of the best ways of reducing the risk of your child developing an allergy in later childhood.

- ✔ **Don't smoke:** Avoid smoking not only in your child's bedroom but any-where in the house. Don't kid yourself that doors keep smoke out – they don't. Some allergic conditions, such as asthma, can be made much worse by exposing your child to smoke.

- ✔ **Keep pets out:** Don't let pets into your child's bedroom, and bath pets regularly if possible.

- ✔ **Remove carpets and rugs:** Hard floor surfaces don't collect dust as much as carpets do, so try to opt for hard flooring in your child's room.

- ✔ **Avoid dust traps:** Don't hang heavy curtains and keep soft furnishings to a minimum, as they allow dust to accumulate.

- ✔ **Clean frequently:** Vacuuming and dusting regularly helps to get rid of dust mites.

- ✔ **Cover pillows and mattresses:** Ask your health visitor for advice on special covers to seal pillows and mattresses if your child's allergic to dust mites.

- ✔ **Shut the windows:** If your child's allergic to pollen, keep your windows closed when the pollen season's at its peak, change your child's clothing after she's been outdoors, and don't let your child mow the lawn.

- ✔ **Watch out for damp:** Keep your child away from damp areas such as basements if she's allergic to mould, and keep bathrooms and other mould-prone areas clean and dry.

Considering complementary therapies

Several complementary therapies have been shown to be useful in managing allergies. You may perhaps consider the following:

- ✔ **Homeopathy.** Following the principle that like cures like, homeopaths agree that any substance that produces symptoms should, in minute doses, cure those symptoms. Homeopaths tailor treatment to the indi-vidual patient rather than to the symptoms. Hayfever may respond well to homeopathy.

 ✔ **Herbal medicine.** Traditional Chinese herbal tea has proved successful
 in the treatment of atopic eczema – but the tea is pretty unpalatable and
 it can be difficult to persuade your child to drink it. Some traditional
 Chinese remedies contain steroids – which accounts for their benefits in
 eczema – and you should avoid giving your child steroids without seeking advice from your GP.

Always consult a registered qualified practitioner before embarking your
child on a course of complementary medicine. You can find details of how to
find a registered practitioner in Chapter 18, together with information about
various forms of complementary medicine.

Taking a Closer Look at Asthma

There's no question that asthma – reversible obstruction of the airways
caused by a combination of spasm of the muscles in the small airways of the
lungs, and mucus and inflammation blocking the airways – is on the increase
in the UK. Asthma affects about one in ten children in the UK, and the UK has
one of the highest incidences of severe asthma in the world.

About 1 in 70 children in the UK under the age of 15 years is admitted to hospital every year because of asthma. Many more children lose time from
school or attend their GP or hospital emergency department because of
asthma.

Naturally, you worry if your child starts to wheeze, but don't just assume that
she has asthma. Always ask a doctor to check out your child if she's coughing
and wheezing, but don't panic: Wheezing and coughing are very common in
babies and toddlers because they have narrow airways, and most young children stop wheezing and coughing as their lungs and airways mature. For this
reason, your doctor's unlikely to diagnose asthma until your child's at least
1½–2 years old. If your young baby wheezes or coughs a lot, the doctor may
treat her with asthma drugs.

Even if the doctor diagnoses your child with asthma, the asthma may well
disappear as she grows up. The majority of youngsters diagnosed with
asthma stop having any symptoms by the time they reach school age.

Sussing out the symptoms and triggers

A persistent night-time cough, with or without a cold, and wheezing or coughing, perhaps on contact with common allergy triggers such as furry pets or
dust mites, are indications of asthma. In children under 2 or 3 years old, a

persistent night-time cough without obvious wheezing tends to be more common. As your child gets older, wheezing and breathlessness become more common symptoms.

The most common trigger of asthma is a cold or other viral infection, but many other things can also set off asthma, such as pollutants and dust mites. Once your child's airways have become inflamed, the airways remain very sensitive. Lots of things can make the symptoms of asthma worse or even bring on an attack, including car fumes, running, crying, and breathing in cold air.

Studies pinpoint various possible causes of childhood asthma, including smoking in pregnancy. One report suggests that smoking in pregnancy can increase the risk of your child developing asthma by as much as 50 per cent.

Asthma often runs in families: Having any allergy, asthma, eczema, or hayfever all count as a family history of allergy. Babies who have one allergic parent have around a 25 per cent greater chance of developing asthma than other children. If both parents are allergic, the baby has a 50 per cent of developing asthma.

Treating asthma

Asthma can't be cured, but it can be controlled by modern treatments that allow your child to lead a healthy active life. Treatment's usually in the form of medicine that your child breathes in via a device called an inhaler. Your baby or toddler won't be able to use an inhaler on her own, however, and so the doctor will give you a large transparent plastic container called a spacer. You squirt the medicine in the inhaler into one end of the spacer and your child then breathes the vapour out of the other. The following are two types of inhaled medications:

- ✔ **Relievers.** These make your child's breathing easier during an asthma attack. Relievers usually come in blue inhalers and work by relaxing the muscles in the airway walls. If your child has an inhaler, make sure that she always keeps it with her.
- ✔ **Preventers.** These are taken regularly, usually once or twice a day, to prevent attacks. The most common preventers are inhaled steroids, such as beclometasone and budesonide, which usually come in brown inhalers. Preventers protect your child's airways, making her less likely to overreact to the allergens she breathes in.

Many parents worry about the safety of asthma drugs, especially if their child needs to use them long term. Research indicates that long-term side effects are extremely unlikely, as the doses of steroids involved are very low. The steroids used to treat asthma are called corticosteroids, which mimic the steroids produced naturally in the body. They're completely different from the anabolic steroids used by bodybuilders and athletes.

Dealing with an asthma attack

The following are signs that your child may be having an asthma attack:

- ✔ She's breathing fast or having difficulty breathing.
- ✔ She needs her reliever inhaler (see the previous section) more than once every 3 hours.
- ✔ The area around her lips turns blue.
- ✔ She becomes very distressed or very quiet and still.
- ✔ She's too breathless to talk.

If you suspect that your child's having an asthma attack, do the following:

- ✔ Try to stay calm and reassure her. If she panics, her symptoms will get worse.
- ✔ Give your child her reliever inhaler every few minutes.
- ✔ Hold your child upright to help her breathe more easily.

If your child has a serious asthma attack, call your GP or an ambulance, or go straight to your local accident and emergency department.

If the doctor admits your child to hospital, she'll probably receive a high dose of reliever medication through a device called a nebuliser to ease her symptoms. Your child may need to stay in hospital overnight so the doctor can monitor her, and reassess her medication.

Making sure that you don't make it worse

If your child needs treatment for asthma or wheezing, or if you think she may be susceptible to asthma, try the following measures:

- ✔ Don't allow smoking in your home, and keep your child away from smoky atmospheres.

✔ Breastfeed your baby for at least the first 4 months – especially if allergies run in your family.

✔ Don't keep furry animals – they're common triggers of asthma.

✔ Keep dust mites at bay by vacuuming carpets and curtains, and washing bedding regularly. Keep soft toys out of your child's bedroom.

✔ Keep your child active, because regular exercise is good for her lungs. If her asthma treatment is correct, she should be able to lead a fully active life.

✔ If you have a history of allergies in your family, avoid giving nut products to your child until she's at least 3 years old, to hopefully reduce the likelihood of developing a nut allergy.

Itching to Find Out About Eczema

Watching your child itching and scratching can be almost as distressing for you as it is for her. Up to 20 per cent of children suffer at some time from the itchy inflamed skin condition known as eczema or dermatitis. The main form of eczema in children is *atopic (or allergic) eczema*, which tends to run in families and seems to be linked to other allergic conditions, such as asthma and hayfever. Experts agree that eczema is becoming more common, but the reasons for the increase are unclear. Theories include an increase in dust mites, fewer childhood infections, and an increase in food sensitivity.

Spotting the symptoms of eczema

A dry, red, scaly, extremely itchy rash is a sure sign of eczema. The rash commonly occurs on the face, neck, hands, and skin folds. Eczema often starts off as tiny pearly blisters beneath the skin's surface that develop into a rash. In severe cases, the rash weeps. Your child may suffer sleepless nights if her eczema is very bad because of the soreness and itching that eczema causes.

Treating eczema

Although eczema has no cure, you can find plenty of ways to soothe it. Even the worst eczema can be controlled with a combination of treatments. Your doctor may suggest one or more options, depending on the severity of your child's symptoms.

Going gooey over emollients

If your child has eczema, try to keep her skin as moist as possible. Emollients, or moisturisers, are essential in the treatment of eczema – apply them to your child's skin at least twice a day. Emollients replenish the natural oils in your child's skin, prevent moisture loss, and provide a protective barrier that prevents irritating substances getting on to her skin. Emollients make your child feel less itchy and more comfortable. Ask your GP to recommend some emollients suitable for your child; they need to be hypo-allergenic to prevent further irritation. You can also use emollient cream or liquid instead of soap in your child's bath, as soap tends to dry out the skin.

Stocking up on steroids

Steroids are most effective in the treatment of inflamed and itchy eczema, as they reduce itching and scratching. Modern steroid creams and ointments used in the correct strength and quantity are thought to be safe. They can have side effects though, such as thinning of the skin, so always follow your doctor's advice.

Steroid creams should not be used on infected skin, as they may cause the infection to spread. Eczema itself does not scar, but the injury to a child's skin caused by constant scratching does.

Taking antihistamines

Antihistamines in syrup form can help relieve your child's itching. They are available on prescription, although some can also be obtained over the counter for children aged six or more (younger children must have a prescription). Before giving your child medicine of any kind, it's always best to consult your doctor or pharmacist first. If you give your child antihistamines at bedtime, she is going to be less likely to wake in the night to scratch.

With prolonged use, antihistamines can become less effective as the body gets used to them, so reserve them for flare-ups of eczema rather than giving them all the time.

Soaking it up: Wet wraps

Wet wraps help to keep moisture in the skin. After applying an emollient to your child's skin, cover the area with cotton bandages soaked in lukewarm water. Then cover the wet wraps with a layer of dry bandages for up to 24 hours. As well as allowing the moisturiser to thoroughly penetrate the skin, the bandages prevent your child from scratching, reducing the risk of infection. Wet wraps are time-consuming but can be invaluable if your child's eczema is hard to control.

Finding out about herbal remedies

Medical trials have indicated that Chinese herbs can be effective in treating children with severe eczema, but it's important to see a qualified practitioner and ensure that your child is monitored carefully during treatment as some of these preparations may affect the liver. One major problem with herbal treatment is that the remedies taste horrible, making it tricky to persuade young children to take them! (Read Chapter 18 for more on complementary medicines.)

If your child's skin is red and angry, with blisters or a crusty yellow surface, it may be infected. See your doctor, who may prescribe antibiotics for your child.

Keeping eczema under control

The mainstay of eczema treatment for any child is moisturise, moisturise, moisturise! Any other treatment that you try must be in addition to using lots of emollients several times a day. There's no such thing as too much moisturiser. Most parents who find that their child is not getting benefit from moisturisers are not using moisturisers often enough or are not using a moisturiser that provides enough effect. Many children have eczema flare-ups that cannot be controlled with moisturising alone, but adequate moisturising should keep the frequency of flare-ups to a minimum. Make sure that the emollient is free from chemicals, and is hypo-allergenic, because many moisturisers can aggravate the skin.

Eczema often goes away on its own after a few years. As time goes on, you may find that your child needs only moisturisers. However, the tips below can help too:

- ✔ Choose the right clothes. Woollen and synthetic fibres next to the skin can aggravate eczema, especially in hot humid weather and cold dry snaps. These fibres encourage excessive sweating, which exacerbates the eczema. Choose loose-fitting clothes in natural fabrics such as 100 per cent cotton or linen, which allow air to circulate. And always buy your child cotton underwear.

- ✔ Soap and bubble bath can dry out your child's skin, so avoid them unless they're specially formulated for soothing eczema. Instead, use a soap substitute, such as aqueous cream or emulsifying ointment, and a bath emollient designed for eczema.

- ✔ Choose 100 per cent cotton bedsheets and nightclothes for your child. If she tends to scratch at night, get her to wear cotton night-gloves, which, combined with neatly clipped fingernails, should help.

- ✔ Don't let your child overheat, as this can make eczema worse.

✔ Gently rub or stroke your child's skin to help calm the itching. When she's old enough, teach her these techniques as an alternative to scratching. Keep her fingernails short as well.

✔ Reduce the number of dust mites in your house by vacuuming thoroughly, damp-dusting regularly, and washing soft toys at 50°C or putting them in the freezer for several hours. If possible, replace carpets with hard flooring.

✔ Contrary to popular belief, detergents are rarely a significant factor in eczema, unless soap residue remains on your child's clothes, which can be an irritant. Check that the rinse cycle in your washing machine works properly, and consider using an extra rinse cycle. Some parents prefer to use non-biological detergents.

✔ Use a fabric conditioner that has been approved by the British Skin Foundation or a similar reputable organisation. Research shows that the smoothing effect of fabric conditioners, which reduces friction against your child's skin, outweighs any possible irritation from the conditioner itself.

✔ Research shows that food additives may aggravate eczema. Children who have eczema may also react badly to some foods such as citrus fruits, tomatoes, wheat, milk, and eggs, so monitor the introduction of these foods into your baby's diet carefully. Don't remove foods from your child's diet without seeking advice from a dietician or health visitor.

✔ Consider installing a water softener, which reduces the need for detergents and soaps; a UK study shows that hard water may be linked to eczema flare-ups.

Helpful organisations

The following organisations offer help and advice about allergies:

✔ **British Allergy Foundation:** phone 01322-619898); Web site www.allergyuk.org.

✔ **National Eczema Society:** phone 0870-241-3604; Web site www.eczema.org.

✔ **Asthma UK:** phone 08457-010203; Web site www.asthma.org.uk.

✔ **British Skin Foundation:** phone 0207-391-6341; Web site www.britishskinfoundation.org.uk.

Chapter 16

Behavioural Problems and Emotional Health

• •

In This Chapter

▶ Examining your child's emotional development

▶ Developing your child's social skills

▶ Handling hyperactivity and other behavioural disorders

• •

*L*et's get this straight – all children can be horrid at some point, and yours is no exception! As children grow and develop, they need to expand their experiences. They do so by pushing at their existing boundaries and, sometimes, by pushing you to the limit. For the vast majority of kids, their challenging behaviour is perfectly normal and, in some ways, helpful (honest!) because it helps your child find out how far he can go.

Children need to get consistent messages in order to understand about changing boundaries, so you as a parent play an invaluable role. Your child also needs to feel secure to test his boundaries – which is why your little one probably does a fair impression of Dr Jekyll in company, but is Mr Hyde when he's alone with you! This is also perfectly normal, and reflects the fact that he feels secure enough to explore his boundaries with you (it could be considered a compliment to your parenting!).

If your child has a behavioural problem, you may find it helpful to get to the root of what is causing the situation. Your child needs your help to develop emotionally and socially. This chapter considers the normal range of behaviours and behavioural problems and looks at what to do if your child is diagnosed with ADHD/hyperactivity, dyslexia, dyspraxia, or autism.

Exploring Emotional Development

All children experience anxiety and fear at some time or another. The way in which these emotions manifest themselves changes as your child gets older – changes generally mark milestones in your child's emotional development:

- ✔ Babies experience *stranger anxiety* and cling to their parents when faced with a person they don't recognise. Stranger anxiety surfaces when a child realises who does and doesn't 'belong' to him and he becomes much more selective about who holds and plays with him. Stranger anxiety usually peaks at 12–15 months and then reduces.

- ✔ Toddlers aged 10–18 months may have *separation anxiety* and become distressed when separated from their parents. Your child realises from your actions that you're about to leave – he gets anxious because he doesn't know when you're coming back. Screaming at night is an expression of separation anxiety.

- ✔ Children aged 4–6 years are often afraid of irrational (to you) things such as monsters, ghosts, and the dark: Your child's imagination is highly developed, and his bedroom looks totally different to him at night. Your child is probably facing disruptive changes at this age, such as starting school. These irrational fears usually disappear as your child gets older.

- ✔ Children aged 7–12 years are often afraid of real things that may happen to them, such as natural disaster, injury, and underachievement at school or socially. Your child may feel that he has no control over such things.

These fears and anxieties are completely normal in your child and prepare him for handling later life experiences. However, if your child's fear is excessive or intense, it can develop into a *phobia* – and you need to intervene before the problem overcomes him.

Recognising signs of anxiety and phobias

Anxiety's a normal feeling that occurs when you feel threatened or face a difficult situation. Being worried or afraid usually helps you to deal with life and avoid danger, but if the fear lasts too long it can become debilitating. Symptoms of long-term anxiety include feeling worried all the time, tiredness, inability to concentrate, irritability, and not sleeping well. Anxiety may be genetic or a result of life changes and upheaval.

Many childhood anxieties and fears are normal. Your child may be afraid of strangers, heights, dark, animals, blood, insects, or being left alone. Separation anxiety, for example, is common when a child starts school. Generally these anxieties decrease as your child grows comfortable in his new surroundings or gets used to new experiences. Occasionally, however, your child may have a hard time adjusting, and his fears continue. If these feelings persist, they take their toll on your child's well-being.

Anxieties can also be acquired – and every child's biggest role models are their parents. If you're terrified of rats (or spiders, or heights, or, or, or...), consider getting help to conquer your own fear, or at least take steps to avoid letting your child sense your anxiety. Talk to your GP – he may be able to recommend a form of therapy called cognitive behavioural therapy to help you conquer your anxieties (take a look at *Cognitive Behavioural Therapy For Dummies* by Rob Willson and Rhena Branch for more).

Your child may show certain symptoms when he faces an object or situation he's afraid of. He may experience a surge of anxiety and have to get out of the situation that scares him. Look out for the following signs that your child's anxious about something:

- ✔ He's clingy, impulsive, or distracted.
- ✔ He has nervous twitches.
- ✔ He can't get to sleep or he stays in bed longer than usual.
- ✔ His hands are sweaty, or he has feelings of nausea, headaches, or tummy ache.

Generalised anxiety is when your child has unrealistic worries that aren't related to any one thing in particular. He may be self-conscious and tense, experience 'aches and pains', and need reassuring constantly.

If your child's anxieties and fears persist, problems can arise. The anxiety may become a *phobia* – an extreme, persistent fear. Your child may find it difficult to deal with phobias, and you may find it hard to tolerate them.

To determine whether your child has a real phobia, look for patterns such as fearful behaviour occurring at particular times or because of particular things – seeing a spider, for example. An isolated incident that your child resolves isn't usually significant. If your child runs screaming from the room because the pet hamster startles him but he enjoys playing with the hamster at other times, then you're not dealing with a phobia. But if a persistent pattern emerges – say, your child's fearful of the hamster all the time and shudders when he sees his friend's gerbil – you need to intervene to prevent the phobia affecting your child over time.

The ups and downs of hormones

Hormones are chemical substances made by the endocrine glands. The endocrine glands pass hormones into the bloodstream, which carries the hormones around the body. For your child's body to function well physically and emotionally, each gland must produce the right amount of hormone at the right time. Hormones do lots of important things, including controlling your child's weight, growth, metabolism, fertility, moods, and emotions. Some hormones have long-term effects, such as growth and puberty changes; others hormones have short-term effects and act as regulators to keep the body well balanced. Some of the most important hormones include:

✔ **Adrenalin:** Adrenalin's often referred to as the 'emergency hormone' because your child's body produces it when he's frightened or excited. Adrenalin increases the heart rate, narrows the arteries that supply the tummy, and increases blood flow to the muscles. In moderate levels, adrenaline can be productive by helping your child run faster in a race, for example. In excess, however, it can cause anxiety and panic attacks.

✔ **Antidiuretic hormone (ADH):** ADH regulates how much water your child loses in his urine. Your child produces more ADH and thus less urine when he's thirsty or dehydrated.

✔ **Growth hormone:** This hormone controls how much your child grows. Too little or too much growth hormone can affect your child's body development.

✔ **Insulin:** Insulin regulates the amount of sugar in your child's blood. Some children don't produce enough insulin to regulate the sugar in their blood – known as *diabetes*. If your child suffers from diabetes, he may have to inject insulin to control his blood sugar levels.

✔ **Serotonin:** A hormone that regulates your child's mood, sleep patterns, and relaxation. Low levels of serotonin lead to disturbed sleep, loss of appetite, slow speech, and depression.

✔ **Thyroid-stimulating hormone (TSH):** TSH regulates your child's metabolism (how fast he burns up energy), and affects his muscle strength, weight, and overall well-being.

Avoidance behaviour – any form of behaviour that suggests your child is taking active steps to avoid confrontation with the source of their fear – is a particularly important indicator of emerging phobia.

Helping your child deal with fear and anxiety

Unless your child's phobia hinders his ability to function, his phobia will probably disappear as he gets older. Occasionally, children need to see a mental health professional for help with their phobias.

Here are some tips to help your child deal with his fears and anxieties:

- ✔ **Recognise that the fear is real:** Talking about the fear with your child can help, as words take power out of the negative feelings.

- ✔ **Don't belittle or dismiss the fear:** Negative comments won't help your child get over the fear. Don't express your disappointment or make him feel as if he's failed if he reacts to a phobia. 'Never mind, you've done it before and I know you'll manage it again' is a much more constructive way of approaching a minor setback.

- ✔ **Don't cater to the fears:** For example, don't cross the street to avoid a dog if your child's afraid of dogs – this is just going to make him feel there really is something to be afraid of.

- ✔ **Show your child how to rate his fear:** If he can visualise his fear on a scale of 1–10, he may see the fear as less intense than he first thought.

- ✔ **Encourage your child to use coping strategies:** Suggest that he ventures out to tackle his fear and then returns to you, before venturing out again. Encourage him to state positive statements such as 'I can do this' to help him deal with things when he's feeling anxious. Relaxation, deep breathing, and visualisation techniques can also help.

- ✔ **Praise, praise, and praise again!** Children respond extremely well to positive reinforcement. If your child takes even a small step towards overcoming their anxiety – such as sitting still while a dog in the park sniffs the bench they're on, rather than running away – give them lots of praise, and tell others of their success in your child's hearing.

Building Healthy Self-Esteem

Self-esteem's a collection of feelings or beliefs a person holds about himself. Your child's self-esteem affects his motivations, attitudes, and behaviour towards other people.

Patterns of self-esteem develop early in life. When your baby reaches a developmental milestone (discussed in Chapter 2), he feels a sense of achievement, which boosts his self-esteem. His achievement instils a can-do attitude, and your child begins to relish mastering tasks. Your child's self-esteem is also based on interaction with others – which is why your input is so important in helping him build a healthy self-esteem. Your child's self-esteem's also connected to love – a child who feels unloved may have low self-esteem.

Identifying low self-esteem

A child who feels good about himself handles conflict and external pressures more easily. He smiles a lot, enjoys life, and is optimistic and sunny-natured. If your child has low self-esteem, he may find life's challenges a major source of stress and frustration. If your child thinks poorly of himself, he won't be able to solve problems – and if he feels he's no good at anything, he may become passive, withdrawn, and depressed. Look out for the following signs of low self-esteem in your child:

- ✔ He doesn't want to try new things.
- ✔ He speaks negatively about himself and says things like 'I'll never be able to do that', or 'I'm useless'.
- ✔ He gives up easily or lets you take over what he's doing.
- ✔ He's overly critical of himself.
- ✔ He's pessimistic.

Helping your child develop self-esteem

You and your partner can do more than anyone else to help develop your child's self-esteem. Most parents do this unconsciously – but remember your encouragement is not just about lavishing praise on your child: You also need to help your child set goals and achieve them on his own.

Try the following to help your child develop his self-esteem:

- ✔ **Boost your child's independence.** Encourage him to develop enjoyable hobbies that he can do on his own. If he falls out with a friend, don't interfere: Let him sort it out himself.

- ✔ **Be patient and realistic.** Don't take over a task you've given him to do, even if he's taking a long time to do it. That means deciding beforehand if it's realistic to let him start a project (be it laying the table, baking a cake, or weeding the flowerbed) that he may not have time to finish. You're not always going to have time to let him finish tasks at his own rate – so don't try. If he wants to bake a cake for grandma's visit but you need the kitchen to be tidy when she arrives in an hour, you're setting him up to fail. Instead, find (or invent!) a really important, special job that you can't possibly do yourself but which needs completing before her arrival, and save the cake-making for when you don't have a deadline.

✔ **Watch what you say.** Your child's sensitive to your words. Praise him for a job well done, and don't ridicule or criticise him for not achieving a goal. Reward his efforts rather than focusing on the outcome. Encourage him to make positive self-statements such as 'I did my best.' Use clear constructive statements like 'Please clear the table' rather than 'Why do you never clean up?'

✔ **Be a positive role model.** If you're hard on yourself or pessimistic, your child may mirror you. So nurture your own self-esteem.

✔ **Help your child be more realistic in evaluating himself.** Understand your child's feelings, and identify any irrational beliefs such as perfection, physical attractiveness, or ability. After you've done this together, you can challenge his beliefs and hopefully start to change them.

✔ **Be spontaneous and affectionate with your child.** Hug him lots: Your affection boosts his self-esteem.

✔ **Create a safe, nurturing home environment.** A child exposed to parents who argue regularly may well become withdrawn and depressed. Instead, offer your child a home full of laughter, creativity, games, stimulation, conversation, positivity, and warmth.

Developing Social Skills

Good social skills are important for your child in order that he can enjoy relationships with his peers, teachers, and family. How your child relates to other children at school can impact on his relationships in later life. If your child doesn't have friends or playmates, he may get frustrated. And if your child doesn't develop the skills to play and form friendships, he may be excluded from opportunities later in life. Your socially competent child is going to behave positively and be responsive and sensitive to others and the social situation he's in.

Everyday experiences and your child's relationship with you and your partner are fundamental in developing his social skills. Your responsiveness and nurturing are key factors in your child's social competence, helping your child to see the world in a positive way and to expect his relationships with others to be rewarding.

Try the following to help your child develop his social skills:

✔ **Establish rules and standards for acceptable behaviour at home.** Set rules about keeping his room tidy and speaking to other family members with respect – demonstrate respect in the way *you* speak to people. Set routines for bedtime and mealtimes – and try to stick to them.

✔ **Be consistent.** Children need consistency to help them make sense of the world. Talk to your partner about your core values, and try to ensure that you both react in the same way to the same behaviour. For instance, if you've decided never to reward his bad behaviour by buying him things he whines and nags for, stick to that rule no matter how much of a rush you're in, or how embarrassed you are when he throws a tantrum in the middle of the supermarket queue. You may want the ground to swallow you up at the time, but by being consistent you're less likely to get similar tantrums in the future, because he understands they never work.

✔ **Show your child how to respect himself, others, and his possessions.** Encourage him to dress himself neatly, keep his things tidy, and share his toys with his siblings and friends. Invite his friends round to encourage his social skills, interaction, and sharing. Let him help you prepare food and tidy up to show him how to take responsibility. Try to set a good example and shape the way he thinks about and talks to others by being positive and non-critical about other people yourself.

✔ **Demonstrate the behaviour you expect from your child.** He learns by watching, copying, and practising what adults do. So talk kindly to your child to demonstrate the value of talking kindly to others.

✔ **Ask your child to consider other people's feelings.** Ask him how he thinks his behaviour made you (or whoever he was with) feel. Use positive as well as negative examples.

✔ **Encourage your child to respond appropriately to difficult situations.** Rather than telling your child to share things, show him *how* to share things by taking it in turns to play with toys.

✔ **Show your child how to deal with bullies.** Bullying's very common and can seriously affect your child's mental health. If your child's being bullied, listen to him as he talks about it, take him seriously, and don't blame him in any way. Talk about what he can say to the bully to stop the bullying. Words don't always work – but nor does ignoring the behaviour. Encourage your child to ask the bully to stop and then remove himself from the situation.

✔ **Demonstrate how to offer and accept appreciation.** Telling others what you like or appreciate about them is often a hard thing to do. But by doing this, you show your child generosity and awareness of others and help him develop his self-esteem and confidence.

✔ **Give your child the opportunity to play with his peers.** Playing with others helps him develop patience and tolerance and encourages him to share and take turns. However, let your child fight his own battles with friends – if he falls out with one of his friends, don't try to resolve things for him.

> ✔ **Talk to your child about his day.** Ask him what happened at school –
> and if necessary adopt a problem-solving approach. This helps him con-
> sider the various solutions and perspectives and gives your child the
> skills he needs to deal with difficult social situations. Give him feedback
> on how he handles things.

Parents of socially competent children laugh and smile a lot, don't put their
children down, aren't too bossy, and are responsive to their child's ideas.

Homing in on Hyperactivity

Hyperactive children are always on the go and in motion. They touch, talk,
and play constantly, rarely sit still, and fidget a lot. Hyperactive teenagers
may try to keep themselves busy all the time and seem restless and unable
to concentrate for long periods.

Lots of children are hyperactive and easily distracted. If your child has a
mild dose of hyperactive behaviour, it's unlikely to a problem. Hyperactivity
becomes a problem if your child acts impulsively or irrationally, if the behaviour is exaggerated compared with other children of the same age, or if his
actions start to affect his home and school life.

If your child's behaviour is disruptive, if he finds it hard to do a simple task,
if he has mood swings, or if he's extremely clumsy, he may have attention
deficit hyperactivity disorder (ADHD) (discussed in 'Behaving badly:
Attention deficit hyperactivity disorder (ADHD)' later in the chapter).

Identifying a hyperactive child

Most children are lively and full of energy, so how do you tell the difference
between normal energy levels and hyperactivity?

The following may be signs that your baby's hyperactive:

> ✔ Constant crying and screaming but refusing to accept comfort
>
> ✔ Restlessness and persistently little sleep
>
> ✔ Difficulty feeding by breast or bottle
>
> ✔ Excessive dribbling
>
> ✔ Possible extreme thirst

✔ Banging his head or rocking his cot

✔ Not crawling, but running or walking early

✔ Night terrors (check out Chapter 11 for more on night terrors)

In your older child, the following are signs of hyperactivity:

✔ Clumsiness and accident-proneness

✔ Erratic behaviour, screaming fits, and tantrums

✔ Compulsively touching everyone and everything

✔ Constantly moving and wriggling

✔ Aggression and disturbing other children

✔ Lack of concentration and inability to finish tasks

✔ Performing poorly at school

✔ Moodiness

✔ Poor hand–eye coordination

Not all hyperactive children have all of these symptoms.

Coping with hyperactivity

Dealing with a hyperactive child is difficult and draining. You may feel as if your child isn't making any progress at school or home. You may be worried that he is about to do something dangerous and feel you need to watch him all the time. If you have a hyperactive child, your goal is probably to help your child accomplish the things he wants and needs to do to be successful. The following strategies may help:

✔ **Modify your child's behaviour.** Set clear rules on how you expect him to behave at home, and tell him what is and isn't acceptable. Make sure that you agree the rules with your partner. Praise your child if he's done a job well. This way, your child finds out how to develop his self-control.

✔ **Create a routine and plan your child's day.** Spend time with your child on his own. Plan his days and weekends and make sure that he has time to do things he enjoys. Encourage him to follow a routine that offers time to burn off his energy in energetic play. But make it clear that you also expect him to have quiet times and do his homework.

✔ **Considering using medication.** Some drugs such as methylphenidate and dexamfetamine can reduce your child's hyperactivity and improve his concentration, giving him time to develop new skills and feel that he's more in control. But remember that these drugs offer a short-term solution rather than a cure.

✔ **Modify your child's diet.** An American doctor, Benjamin Feingold, suggested that a number of natural substances and artificial food additives affects the brain function of some children. Dr Feingold's food programme is used widely to treat hyperactive children. Log on to the Hyperactive Children's Support Group Web site (www.hacsg.org.uk) for more info on food additives and additive-free products.

Behaving badly: Attention deficit hyperactivity disorder (ADHD)

Attention deficit hyperactivity disorder (ADHD) (also called attention deficit disorder (ADD) and hyperkinetic disorder) refers to a number of behaviours associated with poor attention span. With ADHD, your child may be impulsive, restless, hyperactive, and inattentive. These behaviours may affect your child's ability to absorb information and socialise. About 1.7 per cent of children in the UK have ADHD. The condition is more common in boys than girls.

You may suspect your child has ADHD if he has difficulty keeping his attention focused, he's disorganised, and he's unable to finish what he starts. Your child may also be hyperactive (have a look at 'Dealing with hyperactivity' earlier in the chapter) and have problems with impulse control – for example, he may interrupt conversations with off-topic comments or may take something you told him he can't have.

If your child does have ADHD, you may also be aware of the following:

✔ Temper tantrums, problems with sleep, and clumsiness

✔ Confrontational behaviour, such as losing his temper and arguing with you

✔ Destructiveness, lying, stealing, and breaking rules

✔ Dyslexia and learning difficulties (discussed later on in the chapter)

✔ Severe depression or anxiousness.

Digging deeper for support

Check out the following Web sites for more about hyperactivity:

✔ **Hyperactive Children's Support Group:** www.hacsg.org.uk

✔ **National Attention Deficit Disorder Information and Support Service (ADDISS):** www.addiss.co.uk

✔ **YoungMinds:** www.youngminds.org.uk

About half of children with ADHD outgrow the condition and function normally by the time they reach their teenage years. Other children with ADHD have problems into adult life, such as depression, irritability, antisocial behaviour, and attention problems.

The cause of ADHD is not known, but here are some theories:

✔ Studies of twins suggest a genetic link to ADHD. In 80–90 per cent of identical twins where one twin has ADHD, the other twin also has ADHD. Research shows that there's a greater chance of inheriting ADHD from male relatives.

✔ Studies show that people with ADHD have abnormalities in the *prefrontal cortex* part of the brain, which controls impulsivity and self-control. Drugs that stimulate this part of the brain can be effective in treating ADHD.

✔ The brain structures linked to the development of ADHD are vulnerable to damage during birth. The damage is caused by not enough oxygen reaching parts of the brain if blood flow is reduced.

✔ A poor home environment may increase the likelihood of a child developing ADHD if he is already at risk of ADHD due to genetic factors. Home life can affect the severity of the child's symptoms, how the condition develops, and how long the condition lasts. Family conflict may be a result of the same genes that cause ADHD, rather than a cause of the ADHD.

Diagnosing ADHD

If you suspect your child has ADHD, get a medical diagnosis from your GP, paediatrician, or child psychologist. Other health professionals such as psychologists, speech therapists, health visitors, and teachers may also need to assess your child before a diagnosis is made. No single diagnostic test exists for ADHD, so the diagnosis is based on your child's symptoms, past psychiatric history, educational and medical history, and personality. As part of the diagnosis procedure, you'll probably need to fill out a questionnaire indicating what behaviours you've found in your child. If your child displays certain behaviours for an extended period of time, he may have ADHD. The following are examples of the sorts of things the health professionals ask you about your child in order to make a diagnosis.

Attention difficulties

These may be diagnosed if your child exhibits at least six of the following traits for six months or more:

✔ Failing to pay close attention to detail or making careless mistakes at school or playtime.

✔ Unable to finish tasks or activities.

✔ Not listening to what you say to him.

✔ Not following instructions and not finishing homework or tasks.

✔ Being disorganised with tasks and activities.

✔ Avoiding homework and tasks that call for concentration.

✔ Losing things that are essential to tasks, such as pencils and books.

✔ Easily distracted and forgetful.

Hyperactivity

This may be diagnosed if your child has least three of the following for six months or more:

✔ Running around excessively and climbing over things.

✔ Being very noisy when playing and unable to engage in quiet leisure activities.

✔ Unable to remain seated in the classroom.

✔ Fidgeting with hands and feet or squirming on his seat.

Impulsivity

This may be diagnosed if your child has at least one of the following for six months or more:

✔ Blurting out answers before questions have been completed.

✔ Not waiting his turn in lines and games.

✔ Interrupting others' conversations and games.

✔ Excessive talking.

Treating your child with ADHD

Your child's treatment depends on his diagnosis and takes into account any specific difficulties such as speech, language, and social problems. You need specialist advice and support, as living with a child suffering with ADHD can be difficult. Your local education authority (LEA) can assess your child for special education needs and put you in touch with an educational psychologist, language specialist, and occupational therapist.

Try doing the following to help your child with ADHD:

✔ Create a daily routine for meals, homework, and bedtime.

✔ Be specific in your instructions and requests.

✔ Set clear boundaries around leisure activities, such as how much TV he watches and which games he plays.

✔ Be consistent in how you look after your child. Work with your child's school or nursery to ensure that consistent messages outside, as well as within, the home.

✔ Remove any disturbing elements from your child's daily routine – for example, get him to sit in a quiet room with no TV when he's doing homework.

✔ Work with his healthcare professionals to devise structured programmes to lengthen his attention span and focus.

✔ Communicate with your child on a one-to-one basis.

✔ Use rewards to reinforce your child's positive behaviour, and stop his privileges for inappropriate behaviour and overstepping boundaries.

✔ Talk to the teachers at your child's school or nursery for mutual help.

These techniques may work if your child has mild attention deficit problems. If your child has more advanced ADHD, you may need to consider behaviour-modification strategies, such as reward schemes and positive encouragement, either alone or in conjunction with medication. Treatment includes counselling from a psychologist for both you and your child; behavioural management advice, such as strategies to help your child deal with social problems and develop his self-confidence and self-esteem; and one-to-one help at school.

Trying ADHD medications

Research suggests that a combination of medication and behaviour-modification techniques is the best treatment for ADHD. The three main drugs used to treat ADHD are stimulants, selective serotonin reuptake inhibitors (SSRIs), and non-stimulant medications:

✔ **Stimulants:** These drugs increase the activity of dopamine and nora-drenalin, chemicals in the areas of the brain that control your child's attention and behaviour. These areas of the brain are underactive in children with ADHD. Common stimulant medications include Ritalin, Dexedrine, and Concerta.

✔ **SSRIs:** Your doctor probably won't prescribe SSRI drugs for your child with ADHD unless stimulants don't work for your child. SSRIs are more commonly used for the treatment of depression in adults. SSRIs increase the amount of serotonin in your child's brain. Common SSRIs include fluoxetine (Prozac).

Concerns about ADHD medications

The press gives lots of negative coverage to the widespread use of drugs for ADHD. Some people feel these drugs are over-prescribed and can actually damage children at an important point in their development. Other tales have related that these drugs turn children into 'zombies'. Behind such claims is the concern that drugs for ADHD are a shortcut to dealing with overactive children. If you're in doubt about the sort of treatment your child needs, ask your doctor to refer you to a specialist who can discuss it further.

✔ **Non-stimulant medications:** Types of drugs, such as Strattera, work by increasing the levels of the chemical noradrenalin in your child's brain. Noradrenalin regulates attentiveness, impulsivity, and activity levels. Your doctor probably won't prescribe non-stimulants unless stimulants don't work for your child. Discuss with your child's specialist whether they consider medication to be the only option. Even if they do recommend it as essential in your child's case, always get as much information as you can about behaviour modification and other treatments that may be available to your child, and which may reduce the amount of medicine he is taking or help it to work more effectively.

Modifying your child's diet

Some research indicates that diet isn't a significant factor in most children with ADHD, although other experts suggest that it can be a contributory factor. For example, your child may not be able to metabolise certain substances in food or drugs, especially artificial colourings and preservatives. A few children improve when the culprits are removed from their diets. However, your child with ADHD may have food allergies or intolerances that you need to monitor (head to Chapter 15 for the low-down on food intolerances and allergies). If you suspect your child's diet is causing behavioural problems, ask your doctor or nutritionist for advice.

Trying other treatments

You may consider other forms of treatment for your child with ADHD, such as the following, all of which can be organised for you by your GP:

✔ **Anxiety management:** You and your child's teachers create a daily routine for your child, such as setting homework schedules, sticking to agreed bed- and mealtimes, setting boundaries, and giving clear instructions. Following a routine and being consistent with your child helps to remove disruptive elements from his life.

✔ **Cognitive therapy:** This behavioural therapy helps your child develop problem-solving techniques. Cognitive therapy helps your child work out how he feels about himself and how he acts and behaves.

✔ **Psychotherapy:** This form of counselling may limit your child's difficult behaviour, provide him with a sense of self-worth and achievement, and reduce your own frustration.

✔ **Social skills training:** Social skills training can help your child to perform better at school. You and your child's teachers work together on techniques to develop your child's self-control and self-esteem and improve his academic achievement.

Diagnosing Dyslexia and Dyspraxia

Dyslexia is a learning disability rather than an emotional or behavioural problem. If your child is dyslexic, he has a reading disability and has problems understanding written symbols. Just because your child has dyslexia doesn't mean he has a mental handicap, brain damage, or any speech or visual problems. About 90 per cent of children with dyslexia are boys. Dyslexic children have normal or above-normal intelligence and normal development – parents and doctors only identify the problem when the child starts reading.

Your dyslexic child's reading skills may fall behind that of other children of the same age. Your child may reverse letters and words when writing, and so he probably makes lots of spelling mistakes. A mismatch between his performance in verbal tasks and written tasks is a useful indicator that dyslexia may be a problem. If your child has dyslexia, special needs or an individual education plan may help him overcome his difficulties. Contact your local dyslexia association for a list of special teachers, or ask your child's school to refer him to an educational psychologist. The British Dyslexia Association (www.bdadyslexia.org.uk) provides lots of useful info about dyslexia.

Dyspraxia is the medical term for clumsiness. This condition used to be called 'clumsy child syndrome.' Some 10 per cent of the population in the UK has dyspraxia – most are male. Signs of dyspraxia include poor body awareness and posture; difficulty holding a pen, writing, or reading; inability to catch a ball, ride a bike, skip, or run; and a poor sense of direction. Children with dyspraxia often benefit from the same therapeutic approaches as for dyslexia. You may consider physiotherapy, special exercises, coordination practice, and hand–eye coordination techniques. As your child's brain develops and he gets older, he becomes more capable. For further info, contact the Dyspraxia Foundation (www.dyspraxiafoundation.org.uk).

Understanding Autism

Autism is the result of several changes to the brain, leading to three areas of impairment. If your child has autism, you may notice the following:

- ✔ Your child has difficulty communicating.

- ✔ Your child finds it hard to develop relationships with other people.

- ✔ Your child has a limited imagination when it comes to seeing other people's points of view.

If your child is autistic, he may have a fixed mindset and see things only from his own literal point of view. So, for example, if a bus conductor asks to see your child's ticket, your child may reply: 'No, it's in my pocket.'

People have always considered autism a lifelong condition with no cure. Researchers haven't found any drugs to treat autism fully and successfully. However, a number of treatments now exist that help some children with autism:

- ✔ **Lovaas method for children:** Created by Dr Lovaas, a US expert, this treatment involves understanding your child's mind and finding ways to interact and communicate with him.

- ✔ **Picture exchange communication system (PECS):** A treatment that is a behaviourally based programme, which instructs pre-verbal children in how to express their needs.

- ✔ **SPELL system:** SPELL stands for Structure, Positive, Empathy, Low arousal, and Links, and treatment aims to provide your child with a structured environment and a positive attitude to reduce his stress. The treatment encourages you to see the world from your child's point of view.

- ✔ **Treatment and Education of Autistic and Related Communication Handicapped Children/Adults (TEACCH) programme:** This treatment is based on the fact that people with autism find it easier to process visual information than verbal. For example, rather than asking your child whether he wants to go for a swim or walk, place a picture of the activities in front of him and let him choose. Letting him choose gives your child the power of making a choice and a clear idea as to what happens next.

If your child is diagnosed with autism, consider joining the National Autistic Society's Early Bird Programme. The programme gives both you and your child emotional support helps you make choices about your child's treatment and education. Find out more from `www.nas.org.uk/earlybird`.

Communication is key when it comes to dealing with your autistic child. Reducing anxiety and stress help your child communicate and develop learning skills. Your child's difficult behaviour may disappear when he feels that you understand and he no longer needs to 'act out'.

Other forms of treating and controlling autistic spectrum disorders include Auditory integration training (AIT): Your child listens to specially adapted music through headphones for two sets of 30 minutes each day for ten days. Autistic children hear some sounds well but other sounds only faintly. Distortions are analysed and amended to retrain the ear – this may help speech and behaviour.

Since the 1960s, children with autism have been given vitamin therapy. Studies show that treatment with vitamins A, B6, and C helps some people with autism. Remember that excessive doses of vitamins can be harmful so do not embark on this sort of therapy unless you are under close supervision by a qualified doctor with specialist qualifications in the area.

For further info, contact the National Autistic Society (www.nas.org.uk).

Part V
Playing Doctors and Nurses: Looking After a Sick Child

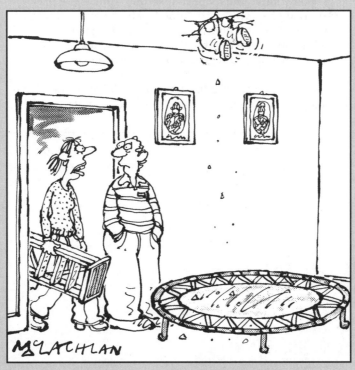

"I know all young children benefit from
excercise but the trampoline should really be
used outside."

In this part . . .

Don your stethoscope and scrubs – this is the part that gives you all the practical help you need when you're caring for a poorly child. From taking your little one's temperature to administering medicines, this part will ensure you're a regular Florence Nightingale.

This part also covers admitting your child to hospital, and some first aid basics for when things get serious.

Chapter 17

Caring for an Ill Child

• •

In This Chapter

▶ Becoming a nurse in your own home

▶ Controlling high temperatures and fevers

▶ Coping with febrile convulsions

▶ Taking your child to hospital

• •

You may not be a trained medical practitioner, but you probably sense instinctively when your child's ill. You soon learn to spot the subtle early signs of illness in your child: She may have a particularly restless night or lose interest in her food or the world around her. She may look pale or flushed or have a sunken appearance around the eyes. She may be whiny, clingy, and irritable, and generally out of sorts – just like *you* are when you're ill.

With a poorly child on your hands, you may find it difficult not to panic. But most childhood illnesses don't need specialist nursing care. In fact, the vast majority of common childhood ailments respond well to treatment at home, not least because that's where your child is happiest. Cuddles and lavish attention are a great form of medicine, so give plenty, along with the recommended dose of infant paracetamol if necessary. Lots of rest and fluids are also essential.

This chapter tells all you need to know to nurse your little one back to health. To find out about the symptoms of some common childhood illnesses, have a look at Chapter 14.

Looking After Your Child at Home

Even though you probably don't have the uniform, you'll be amazed at how quickly you take on the role of a nurse when you're looking after a poorly child. And yes – it can be a full-time job.

Taking your child's temperature

A common symptom of many childhood illnesses is a fever (more about this is in the section 'Fighting a Fever', later in the chapter). One of the first things you need to do when your little one is ill is take her temperature.

If you don't have a clinical thermometer, don't panic. You can tell whether your child has a fever simply by feeling her skin. If her tummy feels burning hot, she's probably got a fever. A hot, clammy forehead is another sign, especially if your child also has other symptoms, such as a runny nose, cough, or earache.

Using one of the many types of thermometer, take your child's body temperature reading from her mouth, armpit, ear, or skin surface. A reading of 38°C or more is considered a fever.

Many different types of thermometer are available. Whichever type you choose, practise how to use it correctly before your child gets sick. And always keep and follow the manufacturer's instructions. The following are the most common types of clinical thermometer:

- **Digital thermometers:** These usually provide the quickest, most accurate readings, and are really easy to use. They're available from most pharmacies and come in many sizes and shapes. They can be used as oral or underarm thermometers. Your child needs to stay still as you take the reading, so this sort of thermometer can be a bit tricky to use, especially in younger children.

- **Ear thermometers:** These measure the temperature inside the ear canal. They're quick, accurate, and easy to use in older children, although some experts say they're not accurate in babies as the ear hole is so small.

- **Forehead strips:** These small plastic strips, which you press against your child's forehead, tell you whether your child has a fever, but they're not reliable for taking an exact measurement. They're good to use as a rough guide, especially in infants and children.

- **No-touch thermometers:** These are battery-operated thermometers that you hold over your child's forehead. A number of experts worry about their accuracy, and they can be expensive, but they're non-invasive so you don't have to disturb your child if you want to check on her.

Don't use a mercury thermometer on your child. They are being phased out because mercury is a highly toxic substance. If you have a mercury thermometer in your home, dispose of it and get a new, safer thermometer. Your local council can give you details of how to dispose of it safely. We don't recommend a rectal thermometer either, because you may damage your child's rectum if you don't use the thermometer properly. Some hospitals use rectal thermometers for accuracy, but such accuracy isn't necessary at home.

Nursing care 101

Working out how to keep your poorly child happy can be tough – she's likely to want constant attention from you. Even you need a break sometimes, so try to soothe her or distract her with the following:

- ✔ **Make sure that your child's as comfortable as possible, if only to give you a little peace.** You may find your child more demanding than usual when she's ill, although if she's feeling particularly rough she may just want to be left alone. The best thing is to take the lead from her. Most children prefer to lie on the sofa rather than be banished to the bedroom during the day, so let her be where she's comfortable.

- ✔ **Give your child things to occupy her.** Boredom's a real problem for ill children, especially after they hit the road to recovery. Sort out a box of toys and activities for your child, including a few of her older things: She'll probably have a much shorter attention span than normal, and won't want to play with anything that's too taxing.

- ✔ **Consider turning on the telly.** You'll probably want to relax your standards about watching television when your child's ill: TV can work wonders as a distraction from her aches and pains.

- ✔ **Make sure that your child drinks plenty of fluids.** In the first day or two of an infection, your child is likely to lose her appetite. Going without food for a couple of days is fine, but fluids are absolutely crucial, as dehydration is dangerous. Fruit ice-lollies are a good alternative to drinks to maintain fluid intake.

Cut the risk of vomiting by giving your child small amounts of fluid, very frequently. If your child is very young and finds it hard to stick to a few sips at a time, put just a small amount into a glass or beaker, and top it up each time you offer her a drink. Rehydration fluids, which you can get from your pharmacist, will help.

As well as these suggestions, you can help to lessen your child's aches and pains associated with particular illnesses. For more, read on.

If you've tried everything possible to make your child feel more comfortable but nothing seems to be working, phone your local surgery. If the surgery is closed, you're connected with the out-of-hours service: A trained health professional then talks you through your child's symptoms and advises you on how to care for her, organises for a doctor to visit your home, or recommends that you take your child to hospital (see 'Taking Your Child to Hospital' later in the chapter). Alternatively, call NHS Direct on 0845-4647 for a similar service (see Chapter 21 for more about NHS Direct). Nobody understands your child better than you do: If you're worried about your child, call the doctor.

Common cold

If your child's nose is blocked, encourage her to blow and wipe it frequently with soft tissues. Dab a little petroleum jelly around her nostrils to stop them getting sore. Keep her warm, but don't let her overheat. Let her lie somewhere quietly – she's going to need more sleep than usual, but she'll probably still want to play.

Cough

Sit in a steamy bathroom with your child to help clear her airways. Raise the head of her bed or cot to help drain away mucus. Stop the air in her bedroom drying out by placing a damp towel or a bowl of water over the radiator.

If you don't have radiators (or they're not on), boil a kettle of water in her room. Leave the lid off so that it doesn't turn off automatically, and it produces plenty of steam – but keep small children well clear, and keep an eye on it so it doesn't boil dry!

All coughs tend to get worse at night. That needn't be a worry in itself, even if it's particularly exhausting! But if your child is having difficulty breathing; is breathing very fast or wheezing; or looks blue or floppy, call a doctor.

Earache

Earache is one of the commonest childhood illnesses. Earache is usually caused by a problem with the normal drainage in the middle ear (called Eustachian tube dysfunction) or by an infection.

Eustachian tube dysfunction happens when the mucus from a cold blocks the Eustachian tube, which connects your middle ear with the outside world via your throat. This blockage means that you can't equalise the pressure in your middle ear, and can be painful. Fortunately, it doesn't cause any lasting damage and settles on its own.

Ear infections are usually caused by virus infections, which can't be cured with antibiotics. If your child's ear starts discharging, or if the earache goes on for more than a day or so, go and see your GP.

Infant paracetamol can help enormously in relieving the pain of earache, and can reduce the fever that often goes with it. Try to keep your child upright, supported by pillows, which may help to drain off fluid in the middle ear, which is often what is causing the pain. Older children (but not babies, because they can easily become overheated) may find it comforting to hold a warm covered hot-water bottle over the affected ear.

Vomiting and diarrhoea

Offer your child frequent drinks to prevent dehydration. If you're breast-feeding, feed her frequently and give her water as well – from a sterilised teaspoon if she won't take a bottle. If your child's bottle-fed and under 12 months old, give her normal feeds. Oral rehydration solution can be useful for older children but don't give it without medical advice, and don't give your child flat fizzy or sweetened drinks. When your child feels hungry again, offer her dry toast or plain boiled rice, but avoid fatty foods. Give your child a light diet rather than not giving her any solid foods.

Never give anti-diarrhoea medicines to children because some of them can have dangerous side effects for your child.

Surviving at night

Night-time nursing is harder than the day job. Illness always seems worse in the middle of the night, and it can be scary if you feel you've got no one to help you. To help you make it through 'til dawn, here are a few suggestions:

✔ Have plenty of infant paracetamol to hand. Keep up the doses through the night if your child's temperature is high – even if you have to wake her up to medicate her. Remember: Never exceed the recommended dosage.

✔ Keep your GP's phone number handy – the answering message directs you to your out-of-hours GP service. It's amazing how hard it can be to find the phone book at 3 a.m. with a screaming child!

✔ If you want to stay close to your child, put her cot or a temporary bed near yours, or take up residence in her room. You may be tempted to let your sick child sleep with you in your bed, but if she's feverish she may overheat, so be careful. You probably won't find it much fun sleeping next to a burning, wriggling, moaning little furnace – try it and see! And remember: If you do let her sleep with you when she's ill, you may need to be firm about getting her to return to her own bed after she's better.

The Foundation for the Study into Infant Deaths advises parents not to share a bed or sofa with babies under a year old because of the risk of cot death, which may be caused by overheating.

If you and your child stay in your own bedrooms at night, consider using a baby monitor to alert you if she's restless or coughing at night.

Get thee to a doctor! Emergency situations

Most childhood illness are of the run-of-the-mill variety and safely cared for at home. But occasionally you'll come up against a situation that calls for a doctor's attention.

Seek immediate medical help if your child:

- Is choking, or has been burnt, stung, or bitten, or has had any other accident that requires immediate expert first aid.

- Has a febrile convulsion, or fit, especially if the convulsion is her first. Have a look at the later section 'Dealing with febrile convulsions' for more information.

- Shows symptoms of meningitis, such as fever, frequent vomiting, a high-pitched or moaning cry, irritability, an aversion to bright light, drowsiness, a bulging fontanelle, blotchy or pale skin, a limp body, or a purple rash that doesn't disappear when pressed with a glass.

- Is vomiting all the time and refusing to drink or eat.

- Is dehydrated – symptoms of dehydration include listlessness, sunken eyes, and dry nappies and/or no bowel movements for 12 hours or more.

- Is breathing very fast or finding it difficult to breathe and/or has blue lips.

- Becomes unconscious or is difficult to rouse – when you handle her or talk to her, she doesn't respond.

- Turns very pale or blue or you notice a bluish tinge around her mouth or tongue.

- Becomes unusually quiet and lethargic or droopy and hot.

- Is running a temperature over 39°C that doesn't respond to paracetamol.

- Has difficulty breathing or has noisy, grunting breath.

- Is in severe pain and cannot be comforted.

- Cannot keep drinks down.

- Is vomiting and has a swollen stomach.

- Has blood in her stools or vomit.

- Vomits constantly for over an hour.

Another perfectly justifiable time to seek medical care is if you're worried about your child, even if you can't explain exactly why. You know your child better than anyone. If your instincts tell you something's seriously wrong and it's too late to go to your GP, don't hesitate to take her to your local casualty department. See the section 'Going to A&E' for what to expect.

Fighting a Fever

A fever isn't an illness in itself but a sign of other problems in the body – usually a viral or bacterial infection. Fever is thought to be the body's natural defence mechanism: The body tries to reach a temperature that the virus or bacterium cannot survive in. As well as a high temperature, your feverish child may have clammy skin and feel achy. Take measures to bring down her temperature, not only to help her feel more comfortable but also to stop her body overheating, which increases the risk of having a convulsion (more about convulsions in the section 'Dealing with febrile convulsions', later in the chapter).

Cooling down

Try some of these techniques to bring down your child's fever. They are suitable for babies and children of all ages, unless stated otherwise.

✔ If your child's over 3 months old and her temperature is above 37.5°C (99.5°F), give her the correct dose of infant paracetamol or infant ibuprofen to help bring down the temperature. If necessary, give both infant paracetamol and infant ibuprofen, spaced at regular intervals. But never exceed the recommended dosages.

Never give aspirin to children under 16, because it can occasionally cause a serious complication called Reye's syndrome.

✔ Strip down your child and sponge her with tepid water to help open the blood vessels in the skin and cool down her body. Don't use cold water, because it constricts the blood vessels in the skin and less heat is lost.

Sponging down your child is better than putting her in a bath of tepid water. The cooling effect of sponging is the result of evaporation of water off her skin – sitting in the bath won't have the same effect. Try fanning your child after sponging her to dry the water off: This is an extremely effective way of cooling her body temperature quickly.

> ✔ Give your child plenty of cool drinks to avoid dehydration. She should urinate at least every six to eight hours, and the urine should be the colour of pale straw. Dark urine is a sign that your child's not getting enough fluids, which can be dangerous, especially if she has diarrhoea or vomiting. Offer your child lots of water or diluted fruit juice to prevent dehydration and help flush out toxins from her body.
>
> ✔ When you put your child to bed, leave her in her underwear or nappy and cover her with a light sheet rather than a blanket or quilt. Keep the room cool – it shouldn't be warmer than 20°C.

These measures should start to bring your child's temperature down within a few minutes, and paracetamol or ibuprofen should work within half an hour. If you can't reduce your child's temperature or are worried about her in any way, contact NHS Direct (0845-4647) or your GP.

Dealing with febrile convulsions

Sometimes a high fever causes a febrile convulsion. These fits are normally triggered by the body becoming rapidly overheated, causing unusual electrical activity in the brain. If your child's running a very high temperature (38°C or above), she's more at risk of having a febrile convulsion, which is why you must try to control her temperature. Children are far more prone than adults to febrile convulsions: About 1 child in 30 has a febrile convulsion at some point during her first 6 years.

If your child has a high temperature, she may experience extreme shivering, or rigours, that makes her whole body shake. Unlike a convulsion, your child remains conscious during rigours, although she may seem delirious. If you don't bring down your child's temperature, rigours may turn into a convulsion, so cool her down as quickly as possible.

Looking at what happens

At the beginning of a febrile convulsion, your child loses consciousness and her body becomes momentarily stiff. She may cry out or become incontinent. Within about 30 seconds, she starts to jerk her arms and legs uncontrollably. She may roll her eyes and stop breathing.

Try to stay calm. Hold your child gently. If possible, turn her head to one side to prevent choking (although this is most unlikely to happen). After a few minutes, the jerking movements usually stop and your child drifts off to sleep, although she may wake up briefly first. She'll probably wake up and recover completely within an hour, although she may be a little disoriented to begin with. During the fit, your child is unconscious and isn't in any distress. When she wakes up later, she'll have no memory of what's happened.

Your child, especially if she's very young, will probably be admitted to hospital after her first febrile convulsion so the doctors can identify the cause of, and bring down, her high temperature. The hospital doctors will advise you on how to prevent and treat further febrile convulsions. If your child has a fit that isn't the result of a high temperature, the doctors will investigate for another cause, such as epilepsy.

Watching your child have a convulsion can be absolutely terrifying, but the convulsion's extremely unlikely to damage your child. She won't be in pain or remember anything about it afterwards. Many doctors say it's worse for the parent to watch a convulsion than for the child to experience one. A convulsion must be taken seriously, however, and if it's your child's first one you must get medical help immediately.

Preventing further fits

If your child has already had a febrile convulsion, try to keep her temperature down whenever she's ill or after a vaccination, as she may have another convulsion (see Chapter 3). (About one child in three goes on to have a further convulsion.) If your child's particularly prone to febrile convulsions, her doctor may prescribe a tube of diazepam. If your child has a convulsion, you squirt diazepam into her anus during the jerking stage of the convulsion, which stops the fit quickly. Occasionally, children who are prone to frequent febrile convulsions are prescribed anti-epileptic drugs to stabilise the brain's electrical activity. Your child should take these anti-epileptic drugs until she's old enough to have grown out of having febrile convulsions (usually before the teenage years).

A febrile convulsion's unlikely to have any long-lasting effects. Even children prone to convulsions normally stop having them by the age of 6 or 7 years. Only about 1 in every 100 children who experience febrile convulsions turns out to be epileptic.

Taking Your Child to Hospital

Nobody likes the idea of going to hospital, but the thought of your child going is even worse. Every year, however, thousands of young children are admitted to hospital for an operation, or as the result of an accident or illness. Not being familiar with what to expect at hospital makes things harder: Fortunately, though, doctors and nurses realise just how frightening the experience can be for parents and children, and most do all they can to put you at ease. You can do plenty as well to make the trip as stress-free as possible.

Going to A&E

Your local accident and emergency (A&E) department is the place to go if your child suddenly becomes seriously ill or needs immediate medical attention. If your child's condition isn't life-threatening (for example, if she has hurt a limb after a fall) it can be quicker to get to hospital under your own steam. In an emergency, calling an ambulance is a better option. In certain circumstances, you should always call 999 – for example, if your child is having difficulty breathing, is so short of breath that she can't talk, has a convulsion (fit) for the first time or a convulsion that lasts more than a minute, or becomes unwell after swallowing something poisonous or harmful (remember to take the packet or bottle that contained the poison to hospital with you).

Not all hospital have A&E departments, and some A&E departments don't see children, so always find out the arrangements as soon as you move to a new area. Having a sick child is quite stressful enough without being turned away from A&E when you get there!

At A&E, go to reception and book in your child. A triage nurse will see your child quickly and make a brief assessment of her condition. A&E doctors try to see children as soon as possible – children often have priority over adults at A&E, and some hospitals even have dedicated children's A&E departments.

Waiting in A&E can be tiring and stressful, but most hospitals are geared up to keeping children amused. If you have time before you leave home for A&E, remember to take a puzzle book or toy to distract your child while she's waiting.

Most childhood injuries can be treated within the A&E department and you can take your child home after treatment. However, your child may need to be admitted on to a children's ward for ongoing treatment or observation. If this happens, you may be able to stay with your child overnight.

Going to hospital is a frightening experience for anyone. All hospitals have patient advice and liaison services (PALS), whose staff can give you useful information about what will happen to your child and the sort of care she'll receive. They can also refer you to the right departments to help. Ask at the hospital reception for more details about the service.

Planned admissions

If your child's going to hospital for a routine minor procedure – for example, to have tonsils removed or *grommets* (small tubes in the ear to prevent recurrent infections) fitted – her GP or paediatrician will have referred her to the hospital. Many minor operations are now carried out on a day basis (for more information about grommets, have a look at Chapter 13). The doctor will let you know in advance whether your child needs to stay overnight. Call the hospital on the morning of the planned admission to make sure that a bed is available – your child needs a bed, even if she's in only for the day. When you take your child in, take her to the ward stated in the admission letter.

Preparing your child for hospital

If she's old enough to understand, help your child prepare for her trip to hospital so she knows what to expect. To make the trip less frightening, try the following:

- ✔ Talk to your child about what may happen in hospital, and reassure her that she'll be in the best possible hands.

- ✔ Be honest but reassuring – don't pretend something won't hurt if it is going to. Emphasise that the pain only lasts for a short time, and share your own experiences of visits to hospital.

- ✔ Encourage your child to ask questions about her hospital trip.

- ✔ Look at picture books about going into hospital, and play doctors and nurses with your child's favourite soft toys.

- ✔ If the hospital offers pre-admission visits, take your child round the ward beforehand so she becomes familiar with the surroundings, and meets some of the staff who'll be involved in her care. To arrange a visit, call the phone number on your child's admission letter and ask to speak to the play specialist – all children's wards have specially trained members of staff.

Younger children and babies don't have an accurate concept of time, in which case, don't tell your child about her planned hospital trip until a day or two before she's due to be admitted.

If your child's old enough, let her help to pack her hospital bag. This is a good way of helping her take on board her visit to hospital, and may bring up questions she wouldn't have asked otherwise. As well as essentials such as toiletries, nappies, and clothes, pack a few favourite toys, books, or games. For younger children, check with the hospital to see whether you need to take your own baby food and nappies. If you're breastfeeding, the hospital should supply a breast pump for expressing and a fridge for storing your milk.

Don't forget a bag for yourself. Most parents are allowed to stay in with their child. The hospital may give you a bed, but you may just have to doze in an armchair.

When you're there

Usually, you're responsible for routine care such as feeding and washing your child in hospital. Try to stick to your normal routine for mealtimes and bedtimes as much as possible to help your child feel more secure. If your child's having surgery, the anaesthetist will visit you and your child in the ward to run through how she'll put your child to sleep. You can usually stay with your child in the anaesthetic room until she's asleep and then be with her in the recovery room when she awakens.

Needle phobia is a common fear in both adults and children. If your child is frightened of needles, talk to the hospital play specialist, who'll help both you and your child deal with your fears. Using a special teddy as you describe the process can help. Simple distraction also works, so try singing a song with your child while the nurse does her job. When taking blood tests or giving an injection, the nurse usually puts a little local anaesthetic cream on your child's hand or arm to reduce the pain your child feels during the injection. The cream can take about half an hour to work, however, so ask the nurse in advance. If you have a fear of needles, you don't *have* to stay with your child – after all, you don't want to influence your child's reaction.

After the operation

After your child's operation, the consultant or registrar will visit you at your child's bedside and talk you through how things went, which gives you a chance to find out what happened during the operation, whether it was successful, and what follow-up treatment your child needs. A nurse will talk to you about your child's aftercare, for example looking after stitches, give you a prescription for any medications that your child needs, and tell you who to contact if you have any worries about your child after her operation.

Most operations are short and routine, but if your child needs to stay in hospital, encourage family and friends to visit, both to make your child feel comfortable, and to give you a break. Children's wards usually have open visiting hours.

Your child's hospital visitors must be fit and well. Ask all her visitors to wash their hands properly with anti-infection gels, usually by the ward entrance, before coming on the ward to avoid spreading infections.

Staying Sane

Whether your sick child is at home or in hospital, caring for her for more than a couple of days can be tremendously draining on you. Children often become much more demanding when they're ill, and lack of sleep can take its toll on you. Don't be afraid to ask for help from your partner, members of your family, or friends who are willing to sit with your child while you get some fresh air, do a bit of shopping, or simply take a nap.

Don't forget to look after yourself when you're running around after your poorly child – you don't want to run the risk of getting ill yourself, which makes you of no use to anyone! If your child sleeps during the day, take a nap at the same time to catch up. And look after your diet – even if your child's not interested in food, make sure that you get nourishment and energy.

If you're worried about your child in any way, seek reassurance from hospital staff or your child's doctor. Most importantly of all, remember that your child's illness will pass and life will get easier.

A word about special-care babies

One in 10 newborn babies spends at least a few days in a special-care neonatal unit because they're born prematurely, are very small, or are extremely sick. Your special-care baby will be placed in an incubator for warmth. Depending on her problems, she may be attached to various monitors and tubes. They can look a lot worse than they really are, so ask a doctor or nurse to explain what they do. You can visit your baby at any time, although not all hospitals provide overnight facilities for parents.

To start with the nurses do most of the work, but after a few days the special-care team will show you how to handle and breastfeed your baby, and encourage you to become as involved as possible. Even if you can't be there all the time, other family members are welcome – although some hospitals don't allow children to visit in case they have an infectious illness.

For help and advice on premature or special-care babies, contact Tommy's (www.tommys.org; phone 0870-777-30-60) or BLISS (www.bliss.org.uk; phone 0500-618140).

Chapter 18

Knowing Something about Medicines

In This Chapter

▶ Using medicines safely

▶ Giving your child painkillers and antibiotics

▶ Looking at alternatives to mainstream medicines

*M*any new parents – and, to be honest, most experienced ones too – panic when it comes to giving medicine to their child. If you're struggling, try to remember that you're giving medicine to help your child get better. Be confident and determined, because your child may be remarkably good at picking up on your doubts and may resist no matter what you do. If you're not convinced that your child needs medication, first get reassurance from your doctor.

Giving Medicines Safely

When it comes to giving medicine to your child, the most important thing is vigilance. Medicines can be powerful and potent, so you need to give the right medicine, of the right strength, at the right time, and in the right dose. Whether you're using a prescribed drug or an over-the-counter remedy, we cannot overemphasise the importance of dispensing medicine properly to your child. Given incorrectly, drugs are at best ineffective and at worst extremely harmful. Before accepting a prescription from your child's doctor or buying an over-the-counter remedy at the pharmacy, make sure that you have found out enough about the drug. If you're not sure, don't be shy to ask. Your pharmacist or doctor can tell you:

✔ What the medication is and what it's for

✔ Whether there may be a problem with other drugs your child is taking; sometimes, different drugs may interact, stopping them working properly or causing dangerous side effects.

✔ How often and for how long your child needs to take the medicine

✔ What to do if your child misses a dose

✔ Whether there are likely to be any side effects

✔ How quickly the medicine starts to work

Measuring up

Always use the proper kit when dispensing medicine. Never use a regular kitchen spoon: One teaspoon may be twice the size of another and your child won't receive the correct dose. Instead, try the following:

✔ **Dosage cups:** These are convenient for children who can drink from a cup without spilling. Be sure to check the numbers carefully on the side of the cup. Measure out liquid medicine with the cup at eye level on a flat surface.

✔ **Medicine spoons:** Use a medicine spoon rather than a kitchen teaspoon to ensure that your child gets exactly the right amount he needs. If you're using a medicine spoon for a baby under 6 months old, sterilise the spoon first by boiling it or placing it in sterilising solution.

✔ **Oral syringes:** Syringes are convenient for babies who are still breastfed or bottle-fed and are not used to swallowing from a spoon. Hold your baby in the crook of your arm and take up the specified amount of medicine into the syringe. Place the dropper in the corner of your baby's mouth with the 'spout' pointing into the inside of the cheek, and release the medicine gently.

Syringes are also convenient for storing doses of medicine, for example to measure out a dose for the babysitter to use later on. Some syringes come with caps to prevent the medicine leaking out. The caps are usually small and are choking hazards, so be sure that your baby doesn't get hold of one.

Getting your child to take the medicine

Gone are the days when children were given a spoonful of sugar to help the medicine go down – Mary Poppins obviously never took her charges to the dentist. These days, nearly all children's medicines are sugar-free to help prevent tooth decay. Most medicines contain artificial sweeteners and colourings to make them more palatable and attractive – although your child may not agree!

It takes two, baby

Babies love to wriggle, especially when you really don't want them to. Giving your little bundle of joy his medicine may mean you end up with more of the sticky stuff on your clothes than in his mouth. If possible, enlist the help of another adult or an older sibling to do some gentle head-holding. Position your baby so his head is raised slightly – don't lay him down flat because he could inhale the medicine into his lungs. If you're on your own, wrap a blanket around your baby's arms to stop him struggling and hold him steady.

Try to give medicine to one side of the mouth, near the middle of the tongue. Medicine falling directly on the centre of the palate triggers gagging. Put tablets at the back of your child's tongue.

Using an oral syringe (details in 'Measuring up' earlier in the chapter) is much easier than using a medicine spoon because you have a lot more control. Put just a little of the medicine in your child's mouth at a time. If he spits it out, persevere – gently scoop the medicine back in while talking to your child and trying to keep him calm. If you can, get another person to hold your child's mouth open.

Older and wiser

Older children usually don't mind taking medicine too much, but try to have a few tricks up your sleeve in case you're faced with opposition. The oldest trick in the book is to disguise the drug – try crushing tablets and mixing them with food. But *never* do this with capsules.

Don't add liquid medicine to drinks: The drug just sinks to the bottom of the glass and stick to the sides, and you won't be sure that your child has taken the whole dose. Instead, consider giving him his favourite sugary drink as a treat to wash away the taste of the medicine.

Try giving your child some control over the proceedings: Ask him to pour out the medicine himself and find out what he'd like afterwards to wash away the taste.

Help your child clean his teeth after he's taken any liquid medicine to prevent syrup sticking to his teeth.

Giving drops

Your child's doctor may prescribe drops to treat infections of the ear, eye, or nose. To give drops to your baby, let gravity help you: Lay your baby on a flat surface before you begin. Try to enlist the help of someone to keep your baby still and hold his head steady. An older child will probably be more cooperative: Just ask him to tilt his head back or to the side as you put the drops in.

Don't use over-the-counter drops for more than three days without consulting a doctor, because your child may need to be prescribed something stronger to fight the infection.

If your doctor prescribes eye, nose, or ear drops, ask for ones that need to be given as few times a day as possible! Eye drops especially can be tough to get in, but these days, some eye drops come in a viscous form that you only need to give twice a day.

Don't let the dropper touch your child's nose, ear, or eye, otherwise you'll just transfer the germs back to the bottle. If the dropper does touch your child, wash the dropper thoroughly with hot water before putting it back in the bottle.

Ear's hoping: giving drops

Ear drops (such as those containing olive oil) can help to unblock your child's ear canal. But don't be tempted to use them without consulting your doctor or pharmacist, because drops can do more damage than good if the ear is infected. Always seek medical advice before putting anything in your child's ear.

To administer ear drops, lay your baby on his side, with the affected ear uppermost. Let the drops fall into the centre of his ear and hold your baby steady for a while, until the drops have run into the canal. Older children are usually more compliant, but you should still encourage your child to stay still to allow the drops to enter the affected area.

Nosing around

Your child's doctor may recommend saline nose drops to help the nasal passages, particularly if your little one's still a baby. Tilt your baby's head back slightly and gently drop liquid into each nostril.

Count the number of drops as you put them in. Two or three drops at a time is usually sufficient. Any more will just run down your baby's throat and cause him to cough and splutter.

Eyes right

Your child's doctor may recommend eye drops if he has an eye infection such as conjunctivitis. To administer them, tilt your baby's head slightly so that his affected eye is lowermost. This way, no drops run from the affected eye to the other. Try to get someone to hold your baby as you put the drops in. Gently pull down his lower eyelid and let the drops fall between his eye and his lower lid.

Try giving at least one dose a day while your little one is asleep. You can often pull the lower lid down and gently smear the drop along the inside of the lower lid without waking him up. It may be nerve-racking (especially if your child has taken a while to get off to sleep and they stir while you're doing it) but you will find it infinitely easier than the alternative!

Abiding by the golden rules

When it comes to giving medicine, safety is your absolute priority. Medicines can be extremely dangerous if used inappropriately. It's important to make your child understand the dangers of medicines as soon as he is old enough, and, of course, lock them away well out of reach.

- ✔ **Always make sure that the drug is safe for children: Never give adults' medicine to a child.** If the label doesn't mention a child's dose, then the medicine's not safe for your child.

  Some medicines work quite differently in children and adults. Some barbiturates, for example, which make adults feel sluggish, make children hyperactive. Amphetamines, which stimulate adults, can calm children. If you have any questions about a medicine, ask your doctor or pharmacist. Children are more sensitive than adults to many drugs. For example, antihistamines and alcohol – both common in cold medications – can have adverse effects on children, causing excitability or excessive drowsiness. Medicines containing aspirin must be avoided at all costs. Don't give a child under 2 years any over-the-counter drugs without asking your doctor first.

  Never give a child under the age of 16 aspirin or products containing aspirin or other *salicylates* (medicines derived from salicylic acid) without your doctor's advice, because they have been associated with the development of Reye's syndrome, a rare but deadly condition that can affect the liver and brain. Reye's syndrome doesn't affect adults.

- ✔ **When giving a drug to your child, watch closely for side effects while he's taking it.** If you're concerned in any way about your child after he's taken medicine, don't assume that everything's OK. Better to phone the doctor or nurse than have a bad reaction to a drug.

- ✔ **Don't give drugs unless they're truly necessary.** Not every ailment needs medicine. Common viruses run their course in 7–10 days with or without medication. Some over-the-counter medications can make your child more comfortable and help him eat and rest better when he's got a viral infection, but others may trigger allergic reactions or changes for the worse in sleeping, eating, and behaviour.

✔ **Always read the label.** You've probably heard this phrase a million times before, but reading the instructions first is the most important thing you can do to make sure that you're giving your child medicine safely. Medicine labels contain many warnings – for a reason. Don't use the product until you understand what's on the label. Prescription drugs come with precise instructions from the doctor – follow them carefully. Over-the-counter drugs have dosing instructions on their labels – don't ignore them. Getting the dosage right for an over-the-counter drug is just as important as for a prescription drug.

Reactions and overdoses can happen with any drug, whether prescribed or bought over the counter. Overdosing is incredibly easy, especially if you don't read or understand the label or if you measure out the medicine incorrectly. Problems can also occur if you give your child several different medicines containing the same ingredients: Never mix medicines without consulting your doctor first.

Understanding Commonly Used Medications

The number of medications, both prescribed and over-the-counter, is mind-boggling and can lead to a great deal of confusion. If ever you're in doubt about a particular medicine, ask your pharmacist for the information you need – that's what he or she is there for.

Painkillers

Painkillers come in many different forms and varieties, but the two most common for children are paracetamol and ibuprofen:

✔ **Paracetamol** is available for children as a liquid, tablets, soluble tablets, and suppositories (tablets that you put in your child's rectum). Most of these are available at chemists and supermarkets.

✔ **Ibuprofen** belongs to a group of drugs called non-steroidal anti-inflammatory drugs (NSAIDs). In low doses, ibuprofen reduces pain. In higher doses, it also reduces inflammation (swelling and redness). It also brings down temperatures.

Seeing how painkillers work

When your child's in pain, for example with an ear infection, his body produces chemicals to fight off the bacterium or virus that's making him ill. These chemicals cause inflammation in the affected area, leading to swelling and pain. Ibuprofen stops the body making the chemicals that cause pain and inflammation. Paracetamol works by stopping the chemicals from sending such strong pain messages, so the pain fades. But don't worry – painkillers won't stop your child's body from fighting off the infection. They won't speed up your child's recovery either, but they can make him more comfortable while his own immune system fights the infection in its own time.

Worrying about side effects

Some children feel sick, vomit, or have tummy pain after taking painkillers, but these problems are usually mild. If your child does have side effects, you may be able to reduce them by giving him the medicine soon after meals or with food or milk.

If your child's taking paracetamol, don't give him any other medicine that also contains paracetamol – such as some cough syrups – because this can lead to overdosing. Overdosing on paracetamol can damage your child's liver and kidneys and lead to organ failure, so never exceed the recommended dose for his age.

Antibiotics

Two types of germ make your child sick – bacteria and viruses. Although some bacteria and viruses cause diseases with similar symptoms, the organisms multiply and spread illness in quite different ways:

- ✔ **Bacteria** are living organisms. They're everywhere, and most don't cause any harm. In fact, some bacteria are beneficial: Everyone has healthy bacteria in their intestines, for example, to help digest food. But some bacteria are harmful and can cause illness by invading the human body, multiplying and interfering with normal bodily processes. Antibiotics are effective against bacteria: The drugs kill these living organisms by stopping their growth and reproduction.

- ✔ **Viruses** have to invade other living cells to survive. The body's immune system fights off some viruses before they cause illness, but other viruses – such as colds and chickenpox – must simply run their course. Viruses do not respond to antibiotics at all.

Frequent or inappropriate use of antibiotics creates bacteria that are resistant to some antibiotic treatment. Infection with resistant bacteria then calls for stronger or higher doses of antibiotics. Antibiotic resistance is a widespread problem. Bacteria that were once highly responsive to antibiotics have become increasingly resistant. Among those that are becoming harder to treat are pneumococcal infections – for example, pneumonia and meningitis – and skin infections.

Antibiotics are one of the great advances in medicine. But over prescribing them has resulted in the development of bacteria that don't respond to antibiotics that may have worked in the past.

To minimise the risk of antibacterial resistance, follow these tips:

✔ If your doctor or nurse practitioner tells you antibiotics won't work, trust them! Coughs and colds, for instance, are almost always caused by virus infections. That means that no matter how frustrating or worrying it is to have a child with a hacking cough for weeks on end, giving antibiotics won't speed up their recovery. Seek advice from your doctor – and ask questions if you don't understand. Letting milder illnesses – especially those thought to be caused by viruses – run their course to avoid the development of drug-resistant germs is often a good thing.

✔ Never use another person's medication.

✔ Use antibiotics only as prescribed.

✔ Don't save antibiotics for 'next time'.

✔ Always finish the course of antibiotics. Antibiotics are effective only if your child takes the full course for the right amount of time prescribed by the doctor.

Antibiotics often have side effects, including diarrhoea and feelings of sickness. They may also trigger fungal infections such as thrush in the mouth or, in girls, the vagina. If your child suffers from any side effects, see your doctor who can discuss treatments or change your child's prescription if necessary.

Steroids

Two of the most common reasons for your doctor to prescribe steroids are because your child has asthma or eczema. Both of these conditions are known as 'atopic' or 'allergic' conditions (you can find out more about them in Chapter 15).

Steroids in gunk form: Creams and ointments

Steroids in prescribed skin creams and ointments (called *topical steroids*) can be invaluable at reducing the skin inflammation of eczema. If your child's skin becomes too inflamed it can crack, damaging the protective barrier and allowing infection in.

However, do not overuse steroids. Topical steroids can be absorbed through the skin, and the thinner the skin, the more steroids areabsorbed. Too much steroid in your child's system can cause thinning of the skin, unpleasant looking stretch marks (or *striae*) or, in unusually high doses, stunt your child's growth.

Debunking the steroid myths

Many parents worry about giving their child steroids because of all the scare stories they hear – they'll turn your child into a muscle-bound bodybuilder; they thin the skin, letting infection get through the skin barrier; they cause hair to sprout all over; they'll stunt your child's growth.

In fact, your child's body produces its own natural steroids, which are essential for the workings of the brain and other parts of the body. In excessive quantities, steroids can certainly harm your child's health – but if he needs them, avoiding them completely can be even more harmful.

The younger your child, the more susceptible he is to the side effects of topical steroids. The thinnest parts of your baby's skin (his face, his genitalia, and his skin folds) are the most likely to be affected by steroids. Always check with your doctor about whether to avoid using the topical steroid on these delicate parts.

When you're using topical steroids for a flare-up of eczema, use them in the mildest form possible, over the smallest area possible, to bring the inflammation under control. After the worst of the inflammation has settled, you can use a milder steroid, or stop using it until he suffers another flare-up. That way, your child gets the benefits of steroids completely safely.

If your doctor recommends steroid cream, ask if the mildest strength will work successfully. Your doctor will be happy to tell you why he considers the particular steroid cream is necessary, and whether a milder steroid can be given once the inflammation settles.

Breathe deeply: Steroids for asthma

One of the most common and effective treatment for childhood asthma is inhaled steroids.

Most steroid inhalers given to children are quite safe, even if your child needs to take them every day. But your child shouldn't take more than they need, which is why regular check-ups with your GP or practice nurse are so important. If your child needs his 'reliever' inhaler less than once every couple of days, your GP may suggest reducing the dose. Higher doses of inhaled steroids over a long period are likely to have an effect on your child's growth, but having lots of illness (such as poorly controlled asthma) can also severely restrict your child's growth. However, your child may catch up on growth when his asthma is less severe.

Looking at Complementary Medicines

Complementary medicine is no longer the realm of hippy-dippy tree-huggers. It is becoming increasingly popular among even the most conservative of parents and professionals – and the industry is growing rapidly to keep up. Many parents want to take more responsibility for their children's (and their own) health without recourse to traditional drugs such as antibiotics.

A world of difference often exists between 'complementary' and 'alternative' health practitioners. Complementary practitioners often work closely with mainstream medicine, offering treatments that complement or add to those provided by doctors. Certain alternative practitioners, on the other hand, don't accept part or all 'mainstream' medicine, and actively encourage their patients to stop using medication prescribed by their doctor. Stopping prescribed medicine without medical advice can be extremely dangerous and occasionally fatal.

Complementary therapists practise holistic – whole-person – health. This means that the therapist considers all aspects of your child's physical and emotional wellbeing, even if the problem seems to be located in only one part of your child's body. Loads of alternative therapies exist, but nearly all of them concentrate on treating your child by restoring his body's natural balance and maximising his ability to heal himself.

Although most complementary medicines work alongside conventional treatments (hence the term 'complementary'), seek advice from your doctor *and* your complementary practitioner if you want to mix remedies, because certain drugs – particularly herbal medicines – interact with each other.

Considering homeopathy for your child

Homeopathy is one of the most popular, and one of the fastest growing, of the natural therapies. Homeopathy can be a really effective natural form of treatment for common childhood ailments.

Homeopathy is based on the theory that like cures like: The homeopath chooses remedies that in much larger quantities produce similar symptoms to those being treated. For example, if your child suffers from hay fever caused by pollen, the homeopath may treat him with a remedy called 'mixed pollen'. The remedy acts as a catalyst, kick-starting the body's natural healing process. Homeopathic remedies are very dilute – so weak, in fact, that no measurable molecules are left in the original substance.

Homeopathic remedies are based mainly on animal, plant, and mineral substances, although some make use of human secretions or tissues and a few are based on micro-organisms. The remedies are given in a dilute form, which is made by dissolving the substance in a solvent such as alcohol and then diluting it by a factor of 100. The process of dilution is repeated many times, so that each successive dilution has one-hundredth the strength of the previous dilution. The first dilution has a potency of one centesimal (1c), the second two centesimals (2c), and so on. As the number of dilutions increases, the smaller the amount of the original substance that remains. The higher the number of dilutions, the more potent the remedy. So, for example, a remedy of 30c is more potent than a 6c remedy.

Going for a consultation

If you want to treat your baby or child using homeopathic remedies, get a consultation with a registered practitioner. The first consultation is likely to last for an hour or more, because the homeopath wants to find out every detail of your child's physical, emotional, and behavioural state in order to find the right treatment. The questions the homeopath asks are varied and far-reaching and may seem to have nothing to do with the problem – for example, the homeopath may ask you what position your child sleeps in or whether he concentrates at school. Your answers give the homeopath a complete picture of your child so that he can prescribe the correct remedy. Some homeopathic treatments work by simulating the original symptoms: Therefore, your child may get worse before he begins to recover.

Administering the remedies

Homeopathy treats a wide range of ailments, from allergies to gastric problems. Remedies usually come in the form of pills or granules (great for babies) that dissolve on the tongue. Follow these tips when giving your child a homeopathic remedy:

- ✔ Try not to touch the remedy, as you may contaminate and weaken it. Drop it from the lid of the container into your child's mouth – preferably under his tongue – and allow it to dissolve.

- ✔ Don't let your child eat or drink anything or clean his teeth for half an hour before or after taking a remedy, as this can interfere with the healing action of the remedies. You can crush or dissolve remedies in water though.

- ✔ Give one dose and wait to see what relief it brings your child. Repeat the dose (after leaving the recommended gap) if your child's symptoms are unchanged. But never give more than three doses a day. If your child is no better after three days, or becomes worse, talk to your practitioner, as your child may need a different remedy.

Although you find many first-aid homeopathic remedies in health shops and pharmacies, see a qualified homeopath first to make sure that your child gets the most accurate treatment and dosage. The usual recommended potency is 6c, but for chronic conditions and first-aid treatment the homeopath may recommend 30c remedies.

Finding a homeopath

The medical establishment is slowly coming round to the idea that homeopathic treatments can be beneficial, and many orthodox doctors no longer consider that homeopathy and orthodox medicine are mutually exclusive. The NHS now employs some doctors who practise homeopathy, several NHS homeopathic clinics exist. Your GP can give you more information about them, or you can visit www.trusthomeopathy.org.

Before choosing a homeopath, check the practitioner's credentials. Try the Society of Homeopaths (www.homeopathy-soh.org; phone 0845 450 6611) and the British Homeopathic Association (www.trusthomeopathy.org; phone 0870 444 3950).

Using herbal medicine for your child

Herbalism is one of the oldest natural treatments. It flourished in the 16th and 17th centuries until it was overshadowed by developments in science and the rise of orthodox medicine. Modern herbalism is based on the belief that plants have a vital energy that can be beneficial to the body by encouraging it to heal itself.

Herbal remedies are prepared from the leaves, flowers, and other parts of plants. Herbs have proven medicinal properties: many of the most effective drugs used in orthodox medicine originated in herbalism (aspirin, for instance, originally came from the bark of the willow tree). However, remember that, as with all other effective medicines, they carry risks as well as benefits. Digitalis, for instance, which comes from the foxglove and is widely used in hospitals to treat heart failure, is potentially lethal in quite small excess (don't worry, no herbalist would give your child digitalis!). Orthodox medications have to undergo extremely stringent safety procedures, and their dose is extremely accurately controlled.

Use only those herbs specifically recommended for babies and children, and even then only under the supervision of a trained medical herbalist.

When choosing a medical herbalist, by personal recommendation always ensure that you pick a herbalist who's a member of the National Institute of Medical Herbalists and with the initials NIMH (National Institute of Medical Herbalists) or FNIMH (Fellow of the National Institute of Medical Herbalists) after his name.

Osteopathy and chiropractic

Osteopaths and chiropractors are skilled practitioners of hands-on techniques that diagnose and treat disorders of the spine, joints, and muscles. Chiropractors view the spine as the key support that protects the nervous system and links the brain to the body. Osteopaths are most concerned with the body's framework and how well it functions. Both chiropractors and osteopaths manipulate the spine, which may produce a sudden popping feeling as a joint stretches and relaxes.

Osteopathy and chiropractic in adults are used mostly to treat muscular or skeletal problems. In children, however, osteopathy is widely used to treat such diverse conditions as colic, sleeplessness, and glue ear. *Cranial osteopathy*, which involves manipulation of the skull and neck, is often used in babies and children with these types of problem. In the right hands (sorry about the pun!) cranial osteopathy is safe, and many parents of colicky babies bless it on a daily basis!

Always use a registered osteopath or chiropractor. The General Osteopathic Council keeps a register of osteopaths, all of whom have to have a recognised qualification in osteopathy, and be insured and vetted. You can find out more from their Web site at www.osteopathy.org.uk. Find a registered chiropractor at www.gcc-uk.org.

Aromatherapy

Aromatherapy is one of the most widely used complementary therapies. As well as helping to lift the spirits, aromatherapy can be a particularly powerful treatment for a range of ailments and conditions associated with stress, such as sleep and digestive problems.

Aromatherapy oils are produced commercially from herbs, flowers, bark, roots, and other plant material.

Babies, toddlers, and older children may benefit from aromatherapy during difficult phases of normal growth and development and if they're suffering from a physical complaint such as recurrent coughs or colds. Many essential oils have strong antibacterial or antiviral properties and are particularly beneficial for treating infections.

Although a number of aromatherapy oils are safe to use at home without the advice of a practitioner, it is best to first consult an aromatherapist, especially if you're treating a baby or toddler. Some essential oils are toxic if they're not prepared properly or taken in large doses, while others can irritate the skin. Use only those oils specifically recommended for children.

Essential oils are potent and must first be diluted with a carrier oil such as apricot kernel or grape seed. The usual recommended dilution for children is three to five drops of essential oil to every 30 ml/2tbsp of carrier oil, although you ought always to consult your aromatherapist or label on the bottle.

You can find our more about aromatherapy or track down an aromatherapist in your area by contacting the International Federation of Professional Aromatherapists (`www.ifparoma.org`) on 01455 637987.

Chapter 19

Knowing Something about First Aid

. . . .

In This Chapter

▶ Taking control of emergencies

▶ Resuscitating your child

▶ Dealing with choking and other emergencies

▶ Tackling poisoning and insect stings

. . . .

*N*o one wants to think about an emergency happening at home – or any-where else for that matter – but better to face the possibility than to be unprepared. Children are naturally adventurous, and one thing's guaranteed: You'll become an expert at dealing with bumps and bruises as soon as your child's on the move. Although you can prevent many serious accidents from happening in the first place by taking sensible safety measures, you should be familiar with the basics of first aid when you're looking after little ones. By far the best way to learn first aid is to attend a recognised training course – and then update your training regularly. Organisations such as St John's Ambulance and the British Red Cross run these courses and are well worth the time and money invested: The skills you develop on the course are so important that they could save a child's life. Take a look at www.sja.org.uk/training or www.redcrossfirstaidtraining.co.uk.

This chapter explains what to do for your child in an emergency, and covers the basics of first aid. With any luck, you'll never need to use this informa-tion, although it's essential to read it through to familiarise yourself with the basics.

Staying Calm in an Emergency

The golden rules when you're faced with an accident involving your child is to stay calm and not put yourself in any danger. Not panicking can be very difficult, but losing control may make the situation worse for both you and your child. People often become distressed and disoriented in the face of an accident, so take these simple precautions *before* an accident happens:

✔ Keep important contact details of emergency phone numbers such as your child's doctor and dentist close to hand and by the phone. That way, they're in easy reach for anyone who's looking after your child.

✔ Show your child how to call for help if she's old enough. She should know how to dial 999 and be able to state her address and phone number, so practise these with her regularly and talk about what she should do if she ever needs help. Keep the house phone number and full address by the phone so that your child or the babysitter (who may not know this info off by heart) can access it easily.

✔ Keep a first aid kit handy and make sure it's fully stocked. See the Cheat Sheet at the front of this book for a list of essentials.

Some Common First Aid Emergencies

Children bounce back remarkably well from all sorts of scrapes, but sometimes things get a bit more serious. This section prepares you for the more everyday emergencies like trapped fingers and nosebleeds.

A knocked-out tooth

Children often lose teeth when playing contact sports or riding bikes. Losing a baby tooth isn't too much of a problem, but a knocked-out permanent tooth is a dental emergency. Quickly put the tooth back into its socket – this is vital in order to preserve the tooth, but make sure your child doesn't swallow it. Every minute a tooth's out of its socket reduces the chances of it surviving. Ideally, you should put the tooth back in its socket within half an hour of it coming out.

If your child knocks out a tooth, take these steps:

1. **Find the tooth.**

   If you're not sure whether its a baby tooth or an adult one, look at the edge: Adult teeth have rough edges and baby teeth have smoother edges. If you're in doubt, call a dentist immediately.

2. **If possible, rinse the tooth immediately with saline solution or milk.**

   Don't rinse in tap water, because it contains chlorine, which can damage the root of the tooth.

3. **Stop the tooth from drying out by inserting it back into its socket in your child's mouth, if she can hold it in place.**

   Keeping the tooth from drying out is crucial until you get to a dentist. If your child can't hold it in place – for example, if she's too frightened or too young – store the tooth in milk or salt water or place it between your own cheek and lower gum.

4. **Head to your child's dentist or go to A&E immediately.**

A nosebleed

Nosebleeds look scary, but they're very common in children and usually aren't serious. Most nosebleeds stop of their own accord. The most common causes of nosebleeds are nose-picking and dry air. If your child's susceptible to nosebleeds, keep a humidifier in her room. And make sure her fingernails are short!

If your child does get a nosebleed, follow these steps:

1. **Get your child to sit upright, with her head tilted slightly forward.**

   Don't let your child lean back, as this encourages the blood to drip down her throat, leading to gagging or vomiting.

2. **Pinch the soft part of the nose (near the tip) for at least ten minutes.**

If your child has frequent nosebleeds, has recently started medication and then gets a nosebleed, or has put something in her nose, see a doctor. Seek medical help if your child gets dizzy with the nosebleed, if the nosebleed doesn't stop after applying pressure for more than 20 minutes, or if the nosebleed follows a blow to your child's head or a fall.

Trapped fingers

Small children are very good at trapping their fingers in doors. The first thing you need to do is release your child's fingers quickly, causing as little extra pain as possible. After you've extricated your child's digits from the offending door, follow these steps:

1. **Hold your child's hand under running cold water to reduce swelling.**

2. **Clean the wound and apply a plaster to any cuts.**

3. **Raise your child's injured hand in a sling to reduce the pain and swelling. If the pain or swelling persists, apply a cold compress.**

If you don't have a sling in the house (most families don't!) use a headscarf folded in half diagonally, tied around the arm and over the shoulder and pinned to keep it in place.

If your child's fingers are still swollen or she finds it difficult to move them after half an hour, take her to hospital so the doctor can check for fractures.

If your child's fingers are severed, stay calm. You must act quickly and with control. Severed digits and limbs can now be reattached successfully in many circumstances. The quicker your child and the severed part get to hospital, the better the chances. So follow these steps:

1. **Stop the bleeding.**

   Place a clean pad or sterile dressing on the injury and press firmly. Then raise the injured part if possible.

2. **Wrap it up.**

   Cover the severed part with cling film or place it in a clean plastic bag. Then wrap in soft material and place it inside another plastic bag containing ice. Never put ice directly on the severed part, as this could burn and damage the area further.

3. **Take your child and the severed part to hospital immediately.**

Splinters

Even if you don't have a drama queen for a child – and most people do! – you can pretty much guarantee that your child will react as if removing a splinter is on a par with major brain surgery without the anaesthetic. Faced with this sort of reaction, it can be tempting to take the easy option and leave the splinter where it is. But do get it out – even small splinters can cause nasty infections if they aren't removed.

If your child is very young, sit her on another grown-up's lap and cuddle her firmly to stop her wriggling. If possible, have a couple of grown-up assistants on hand – one to keep your child still and one to hold the limb with the splinter – it's amazing how strong even a toddler can be when she's het up!

If your child gets a splinter, remove the splinter with tweezers. Follow these steps:

1. **Sterilise the tweezers by holding them under a match flame. Let the tweezers cool, but don't wipe off the black part.**

2. **Grasp the end of the splinter firmly and pull it out along the line it went in.**

   Don't try to pull straight up: the splinter is more likely to break and it will hurt like mad.

3. **After you've removed the splinter, encourage the wound to bleed by squeezing the flesh around it.**

   Doing so washes out any remaining dirt.

4. **Clean the wound and cover it with a plaster.**

If you can't get the splinter out or the splinter breaks under the skin, take your child to the doctor in case of infection.

Blisters

Blisters occur when the skin surface is rubbed or burned but not broken. They're like pockets filled with clear fluid. This fluid is not the same as pus – it's not infected, and it actually protects the sore area underneath.

Never burst a blister, because this can introduce an infection. Keep the area surrounding the blister clean and dry. If the blister's likely to get rubbed or broken, cover it with a non-adhesive dressing. It will disappear on its own within a few days.

If the skin around the blister gets red, hot, and very tender, an infection may have set in. If this happens, make an appointment with your GP.

The ABC of Resuscitation

This is probably the last thing you want to think about, but the airway–breathing–circulation check, known as the ABC of resuscitation, is the most important principle of emergency first aid for an unconscious baby or child. If the worst happens, by knowing how to resuscitate your child you can supply her vital organs with enough oxygen until medical assistance arrives.

Never, ever shake your baby, even if she appears to be unconscious.

Resuscitating your baby or child

Throughout this section, we use the term 'baby' for infants under 1 year, and 'child' for anyone from 1 year to puberty.

If your baby or child falls unconscious, try to get some kind of response from her by calling her name or tapping the sole of her foot. Shout for help if necessary, and call an ambulance on 999, but try to stay calm and follow this sequence:

1. **Check the airway.**

   Open your baby or child's mouth and check to see if she's breathing. Lay her down on a flat surface and tilt her head back slightly with one hand on her forehead, and the fingertips of the other hand under the bony tip of her chin. Remove any obvious obstacle from the mouth, but don't put your fingers into her throat. With one finger, gently lift her chin. Check for signs of breathing by looking along the chest for movement, listening for breathing sounds, and leaning over and feeling for any breath on your cheek.

2. **Check for breathing.**

   If your child is breathing, put her in the recovery position (see the section 'Putting your child in the recovery position' later in this chapter and Figure 19-1, or Figure 19-2 for a baby).

   If you haven't seen evidence of breathing after checking for 10 seconds, take a deep breath, seal your lips over her mouth and nose, and blow steadily into her lungs for 1 or 1.5 seconds. Watch her chest rise. Remove your mouth and let her chest fall. Give five of these rescue breaths, taking fresh oxygen yourself after each one. The air you exhale contains enough oxygen to sustain your child's vital organs.

3. **Check for circulation.**

   Circulation means blood flow: you need to check to see if your baby or child has a pulse. The best place to feel a child's pulse is with your index and middle finger placed gently on the neck, just to the side of the airway that you can feel as a firm 'tube' in the middle of the neck. For a baby, feel a pulse by pressing the same two fingers against the inner aspect of the top of the arm, just below the armpit. Look, listen (with your ear on her chest), for movement. A normal colour to the skin is a good sign that her circulation is functioning. If her circulation appears to be functioning, continue rescue breaths and recheck her circulation every minute. If your child shows no signs of circulation, begin CPR (see 'Performing CPR on Your Child' later in this chapter).

If you cannot get your breaths into your baby, and you know that she has choked, go straight to CPR and give chest compressions.

Putting your child in the recovery position

If your child's breathing, put her in the recovery position and call for help. To put her in the recovery position, lay her on her left side with one hand under her cheek and her right leg bent to stop her rolling over, as shown in Figure 19-1. Before you begin to turn your child, make sure her airway is clear. Recheck her airway after you've moved her into position.

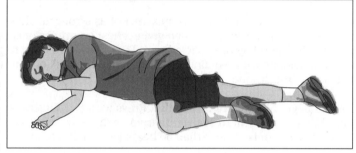

Figure 19-1:
The recovery position for children and toddlers.

If you suspect your baby or child has an injury to her spine, don't move her unless she's in immediate danger or her breathing is obstructed. Don't tilt your child's head to give rescue breaths: Instead, just lift her chin gently.

If your baby is under a year old, cradle her in your arms with her head tilted downwards, as shown in Figure 19-2. This prevents her from choking on her tongue or inhaling vomit.

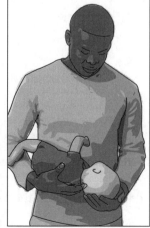

Figure 19-2:
The recovery position for babies.

Performing CPR on Your Baby or Child

Performing cardiopulmonary resuscitation (CPR) means giving chest compressions along with rescue breaths to keep your child's organs supplied with oxygen until medical treatment can be given.

Giving CPR to your baby

Babies are fairly robust, but their bones are not as strong as older children's. If you apply too much pressure when giving chest compressions, you may do more harm than good by breaking a bone. That's why you need to give babies chest compressions with two fingers (rather than the heel of your hands) placed on the breastbone.

Before you begin CPR, check for a pulse. Press with two fingers on the inside of your child's upper arm to see whether you can detect a pulse. If you can't feel a pulse or the pulse is less than 60 beats per minute, follow these steps:

1. **Find the point where your baby's lowest ribs meet in the middle. This is the bottom of the breastbone, or sternum. Put your index and middle fingers over his sternum, with the lower edge of your middle finger about a finger's breadth above the lower end of his sternum (see Figure 19-3).**

   This prevents you doing any harm by pressing down on his stomach.

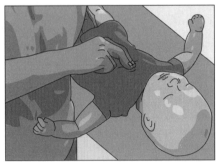

Figure 19-3: Placing your index and middle fingers on your baby's sternum to aid resuscitation.

2. **Press firmly with these two fingers fifteen times and release the pressure without moving your fingers.**

   You should be pressing the sternum down by about one third of the depth of your baby's chest.

   Do this quite quickly: Aim for around fifteen times in ten seconds.

3. **Give two rescue breaths and repeat the chest compressions.**

4. **Repeat this cycle of fifteen compressions to each two breaths until the ambulance arrives or your baby starts to breathe.** If your baby starts to breathe, put her in the recovery position and monitor her constantly until medical help arrives.

Giving CPR to your child

As with a baby, when you perform chest compressions on a child, you'll need to press her breastbone down by about one third of the depth of his chest. Obviously, the pressure you'll need to apply to do this will vary with the size of your child. For younger children, you should use the heel of one hand. For older or bigger children (from 8–10 years upwards) you may need to inter-lock your hands and press down with the heels of both hands together.

If you can't feel a pulse or the pulse is barely noticeable (see earlier section on finding a pulse), follow these steps:

1. **Find the point on your child's chest where her lowest ribs meet – this is the bottom of her breastbone, or sternum. Put the heel of your hand onto her sternum, with the lower edge of your hand about a finger's breadth above the lower end of the sternum. The heel of your hand should be over the bottom one third of her breastbone, with no pressure on the top of her stomach, as shown in Figure 19-4.**

Figure 19-4:
Placing the heel of your hand on your child's sternum to aid resus-citation.

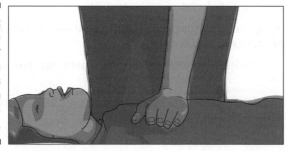

2. **With the heel of your hand, press down to around one-third of your child's chest depth. Do this fifteen times in ten seconds.**

   Keep the fingers of your hand slightly raised (rather than having your hand flat across your child's chest) to avoid pressing down with your fingers on her ribs.

3. **Give rescue breaths.**

   Pinch your child's nose, lift her chin, seal your lips over her mouth, and give one rescue breath.

4. **Repeat chest compressions and breaths in a cycle of 15 compressions to two rescue breaths until help arrives.**

Treating Your Child for Shock

Your child may go into shock after an accident, especially if she has severe bleeding or a serious burn or scald. 'Going into shock' is basically the body's reaction to a huge attack on the system, such as a major accident or trauma. Symptoms of shock include the following:

- Pale, cold, sweaty skin
- Rapid pulse, possibly getting weaker
- Shallow, fast breathing
- Restlessness, thirst, or nausea
- Continual yawning

The most important thing to do is improve the blood supply to your child's brain, heart, and lungs. To do this, follow these steps:

1. **Lay your child flat on the floor, keeping her head flat too (not on a pillow) so that she's less likely to lose consciousness because the blood will keep flowing to the head.**

2. **Support her legs above her heart by placing them on a chair, and turn her head to one side.**

   This also helps to keep blood pumping to her brain and other vital organs and prevents choking.

3. **Loosen any tight clothing that your child's wearing to reduce constriction at her neck, chest, and waist.**

4. **Cover your child with blankets to keep her warm, and call an ambulance.**

   Before the ambulance arrives, keep a check on your child's breathing and pulse.

Coping with Bleeding

Every child has accidents – it's all part of growing up and exploring. Fortunately, most causes of bleeding are quite minor, but they still look very scary. Lips and gums in particular are very well supplied with blood, so even a small cut can produce a surprising amount of blood. Don't worry, though – this good blood supply also helps it to heal quickly.

Massive bleeding can be very distressing and may cause you to panic but remember to stay calm so you can help as much as possible. Blood loss is rarely so severe that it causes the heart to stop, but remember your ABC of resuscitation (refer to the earlier section 'The ABC of Resuscitation'). Bear in mind that your child may go into shock and lose consciousness if she's bleeding heavily.

Minor cuts and grazes

Minor cuts and grazes can easily be treated at home. Always wash your hands with soap and water before treating your child's cuts – and wear surgical gloves if you have any in your first aid box. Sit or lay your child down while you examine the wound. Wash the wound carefully under running water until it's clean, then gently pat it dry with a clean towel. Press gently with a clean pad or cloth to stop any bleeding, and then cover with a non-stick dressing and adhesive tape or a plaster larger than the wound. If the wound is gaping open or the wound is on the head, take your child to hospital.

Any wound can become infected with germs from the cause of the original injury, from spores in the air, or from the hands of people treating the wound. Wash your hands before dealing with any wound.

If your child's wound doesn't heal within 48 hours, or if it increases in tenderness or swelling, or produces pus, cover the wound with a sterile dressing and seek medical help.

Severe bleeding

If your child is bleeding severely, follow this advice:

1. **Don't touch the wound directly, because this increases the risk of infection.**

2. **If anything's embedded in the wound, don't try to remove it, because you may cause further damage.**

3. **Staunch the blood flow.**

   Press on top of the wound using a clean non-fluffy cloth or pad until bleeding eases. If blood soaks through the pad, add another layer. If the wound is on a limb, lay your child down and raise the wounded part above the level of your child's heart. If something is embedded in the wound, try to stop the bleeding by applying pads or rolled bandages either side of the protrusion and applying pressure, being careful not to push the protrusion in further.

4. **When the bleeding eases, cover the pad with a dressing and bandage.**

   Hold the dressing firmly but not tightly in place. Keep the wounded part raised, using a sling if necessary, and take your child to hospital.

5. **If you can't stop the bleeding, put another dressing on top of the first and maintain pressure over the wound.**

   Support your child's legs above the level of the heart. Call an ambulance.

6. **Lay your child down, keeping constant pressure on the wound to reduce the risk of shock.**

   For information about dealing with shock, refer to the earlier section 'Treating Your Child for Shock'.

Dealing with Your Choking Child

If your baby or child chokes on something, her automatic reaction is to cough. Fortunately, this usually works and is more effective than any artificial attempt to get the foreign body out. Sometimes, though, her own body's attempts at coughing don't work, and if the foreign body is completely obstructing her airway, she can become short of oxygen in a very short space of time.

If she chokes, then, let her try and cough it out first. As long as she's coughing 'effectively', you don't need to start resuscitation. Signs that she's coughing effectively include:

✔ The cough is loud

✔ She's crying or can speak

✔ She can take a breath before she coughs

✔ She's fully conscious

✔ She's a good pink or red colour (not at all blue in the face or around the lips)

If, on the other hand, she can't talk or make a noise; can't take a breath before she coughs; goes blue or is coughing silently, you need to take the steps below promptly.

Call an ambulance at once if your baby or child loses consciousness when choking. As you wait for the ambulance, follow the ABC sequence explained in the section 'The ABC of Resuscitation'.

Treating your choking baby

If your baby's choking, follow these steps after calling for an ambulance:

1. **Lay your baby face down along one of your arms, with her head lower than the body. Support the bony tip of her chin between your fingers, as shown in Figure 19-5. Carefully but firmly give five sharp slaps on the middle of her back using the heel of your hand.**

   Never press on the soft flesh below your baby's chin when you're supporting her in this position because this could worsen the obstruction to her airway.

2. **Check your baby's mouth. If necessary, use one finger to remove any obvious obstruction.**

   Don't feel down your baby's throat, because doing so could push an object further down and block the airways even more.

3. **If back slaps don't work and your baby's still choking, give five chest thrusts as follows:**

   Turn her over to face you and put two fingers on her breastbone, below her nipple line. Carefully give inward and forward thrusts – about one every two seconds. These are similar to the chest compressions in baby resuscitation (see earlier section) but they are sharper.

4. **Check your baby's mouth again and remove any obvious objects.**

5. **Repeat Steps 1–4 three times if your baby's still choking.**

6. **If the obstruction hasn't cleared after three repetitions, keep your baby with you and phone for an ambulance.**

7. **Repeat Steps 1–4 until help arrives.**

Figure 19-5:
If your baby chokes, lay her along your arm and use the heel of your hand to slap her back. Support the bony tip of her chin between your fingers.

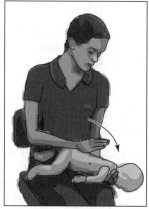

Treating your choking child

Follow these instructions to treat a choking child:

1. **Put your child in the appropriate position (see below). With the heel of your hand give five sharp slaps between the shoulder blades.**

   With a child over 12 months, lean her forwards, supporting her with one hand. Use your other hand to give the five sharp slaps.

   With a baby, lay her across your lap and support her head lower than her body.

2. **Check your child's mouth and remove any obvious objects.**

   Don't feel down your child's throat because doing so could push an object further down and block the airways even more.

3. **If back slaps don't work, give chest thrusts, as follows:**

   1. Stand or kneel behind your child and put your arms around her.

   2. Make a fist against the lower half of her breastbone.

   3. Grasp your fist with your other hand, and pull sharply inwards and upwards.

   4. Repeat five times, every three seconds.

   5. Remove any objects from your child's mouth.

4. **If chest thrusts don't work, give your child five abdominal thrusts, as follows:**

   1. Move the clenched fist down to your child's upper abdomen.

   2. Pull sharply inwards and upwards five times.

   Never give abdominal thrusts to a baby because their stomach organs are very delicate and can be damaged this way.

5. **Repeat Steps 1–4 three times.**

   If this is unsuccessful, call an ambulance and continue until help arrives. If your child becomes unconscious, start resuscitation using ABC (see the earlier section 'The ABC of Resuscitation').

Treating Burns and Scalds

Burns can be caused by heat, cold, the sun, chemicals, and hot liquids. Always take burns seriously, because the tissues under the skin may be damaged as well as the surface. If your baby or child suffers a burn larger than an inch in diameter, take her to the doctor's surgery or A&E immediately.

If your child is burned, follow these steps:

1. **Remove your child from the cause of burning without endangering yourself.**

2. **Hold the burned part under cold running water for at least 10 minutes.**

   This is the most effective thing you can do: Skin continues to burn for several minutes after contact with the heat or chemical. By cooling the affected area, you minimise any damage.

3. **If possible, remove any clothing from the affected area – but only if it isn't stuck to the burn and you can do so easily without doing more harm.**

   Do this *after* cooling with water. Loosen tight clothing and remove jewellery immediately after you've cooled it down, because the burned area may swell.

4. **To prevent infection, cover the burn with a sterile dressing.**

   If you haven't got any sterile dressings, use cling film or a clean, non-fluffy cloth, or put a clean plastic bag over a foot, hand, arm, or leg.

Don't apply any lotion, cream, or fat to the burn. Don't try to burst the blisters. And don't use adhesive dressings. All of these can damage your child's skin even further.

Electrical burns and shocks

Children are at risk of electrical burns if they play with flexes, plugs, or sockets, so take measures against this (see Chapter 22). An electrical current can stop your child's breathing or heart. Current can also burn your child's skin at the points where it enters and leaves her body. Electrical burns can be more serious than they first appear, because the tissues underneath the skin can be burned and damaged.

If your child suffers an electric burn or shock, follow these steps:

1. **Separate your child from the source, *but don't touch her* until she is away from the source.**

   Don't get burned or shocked yourself! You need to be there to help your child.

If your child's still in contact with the electrical appliance, switch off the power at the mains. Stand on a newspaper, rubber mat, or large book and remove the source of electricity using a wooden broom handle or chair leg. Alternatively, without touching your child directly, twist a large dry cloth around her ankles and pull her away from the source.

2. **If your child's unconscious, follow the steps for resuscitation and shock.**

   See the earlier sections 'The ABC of Resuscitation' and 'Treating Your Child for Shock'.

3. **Call an ambulance or take your child to A&E immediately.**

Chemical burns

Household chemicals such as bleach, paint stripper, ammonia, and glue are the most common causes of chemical burns in young children. If your child has been chemically burned, she may complain of stinging or burning, and you may see redness, soreness, blistering, peeling, or swelling of the skin.

If your child suffers a chemical burn, call 999 and follow these steps:

1. **Wash the chemical off your child's skin with lots of running cold water for at least 20 minutes.**

   Wear rubber gloves so that you don't get burned yourself.

2. **Remove your child's clothes, being careful not to get any chemicals on others parts of her (or your) body.**

3. **Cover the burned area with a clean non-fluffy material such as a pillow case and take your child to A&E.**

   Keep a note of the name of the chemical so you can tell the medical team at the hospital what caused the burn.

If your child gets chemicals in her eye, wash her eye under gently running cold water for at least 10 minutes, or pour cold water from a jug over her eye. Pull her eye open to ensure that the water goes inside it. Make sure the water drains well away from the other eye. Cover the affected eye with a clean pad and take your child to hospital.

Handling Poisoning

Poisoning's most often the result of a child accidentally swallowing medicine, berries, plants, or household cleaner. Signs of poisoning include burns or redness around your child's mouth, drowsiness, and abnormal behaviour. Unexplained unconsciousness can be due to accidental poisoning. You may also find telltale berries or empty or part-empty containers near your child.

If you think your child has swallowed something poisonous, follow these steps:

1. **Remove any berries, plant pieces, or pills from your child's mouth.**

   If she's old enough, give her water to rinse out her mouth and get her to spit it out. Don't let her swallow this water.

2. **Give your child sips of cold water or milk to alleviate any burning to the lips, mouth, and throat.**

   Don't try to make your child vomit, because this may do more harm than good and burn your child's throat.

3. **Find out what – and, if possible, how much – your child has swallowed.**

   It's absolutely essential for the medical team to have this information so they can know what action to take.

4. **Call a doctor.**

   If your child becomes unconscious, check her breathing and be pre-pared to resuscitate her (see the earlier section 'The ABC of Resuscitation'). Place her in the recovery position (refer to the section 'Putting your child in the recovery position') and call an ambulance.

Almost every household contains potentially poisonous substances. Keep anything remotely dangerous locked well away from your child.

Looking After Bites and Stings

Most stings cause your child a bit of pain but aren't serious – although you'd never know it from listening to her wails! You may notice a red swollen lump in the stung area, which is the body's natural response to fighting it. If your child is stung inside her mouth, the mouth can swell and cause breathing dif-ficulties, which requires emergency treatment. Rarely, your child may develop an allergic reaction, called *anaphylaxis*, to an insect sting: This requires emergency medical treatment (see the section 'A word about ana-phylaxis' in Chapter 15).

Wasps never leave their sting behind, but bees sometimes do. If you can see the sting in your child's skin, follow these steps:

1. **Remove the sting as quickly as possible using a credit card, the blunt edge of a knife, or your fingernail.**

   Don't use tweezers to remove a sting, because this can cause the sting to release even more venom into your child's bloodstream.

2. **Rinse the area under cool running water or put a cold compress on it for a few minutes to reduce the pain and swelling.**

3. **If the sting's inside your child's mouth, give your child an ice-cold drink to sip or some ice cubes to suck.**

   If the swelling gets worse or your child's breathing becomes affected, call an ambulance and if necessary use the resuscitation techniques described in the section 'The ABC of Resuscitation'.

Anaphylactic shock

Very occasionally a sting produces a severe allergic reaction called anaphylactic shock or anaphylaxis. The face and neck swell up, the airways constrict, and breathing becomes difficult. This requires urgent treatment. Anaphylaxis can also occur if your child eats something to which she is particularly sensitive, such as a peanut. If you think your child has anaphylactic shock, call an ambulance immediately. As you wait for help to arrive, support your child in the way that makes it easiest for her to breathe – a semi-sitting position is usually good. Loosen any clothing around her neck and waist. Reassure her, because panic can make her breathing even worse. If your child loses consciousness, check her breathing and be prepared to resuscitate following the techniques described in the section 'The ABC of Resuscitation'.

Part VI
The Part of Tens

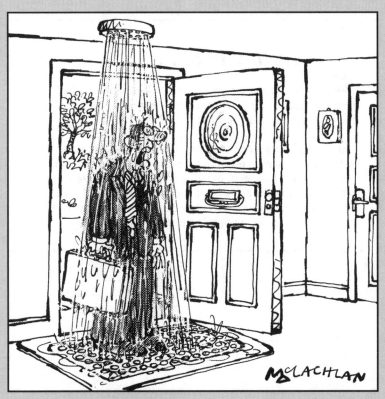

"Samantha!! – Aren't we taking this germ-free
environment for the baby a little too far!?!"

In this part . . .

Every *For Dummies* book has a bunch of useful little chapters in the very last part – and *Children's Health For Dummies* is no exception!

This part gives you a condensed look at keeping your kids healthy while on holiday, and includes tips on child-proofing your house, car, and garden. We also give you ten really useful Web sites offering information about a whole variety of topics related to children's health, from coping with asthma to using complementary medicines.

Chapter 20

Ten Ways to Stay Healthy on Holiday

In This Chapter

▶ Preparing for your holidays

▶ Eating and drinking safely

▶ Surviving in the sun

Gone are the days of packing a little overnight bag and skipping off to the sun for some serious partying. Holidays with children are a completely different experience – suddenly you have a lot more to concern you than how deep your tan will be. Family holidays can be daunting, albeit exiting, because when you're away from home your first concern is the health and safety of your child. But you needn't let this ruin your fun; with a few simple precautions, you can relax and enjoy your special time together.

Ensure You're Insured

Whether your child comes down with a dose of Delhi belly or needs emergency treatment for an accident, the last thing you want to worry about on holiday is medical costs. Taking out good medical insurance for your whole family is an absolute must, even in countries within the European Union (EU). Check that your insurance covers repatriation to fly you or your children home if medical treatment is needed.

All countries in the European Economic Area (the EU, plus Iceland, Liechtenstein, and Norway) have a reciprocal agreement with the UK for the provision of basic healthcare free of charge or for a minimal fee. To be eligible for this reciprocal healthcare, you need to travel with a European Health Insurance Card (EHIC), issued by the Department of Health. You can order an EHIC online at www.ehic.org.uk or by calling 0845-606-2030. Even if you have an EHIC, take out private medical insurance too, because the EHIC may not cover all your medical expenses abroad.

Have the Jabs

Make sure you know about all the immunisations you need well before you go on your trip. Some immunisations need time – up to three months – to take effect. If you're unsure about whether your child needs vaccinations, ask your GP or check out www.fitfortravel.nhs.uk. The most common travel vaccines are hepatitis A, typhoid, and yellow fever. In more high-risk areas, rabies, TB, hepatitis B, and Japanese and tick-borne encephalitis may be recommended. If malaria is prevalent in the area in which you're travelling, you and your children will need to take preventive medicine – usually in tablet form – on a regular basis. Antimalarial medication needs to be taken for at least a week before your departure, for the whole of your trip, and for some time after you return. Many people complain of side effects from antimalarial medication, including stomach cramps and nausea. If you would rather spare your child this experience, consider travelling to somewhere malaria-free.

Take Care in the Sun

Everyone needs some sun exposure: The sun's our primary trigger for vitamin D production, which helps us absorb calcium for strong, healthy bones. But most people get the vitamin D they need pretty quickly, and extended unprotected exposure to the sun's ultraviolet rays can cause heatstroke, sunburn, skin damage, eye damage, and cancer. The sun's rays are particularly dangerous to young children.

Ultraviolet (UV) rays are the most damaging of the sun's rays. UV rays react with a chemical called melanin in the skin. Melanin is our first defence against the sun, absorbing dangerous UV rays before they do serious damage to the body. Melanin is found in different concentrations according to skin colour: The lighter your child's natural skin pigment, the less melanin it contains. But both dark- and pale-skinned children need protection from UV rays because any tanning or burning causes skin damage. Unprotected sun exposure is even more dangerous for children with moles, very fair skin and hair, or a history of skin cancer. You should be especially careful about sun protection if your child has one or more of these high-risk characteristics.

Follow these tips to stay safe in the sun:

- **Keep your baby in the shade.** This one isn't negotiable. Babies under the age of 6 months should be kept out of the sun altogether.

- **Avoid the midday sun.** The strongest rays of the day are normally between 10 a.m. and 4 p.m. If your child is in the sun between these hours, keep him covered up in light-coloured clothing and apply protective sunscreen to his skin.

✔ **Use a sunscreen at all times**. The higher the sun protection factor (SPF) of the sunscreen, the better – use SPF 15 or higher. Avoid sunscreens containing PABA (para-amino-benzoic acid), because this can cause skin allergies. Apply the sunscreen generously to your child's skin about 30 minutes before he goes outside, and then reapply every two to three hours and after swimming, even if the sunscreen is waterproof.

✔ **Protect the skin even on cloudy days.** UV rays pass through clouds. Your child may be unaware that he's burning on cooler or windy days, because the temperature or breeze keeps the skin feeling cool on the surface.

✔ **Don't forget that light reflects.** Remember those panda eyes you see on people just returned from skiing holidays? Light reflects, especially off bright surfaces like snow, and can do every bit as much damage as direct sunlight. Sunlight can reflect off water, sand, or even concrete, so if you're on a sunshine holiday, keeping your little one out of the sun means well and truly out!

✔ **Cover up.** Get your child to wear thick-woven clothes and use umbrellas or a beach tent on the beach. Make sure your child wears a hat – preferably with a flap to protect the back of the neck. Buy a stretchy sun suit for your kids with built-in high protection sun protection. Not only do they look cool (kids usually love them!) but they really work. Kids can wear them in and out of the water, as well, and they're made to dry off quickly. Look for one with a high SPF (25 at least) and check the cleaning instructions to avoid ruining it before the holiday even starts!

✔ **Keep the water flowing.** Dehydration in babies and young children is dangerous and can happen extremely quickly. Carry fluids with you at all times, and encourage your child to drink frequently. If you're breastfeeding, your baby may need more frequent feeds to quench his thirst.

✔ **Look cool in sunglasses.** Sun exposure damages the eyes as well as the skin. Just one day in the sun can result in a burned cornea (the outermost, clear membrane layer of the eye). Cumulative exposure can lead to cataracts later in life, which may result in blindness. The best way to protect your child's eyes is for him to wear sunglasses. Not all sunglasses provide the same level of protection: Darkened plastic or glass lenses without special UV filters just trick the eyes into a false sense of safety. Purchase sunglasses with a label that confirms they provide 100 per cent UV protection.

If your child's skin does get sunburned, bathe the affected area with cool water or cold compresses. Apply calamine lotion and give him infant paracetamol if necessary. If the skin is blistered, keep it dry and cover any burned areas, because they can easily become infected (for more on burns, see Chapter 19). Extensive sunburn in a child can lead to hypothermia, because your child may lose a lot of body heat – so seek medical advice immediately if sunburn is extensive.

Don't Let the Bugs (or Other Animals) Bite

Pesky insects can ruin a lovely holiday, but you can do plenty to avoid the misery. Pack some insect repellent or use natural oils and sprays such as citronella. Make sure your rooms are screened with gauze over the windows and doors (check for holes), spray the room with an insecticide if necessary, and use a mosquito net over the bed. Dress your child in long trousers and socks and long-sleeved clothing after sunset. Go for light colours, as these are less attractive to mosquitoes.

Bites from animals can cause serious (and sometimes fatal) illnesses if not treated promptly. Be extremely cautious of all animals, even those that appear to be tame, and teach your children to be cautious too. If your child gets bitten by an animal, seek medical advice immediately.

Pack Up Your Troubles: The Medical Kit

Pack a small medical first-aid kit, with special thought to children's ailments, to carry on holiday. Remember to pack any medications you may need, including essentials for your child such as his asthma inhaler. Keep your first-aid kit in your hand luggage in case you need it while you're travelling. Your medical kit may include the following:

✔ Infant paracetamol and/or ibuprofen

✔ A thermometer

✔ Insect repellent

✔ Sticking plasters and antiseptic ointment/wipes

✔ Antihistamines for allergies and insect bites

✔ Soothing cream, such as calamine lotion, for bites and sunburn

✔ Rehydration solutions in case of tummy upsets

Water, Water, Everywhere . . .

Tummy bugs are easy to pick up when you're abroad, particularly in countries with poor sanitation and hygiene. If you don't know for certain that the water is safe, *always* assume the worst. Only use bottled water from containers with a serrated seal – not bottle tops or corks, as these bottles may have been filled with tap water. Take care with fruit juice, in case water has been added, and check that milk has been pasteurised. If you cannot get hold of any safe bottled water, the simplest way to purify water is to boil it for at least five minutes. Make sure your child drinks only bottled water, even for cleaning his teeth.

Water doesn't only come in liquid form! Most ice is made from tap water, and the freezing process won't necessarily kill off germs. Packaged ice creams are usually fine, but locally made ice cream or sorbet is a no-no.

Water isn't just a threat for drinking – it's also one of the most common causes of holiday accidents. Most drownings involving children occur on holiday, so be very cautious around swimming pools and on the beach. Don't take your eye off your child even for a minute when he's anywhere near water.

Food, Glorious Food . . .

If you have any doubts about food hygiene in the country you're travelling in, use this rule of thumb: If you can cook it, boil it, or peel it, then you can eat it – otherwise, forget it! Salads and fruit should be peeled or washed with purified water. Beware of buying anything edible from street vendors in developing countries.

Diarrhoea can cause anything from embarrassment and inconvenience to misery that wreaks havoc on your holiday. The best protection comes from choosing and preparing food carefully. High-risk foods include raw or inadequately cooked shellfish and seafood, raw salads, food that's been stored and reheated, and food left out in warm temperatures, such as hotel buffets, where bacteria can multiply fast and flies can settle.

Fly in Comfort

Cabin pressure, combined with the air conditioning in aircraft, can cause dehydration. Children are particularly vulnerable, so take plenty of water on the journey for your little one, and offer him frequent drinks. If you're travelling with a young baby, try to book your airline seat well in advance and ask for a sky cot. During take-off and landing, get your baby to bottle- or breast-feed to help equalise the pressure in his ears; if your child is older, sucking a sweet or lollypop will have the same effect. Crying also helps to equalise ear pressure. If you child has blocked ears due to an infection, ask your doctor to check them before travel – you may have to delay flying to avoid making the problem worse, or damaging the eardrum.

Nip Travel Sickness in the Bud

Just what makes us travel sick is subject to some debate, but apparently it's all in the mind – or, more precisely, the middle ear, which controls our balancing mechanisms and sends signals to the brain telling it we're in motion. The eyes, meanwhile, give the brain a different story – they think you're staying still (which in a way you are, so you can't blame them). Confused? Your body is too – and it's probably not surprising that nausea can ensue.

You can reduce the chances of your child being travel sick when flying by getting seats over the wings of the plane. As the centre of any moving vehicle is the most stable part, in a car give your child the middle passenger seat. If possible, tilt the seat back and get your child to close his eyes to stop those pesky mixed messages getting to the brain. Reading or focusing on anything close up is a no-no. If your child must keep his eyes open, get him to look at something in the distance, because this helps to coordinate the eye and ear signals. For sea-sickness, get your child to focus on the horizon, rather than anything on board ship.

Anti-sickness remedies are aplenty. The most effective for children include acupressure wristbands. Mint sweets and drinks of iced lemon barley water can also work wonders. If you need to resort to drugs, talk to your pharmacist or GP. But be sure to administer them well before your journey begins: When an attack starts, nothing will stay put, and the results won't be pleasant for your child or you.

Watch Out! Children About!

When you're travelling with young children, you need to be constantly alert to possible dangers. This is, after all, the age of exploration. Toddlers get bored easily and can go exploring places that aren't entirely safe.

Apart from keeping your child entertained non-stop, safety's undoubtedly one of the biggest issues when you're away from home. Just as you do at home, make sure medicines and noxious cleaning fluids are out of your child's reach: The most likely time for a toddler to accidentally swallow a dangerous substance is during a visit to someone else's house.

Electrical accidents and falls are the most common hazards on holiday. When you arrive at your accommodation, check out any potential pitfalls and make them as safe as possible: Cover exposed sockets (remembering that plug sockets outside the UK are different) and wires, and keep the balcony door locked, or ask for a room on the ground floor. Marble floors and staircases are particularly hazardous, especially when wet, and can lead to nasty injuries if your child falls against a sharp corner.

Chapter 21

Ten Health Web Sites You Can Trust

In This Chapter

▶ Finding out where to go online for health information

▶ Looking at the best sites about child safety and first aid

*W*hat did we do before the Internet arrived? It's a wonderful creation that enhances our lives in so many ways. But it doesn't come without its hazards. Chances are, the Internet is one of the first places you turn to when a family member falls ill – but this isn't necessarily the best thing to do. Plenty of nonsense is out there, including lots of inaccurate and conflicting advice. Unless you pick your sites carefully, you're likely to end up thinking every sniffle is a sure sign of a fatal illness. These ten reliable sites help you keep in the right company as you surf. But remember: nothing replaces seeing a real-life doctor if you're in any doubt about a health problem.

Asthma UK

www.asthma.org.uk

This Web site is a great source of independent information about the triggers and treatments of asthma, how to help your child control asthma, and what to do when your child has an asthma attack. The site features a useful A–Z of asthma triggers and a downloadable mini movie about asthma. The site also houses a discussion forum for parents and carers about all aspects of asthma, and offers useful info on subjects such as asthma in pregnancy, swimming with asthma, air pollutants, and asthma and emotions. Asthma UK also has a helpline (08457-010203).

British Nutrition Foundation

www.nutrition.org.uk

This charity's Web site offers sound nutritional information and advice to scientists and the public. The site contains key information about your child's nutrition in health and illness. Check out the downloadable resources and the publications section, from which you can order unbiased computer software, videos, and books on nutrition. Let your child look at the companion Web site Food – A Fact of Life (www.foodafactoflife.org.uk), which is full of easy tips about healthy eating, combined with activities and fun advice on things such as nutritious lunchboxes.

Alternatively, the Food Standards Agency (www.food.gov.uk) contains up-to-date guidelines on every aspect of nutrition for you and your child.

British Red Cross

www.redcross.org.uk

This clear Web site, written in non-technical language, explains some quite simple, but lifesaving, first-aid techniques. Video clips demonstrate how to treat burns, bleeding, and choking, and how to perform cardiopulmonary resuscitation (CPR). The site also covers important survival skills for your child, including advice on road safety.

The Web site lists the British Red Cross courses for first-aid training in your area, and features information on how to join the Red Cross's first-aid campaigns across the UK. Check out the fascinating real-life first-aid stories about people who have saved lives by using the techniques they have learned through the Red Cross.

Child Accident Prevention Trust

www.capt.org.uk

The Child Accident Prevention Trust (CAPT) is a national charity committed to reducing the number of children and young people who are killed, disabled, or seriously injured each year as a result of accidents. The Web site includes a whole range of downloadable fact sheets on all aspects of safety, from being safe in the car to preventing bathwater scalds. The site also features activities, quizzes, and games to help children of all ages learn about safety issues, and sets quizzes for parents, and activity sheets for children to help every-one increase their knowledge of child safety in a fun and interactive way.

Children First for Health

www.childrenfirst.nhs.uk

Children First for Health (CFfH) is a partnership between Great Ormond Street Hospital For Sick Children and the Institute of Child Health. The Web site provides comprehensive health information from British medical experts and paediatricians, including health news, features and fact sheets on diseases, advice on health matters and hospital life, and children's own views and experiences. The site's discussion forum is a good way for children to find out about health issues and share their own experiences on everything from chronic illness to staying in hospital.

Complementary Healthcare Information Service, UK

www.chisuk.org.uk

This Web site is a good first port of call if you're interested in finding out more about complementary therapies. If you've ever wondered about the difference between osteopathy and chiropractic, or aromatherapy and massage, this is the place for you. The site provides information on all the popular alternative therapies, from acupuncture to yoga, as well as some that you may not have heard of, such as zero balancing and biofeedback. The site directs you to specific organisations for each therapy and helps you search for health practitioners in your area. You'll find lots of useful articles about complementary healthcare, a news section about the latest research, and a bookshop.

NetDoctor

www.netdoctor.co.uk

Over 250 doctors and health professionals from the UK and Europe write, edit, and update NetDoctor and respond to users' questions and concerns regarding health. On this Web site you can join medical discussion forums, ask a doctor a question online, and look up information on diseases and medicines, medical definitions, news stories, and help organisations. The Web site's doctors, writers, and editors follow the same standards of practice as leading medical journals and are not answerable to sponsors or advertisers. The team of doctors has answered thousands of questions, which you can sift through to find answers relevant to you.

NHS Direct Online

www.nhsdirect.nhs.uk

This is the Web site for the NHS 24-hour telephone helpline, NHS Direct (0845-4647). The site provides information about an extensive range of common health problems and advice on when to call for a doctor. The self-help section covers the most common symptoms that people call NHS Direct about and explains some important preventive measures you can take to reduce the likelihood of your child falling ill. The most helpful sections include the A–Z encyclopaedia of ailments and 'best treatments' (available at www.best treatments.co.uk), which is run in conjunction with the *British Medical Journal* and gives details of the latest research studies of treatments. The main site helps you locate your nearest NHS doctors, dentists, opticians, and pharmacies. Try putting your health knowledge to the test with the interactive quizzes, and find out how to calculate your child's body mass index.

Patient UK

www.patient.co.uk

This Web site, launched by Patient Information Publications, provides a huge range of online leaflets and links to other useful sites. The leaflets take you through pretty much every common (and uncommon!) childhood condition seen in the UK. The site is clearly written, and the Centre for Health Information Quality, which assesses it regularly, praises is as 'very user friendly' and 'a large reliable resource for information on all aspects of medical conditions'.

WellChild

`www.childrenshealth.org.uk`

This is one of the Web sites of the WellChild Trust, the UK's leading charity for improving children's health in the UK. The charity provides support for families with sick children, raises awareness about children's health issues, and funds research into developing better treatments and improving the quality of life of sick children. The Web site contains extensive, accessible information about all aspects of children's health and issues of parenting, from potty training, through starting school, to helping your child get over chickenpox. A fun area of the site lets children share their stories about everything from asthma to hospital stays. The site also runs children's competitions, with 'cool prizes'.

Chapter 22

Ten Ways to Keep Your Child Safe at Home

*E*very year in the UK, thousands of children are admitted to hospital with injuries sustained from domestic mishaps – and many more are treated at home by parents and carers who are counting their lucky stars that it wasn't more serious. Being aware of the causes and knowing how to avoid danger helps reduce the risk of hazards in your home. One of the easiest things you can do to safeguard your child at home is simply to get down to his level and look at things from his point of view: Through your child's eyes, boring old cupboards, fireplaces, furniture, and plug sockets are exciting things to explore. You'll need to re-evaluate your safety measures as your child grows, but as soon as he's able to understand, you can make him aware of potential dangers by explaining in simple terms when things can burn or hurt.

Let the Alarm Bells Ring

Buying and fitting a smoke alarm is one of the most important things you can ever do. If you don't have smoke alarms already, now is the time to invest in a few. House fires are the biggest single cause of accidental death of children in the home, mostly as a result of smoke inhalation.

When you're buying a smoke alarm, look for a Kitemark and/or British Standard Number BS 5446.

Test the alarm regularly – at least once a month – and replace the battery once a year.

Take the following steps to reduce the risk of a fire in your house:

- ✔ Don't smoke at home, and keep matches and lighters well out of your child's reach.

- ✔ Work out an escape plan for you and your family. Your local fire brigade will be happy to advise you if you're in doubt about anything.

- ✔ As soon as your child's old enough to understand, tell him what to do if he discovers a fire or hears the smoke alarm.

- ✔ Keep all your house doors shut at night: Smoke spreads very quickly and closed doors can save you valuable minutes.

- ✔ Keep a fire extinguisher and fire blanket in the kitchen.

- ✔ Repair old or worn electrical flexes, and don't overload sockets. Unplug things when you're not using them.

- ✔ Install a smoke alarm just outside your kitchen, and at least one on every storey in your house.

- ✔ If a fire starts in your home, shut the door on it, leave the building, and call the fire brigade immediately.

A carbon monoxide monitor is a good idea if you have a gas cooker or gas central heating. The monitor alerts you to the presence of carbon monoxide, an odourless gas that can be lethal. Although monitors are helpful, it is still vital to have your gas boiler serviced by a Corgi-registered engineer at least every 12 months as well.

If You Can't Stand the Heat . . .

For a small child, the kitchen is the most dangerous place in the house. Ideally, keep your child out of the kitchen at all times. And if this isn't practical, try at least to keep him out while you're cooking. Installing a stair gate across the kitchen doorway is one solution.

Try the following steps to reduce the risk of accidents in the kitchen:

- ✔ When you're cooking, turn pot handles towards the stove and use only the back burners if possible. Tell older children that the oven is hot and not to be touched, and keep reinforcing this message.

✔ Fridges, freezers, washing machines, and tumble driers can prove fatal if your child climbs inside and becomes trapped. Keep all appliance doors closed firmly.

✔ When you load the dishwasher, place cutlery with the handles pointing up so that all the sharp bits are out of the way.

✔ Store cleaning fluid, bleach, furniture polish, dishwasher soap, and all other dangerous products in a high, preferably lockable, cabinet out of sight and reach.

✔ Never store toxic substances in containers that look as though they hold food or drink, such as water or lemonade bottles.

✔ Keep knives, forks, scissors, and other sharp instruments separate from safer kitchen utensils, in a latched drawer.

✔ Store plastic bags in a drawer or cabinet with a safety catch.

Don't Go Stair-crazy

They may come in useful, but stairs are one of the most child-unfriendly features in your home. Around 60,000 children under the age of five are injured in the UK each year by falling down stairs, so you need to be extra vigilant once your child's on the move. As soon as your child can climb up and down stairs, show him how to do so safely. Children under the age of three often find it easier to crawl rather than walk upstairs and to climb down backwards, as if down a ladder. Never let your child use the stairs unsupervised until you're absolutely sure that he's capable of doing so safely.

If you have a young child, install a stair gate at the top and bottom of your stairway. You can find various types of stair gate in the shops. The top gate needs to be particularly strong, so choose one that screws into the wall. Avoid accordion-style gates or gates that that use pressure or suction for use at the top, as your child can push through them and fall. Don't leave any more than a 5-cm gap between the stair gate and the floor, but do leave the first two or three stairs at the bottom of your stairway free so your child can practise climbing on them.

Keep stairs clutter-free. If you have the habit of leaving things on the stairs ready to take up on the next trip, put a basket in the hallway to accommodate these items.

To prevent your child's neck or head getting stuck, you may need to board up your stair rails if they're spaced more than 10 cm apart. And watch out for horizontal bars and slats – your child may be tempted to use them as a ladder.

Brush Away Toilet Troubles

Your bathroom and toilet house a number of potential hazards for your child. The simplest way to head off trouble is to make these rooms inaccessible to your child unless he's with you. You may need to install a latch or lock on the outside of the door at adult height.

A child can drown in as little as five centimetres of water, so it's not only the bath that poses a threat: Toilet bowels, nappy buckets, and sinks can be just as dangerous.

To reduce the risks of bathroom accidents, try the following:

- ✔ Keep toothpaste, mouthwash, soap, and shampoo high up or in a cabinet with a safety latch or lock. Ensure that you lock away sharp objects such as razor blades, scissors, and nail clippers.

- ✔ Don't keep any electrical items in the bathroom.

- ✔ Never throw used razor blades, toothbrushes, or other potentially dangerous materials into the bathroom wastebasket.

- ✔ Check that shower doors and other surfaces are made of safety glass or shatterproof material.

- ✔ Throw away the soap when it becomes small enough to fit inside your child's mouth.

- ✔ Leave the toilet lid down at all times – you may even want to invest in a safety catch – and never leave cleaning fluid in the toilet bowl to soak. Wash and flush away!

- ✔ Install non-slip mats or strips on the bottom of your bath.

- ✔ Always run the cold water before the hot, and then mix the water so that it feels just warm. Cover the hot tap with soft flannels during bath time so your child can't burn himself.

On occasions when you want to leave cleaning products such as bleach on your loo or bath, to give them an extra clean or to get rid of stains, use a belt and braces approach – leave cleaning products to soak at night or when they children are out of the house, and always lock the bathroom door.

Never, under any circumstances, leave your baby or child unsupervised in the bath: Children can drown in seconds. Many accidents happen when a carer leaves a baby or toddler unattended for just a minute while they answer the door or the phone. If you need to leave the room, take your child with you. Remember that bath seats and rings designed for young babies are bathing aids, not safety aids. They cannot stop your child drowning if you leave him unattended.

Watch Out for Windows

Falls from windows are more common than you may think. Make sure that all of your windows have catches or locks and avoid putting furniture under the windows, where it can tempt little climbers. However, do check that you can still open the windows quickly in case of fire. Keep window keys nearby but out of your child's reach, or tape the keys to the upper frames. If possible open the top rather than the bottom sections of windows, or install safety bars or screens on the lower windows so that only adults and older children can push out from the inside in an emergency.

Be sure to keep curtain and blind cords well out of reach. Tie them around wall brackets to keep them away from tiny hands. Cut cords with loops to prevent your child strangling himself.

Go Get the Gadgets

Falling furniture is a common cause of injury, so fit L-brackets, available from hardware stores, to secure unstable furniture to the wall. Freestanding bookshelves, cabinets, chests of drawers, and tables are particularly lethal, as they may become attractive climbing equipment for your child. Make sure that all your large, heavy furniture is resting solidly on the floor, with no wobbly legs.

A whole array of ingenious safety devices has been designed to help you childproof your home. You can protect your child from nasty knocks by covering sharp bits on furniture with padded corner protectors, available from nursery shops and department stores. Try foam stoppers on doors and drawers to prevent them slamming on to little fingers. Safety catches on cupboards and fridges are also a good idea.

If possible, have mirror and window panels on pieces of furniture made from shatterproof glass. A less expensive alternative is to affix invisible safety film to the glass surfaces, which stops the glass from shattering if it breaks.

Try Not To Be Shocked

The most effective step you can take to minimize the risk of your child getting an electric shock is to put plastic covers on all sockets that aren't being used. Best also to get into the habit of unplugging appliances that aren't in use. Children (strange creatures that they are) may be tempted to chew and tug on power cables, which can be a cause of electrocution. Use cord shorteners to tidy up loose wires, and make sure that cables are held firmly in place behind heavy furniture or stapled to the floor or walls. Check your electric cables frequently, and replace any worn cables immediately. Never run cables under carpets or rugs.

Play it Safe

Playing's what children do best, but making sure that they do it safely is important. Tough government regulations and rigorous testing by manufacturers mean that most children's toys on the market are very safe. But, despite this, thousands of children still suffer toy-related injuries every year in the UK. The following are some of the most common causes of childhood accidents involving toys:

- ✔ **Toys with small parts:** Small bits are choking hazards. Don't give your child any toys that aren't suitable for his age: heed the manufacturer's age guidelines printed on the packaging.

- ✔ **Broken toys:** Something as innocent as a doll or teddy may become hazardous if your child pulls off one of the toy's eyes or buttons.

- ✔ **Toys with loose strings and ribbons:** These can become tangled around your child's neck. Strings and cords on all toys should be no longer than 20 centimetres long (8 inches). Dangling objects such as cot mobiles can be particularly dangerous, so remove them as soon as your baby can pull himself up.

- ✔ **Wheeled toys:** Supervise your child at all times when he's wheeling about to prevent falls and crashes.

- ✔ **Balloons:** More children have suffocated or choked on uninflated or popped balloons than on any other type of toy, so keep them away from children of all ages.

- ✔ **Shooting toys:** Toys that shoot plastic objects are a common cause of eye injury.

Always throw away toy wrappings, as staples and sharp edges spell trouble for young children, who have an unexplained innate fascination for packaging.

Many safety experts warn against the use of baby walkers, those wheeled devices that hold babies in an upright position with their feet on the floor. A baby walker can easily tip over, particularly if your child bumps it into an obstacle such as a toy or a rug. Children in baby walkers are also far more likely to fall down stairs and get into dangerous places and situations that would otherwise be beyond their reach.

How Does Your Garden Grow?

Gardens present a whole array of potential hazards. However, you can still make your garden a safe and fun environment for your child to play in.

Make sure that your garden's secure, so your child can't get out and no one can get in without your knowledge. Check that all gates fasten securely, and replace latches, locks, and hinges as necessary. Locks must be out of reach of your child.

Drowning in garden ponds is one of the most common domestic accidents. Even paddling pools and buckets can be lethal. The safest thing you can do with a pond or any other water feature is to fill it in: You can make it into a temporary sandpit for your children. If you decide to keep your pond, fence it off or cover it with rigid, heavy-duty steel mesh, placed well above the surface of the pond. Be especially vigilant in other people's gardens, where the vast majority of pond drownings occur.

Take the following steps to reduce the number of hazards in your garden:

- ✔ If your gate or fence has horizontal bars that can be climbed on, remove them or board them up. A child can wriggle through the smallest of spaces. Check for exposed nails and loose boards too.

- ✔ Don't leave hosepipes, garden forks, lawnmowers, or other garden tools lying around.

- ✔ If you have a greenhouse, cover the lower panes with safety glass or boards.

- ✔ Don't let your baby or child play in soil, as there is a risk of infection from animal faeces (you can read more about cleaning up your act in Chapter 12). And wash your child's hands straight away after he's been playing in the garden.

- ✔ Keep garden sheds, garages, and basements locked up at all times

- ✔ Familiarise yourself with the plants in your garden so that you can decide which are safe to keep and which to dig up. Common poisonous garden plants include yew, foxglove, ivy, and laburnum.

Take Care in the Car

Every year, more children are killed in road accidents than by any other cause. Many tragic deaths in road accidents can be prevented if proper car-seat restraints are used. The single most important thing you can do to keep your child safe in the car is to buy, install, and use an approved car seat for every journey. This is vital, even on the shortest of trips: Most fatal crashes happen at speeds of less than 35 mph and within 5 miles from home.

Choose your car seat carefully: Not every seat fits every car, so try it before you buy it. Some retailers have experts who can check the fit for you. An incorrectly fitted car seat is useless in the event of a collision.

In the UK, the law stipulates that an appropriate car seat restraint should be used for all babies and children under 1.5 metres *if available*, and it is illegal to carry an unrestrained child in the front seat. There are plans to update the law so that it is less woolly by the end of 2006, but whatever the case, as the driver you are legally responsible for your child's safety in a car. Never let him travel without an appropriate restraint such as a baby car seat or booster seat for an older child.

Never put a rear-facing car seat in the front if your car is fitted with airbags, as they could crush your child. Even if your child's seat faces forwards, she can still be crushed by an airbag, so it is always safer to carry your child in the rear of your car whenever possible,

Index

• C •

• E •

• G •

• N •

● **Z** ●

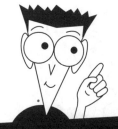

FOR DUMMIES®

Do Anything. Just Add Dummies

HOME ### UK editions

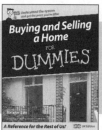

Buying and Selling a Home For Dummies
0-7645-7027-7

Renting Out Your Property For Dummies
0-7645-7016-1

DIY & Home Maintenance All-In-One For Dummies
0-7645-7054-4

PERSONAL FINANCE

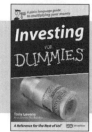
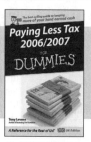
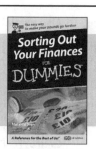

Investing For Dummies
0-7645-7023-4

Paying Less Tax 2006/2007 For Dummies
0-470-02860-2

Sorting Out Your Finances For Dummies
0-7645-7039-0

BUSINESS

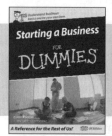
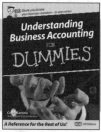
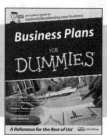

Starting a Business For Dummies
0-7645-7018-8

Understanding Business Accounting For Dummies
0-7645-7025-0

Business Plans For Dummies
0-7645-7026-9

Other UK editions now available:

Answering Tough Interview Questions For Dummies
(0-470-01903-4)

Arthritis For Dummies
(0-470-02582-4)

Being The Best Man For Dummies
(0-470-02657-X)

British History For Dummies
(0-7645-7021-8)

Building Confidence For Dummies
(0-4700-1669-8)

Buying a Home On A Budget For Dummies
(0-7645-7035-8)

Cognitive Behavioural Therapy For Dummies
(0-470-01838-0)

Cleaning and Stain Removal For Dummies
(0-7645-7029-3)

CVs For Dummies
(0-7645-7017-X)

Diabetes For Dummies
(0-7645-7019-6)

Divorce For Dummies
(0-7645-7030-7)

eBay.co.uk For Dummies
(0-7645-7059-5)

European History For Dummies
(0-7645-7060-9)

Gardening For Dummies
(0-470-01843-7)

Golf For Dummies
(0-470-01811-9)

Hypnotherapy For Dummies
(0-470-01930-1)

Irish History For Dummies
(0-7645-7040-4)

Kakuro For Dummies
(0-470-02822-X)

Marketing For Dummies
(0-7645-7056-0)

Neuro-Linguistic Programming For Dummies
(0-7645-7028-5)

Nutrition For Dummies
(0-7645-7058-7)

Pregnancy For Dummies
(0-7645-7042-0)

Retiring Wealthy For Dummies
(0-470-02632-4)

Rugby Union For Dummies
(0-7645-7020-X)

Small Business Employment Law For Dummies
(0-7645-7052-8)

Su Doku For Dummies
(0-4700-189-25)

Sudoku 2 For Dummies
(0-4700-2651-0)

Sudoku 3 For Dummies
(0-4700-2667-7)

The GL Diet For Dummies
(0-470-02753-3)

UK Law & Your Rights For Dummies
(0-470-02796-7)

Wills, Probate and Inheritance Tax For Dummies
(0-7645-7055-2)

Winning on Betfair For Dummies
(0-470-02856-4)

Available wherever books are sold. For more information or to order direct go to www.wileyeurope.com or call 0800 243407 (Non UK call +44 1243 843296)

8821_p1

FOR DUMMIES®

A world of resources to help you grow

HOBBIES

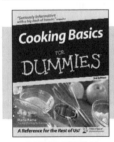

Poker
0-7645-5232-5

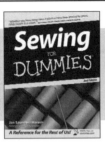

Sewing
0-7645-6847-7

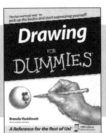

Drawing
0-7645-5476-X

Also available:

Art For Dummies
(0-7645-5104-3)

Aromatherapy For Dummies
(0-7645-5171-X)

Bridge For Dummies
(0-7645-5015-2)

Card Games For Dummies
(0-7645-9910-0)

Chess For Dummies
(0-7645-8404-9)

Crocheting For Dummies
(0-7645-4151-X)

Improving Your Memory
For Dummies
(0-7645-5435-2)

Massage For Dummies
(0-7645-5172-8)

Meditation For Dummies
(0-471-77774-9)

Photography For Dummies
(0-7645-4116-1)

Quilting For Dummies
(0-7645-9799-X)

Woodworking For Dummies
(0-7645-3977-9)

EDUCATION

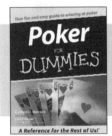

Cooking Basics
0-7645-7206-7

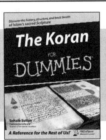

The Koran
0-7645-5581-2

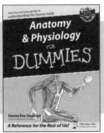

Anatomy & Physiology
0-7645-5422-0

Also available:

Algebra For Dummies
(0-7645-5325-9)

Algebra II For Dummies
(0-471-77581-9)

Astronomy For Dummies
(0-7645-8465-0)

Buddhism For Dummies
(0-7645-5359-3)

Calculus For Dummies
(0-7645-2498-4)

Christianity For Dummies
(0-7645-4482-9)

Forensics For Dummies
(0-7645-5580-4)

Islam For Dummies
(0-7645-5503-0)

Philosophy For Dummies
(0-7645-5153-1)

Religion For Dummies
(0-7645-5264-3)

Trigonometry For Dummies
(0-7645-6903-1)

PETS

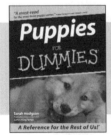

Puppies
0-7645-5255-4

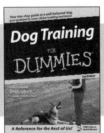

Dog Training
0-7645-8418-9

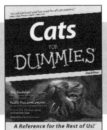

Cats
0-7645-5275-9

Also available:

Labrador Retrievers
For Dummies
(0-7645-5281-3)

Aquariums For Dummies
(0-7645-5156-6)

Birds For Dummies
(0-7645-5139-6)

Dogs For Dummies
(0-7645-5274-0)

Ferrets For Dummies
(0-7645-5259-7)

German Shepherds
For Dummies
(0-7645-5280-5)

Golden Retrievers
For Dummies
(0-7645-5267-8)

Horses For Dummies
(0-7645-9797-3)

Jack Russell Terriers
For Dummies
(0-7645-5268-6)

Puppies Raising & Training
Diary For Dummies
(0-7645-0876-8)

Saltwater Aquariums For
Dummies
(0-7645-5340-2)

Available wherever books are sold. For more information or to order direct go to www.wileyeurope.com or call 0800 243407 (Non UK call +44 1243 843296)

8821_P2

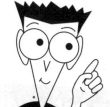

FOR DUMMIES®

The easy way to get more done and have more fun

LANGUAGES

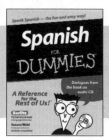

0-7645-5194-9

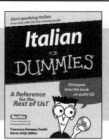

0-7645-5193-0

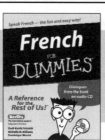

0-7645-5196-5

Also available:

Chinese For Dummies
(0-471-78897-X)

Chinese Phrases
For Dummies
(0-7645-8477-4)

French Phrases For Dummies
(0-7645-7202-4)

German For Dummies
(0-7645-5195-7)

Italian Phrases For Dummies
(0-7645-7203-2)

Japanese For Dummies
(0-7645-5429-8)

Latin For Dummies
(0-7645-5431-X)

Spanish Phrases
For Dummies
(0-7645-7204-0)

Spanish Verbs For Dummies
(0-471-76872-3)

Hebrew For Dummies
(0-7645-5489-1)

MUSIC AND FILM

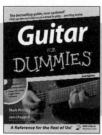

0-7645-9904-6

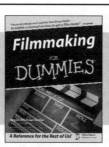

0-7645-2476-3

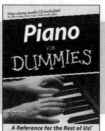

0-7645-5105-1

Also available:

Bass Guitar For Dummies
(0-7645-2487-9)

Blues For Dummies
(0-7645-5080-2)

Classical Music For Dummies
(0-7645-5009-8)

Drums For Dummies
(0-471-79411-2)

Jazz For Dummies
(0-471-76844-8)

Opera For Dummies
(0-7645-5010-1)

Rock Guitar For Dummies
(0-7645-5356-9)

Screenwriting For Dummies
(0-7645-5486-7)

Songwriting For Dummies
(0-7645-5404-2)

Singing For Dummies
(0-7645-2475-5)

HEALTH, SPORTS & FITNESS

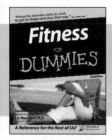

0-7645-7851-0

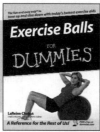

0-7645-5623-1

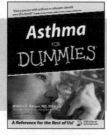

0-7645-4233-8

Also available:

Controlling Cholesterol
For Dummies
(0-7645-5440-9)

Dieting For Dummies
(0-7645-4149-8)

High Blood Pressure
For Dummies
(0-7645-5424-7)

Martial Arts For Dummies
(0-7645-5358-5)

Menopause For Dummies
(0-7645-5458-1)

Power Yoga For Dummies
(0-7645-5342-9)

Weight Training
For Dummies
(0-471-76845-6)

Yoga For Dummies
(0-7645-5117-5)

Available wherever books are sold. For more information or to order direct go to www.wileyeurope.com or call 0800 243407 (Non UK call +44 1243 843296)

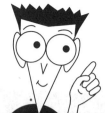

FOR DUMMIES®

Helping you expand your horizons and achieve your potential

INTERNET

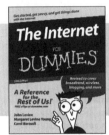

0-7645-8996-2

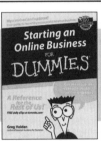

0-7645-8334-4

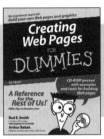

0-7645-7327-6

Also available:

eBay.co.uk
For Dummies
(0-7645-7059-5)
Dreamweaver 8
For Dummies
(0-7645-9649-7)
Web Design
For Dummies
(0-471-78117-7)

Everyday Internet
All-in-One Desk Reference
For Dummies
(0-7645-8875-3)
Creating Web Pages
All-in-One Desk Reference
For Dummies
(0-7645-4345-8)

DIGITAL MEDIA

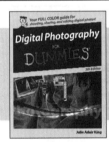

0-7645-9802-3

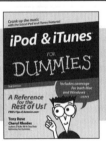

0-471-74739-4

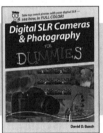

0-7645-9803-1

Also available:

Digital Photos, Movies, &
Music GigaBook
For Dummies
(0-7645-7414-0)
Photoshop CS2
For Dummies
(0-7645-9571-7)
Podcasting
For Dummies
(0-471-74898-6)

Blogging
For Dummies
(0-471-77084-1)
Digital Photography all in
one desk reference
For Dummies
(0-7645-7328-4)
Windows XP Digital Music For
Dummies
(0-7645-7599-6)

COMPUTER BASICS

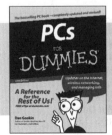

0-7645-8958-X

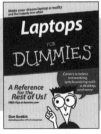

0-7645-7555-4

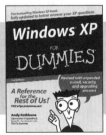

0-7645-7326-8

Also available:

Office XP 9 in 1
Desk Reference
For Dummies
(0-7645-0819-9)
PCs All-in-One Desk
Reference For Dummies
(0-471-77082-5)
Pocket PC For Dummies
(0-7645-1640-X)

Upgrading & Fixing PCs
For Dummies
(0-7645-1665-5)
Windows XP All-in-One Desk
Reference For Dummies
(0-7645-7463-9)
Macs For Dummies
(0-7645-5656-8)

Available wherever books are sold. For more information or to order direct go to www.wileyeurope.com or call 0800 243407 (Non UK call +44 1243 843296)